Radiation Oncology Advances

Cancer Treatment and Research

Steven T. Rosen, M.D., ***Series Editor***

Arnold, A.J. (ed.): *Endocrine Neoplasms. 1997.* *ISBN 0-7923-4354-9.*
Pollock, R.E. (ed.): *Surgical Oncology. 1997.* *ISBN 0-7923-9900-5.*
Verweij, J., Pinedo, H.M., Suit, H.D. (eds): *Soft Tissue Sarcomas: Present Achievements and Future Prospects. 1997.* *ISBN 0-7923-9913-7.*
Walterhouse, D.O., Cohn, S. L. (eds): *Diagnostic and Therapeutic Advances in Pediatric Oncology. 1997.* *ISBN 0-7923-9978-1.*
Mittal, B.B., Purdy, J.A., Ang, K.K. (eds): *Radiation Therapy. 1998.* *ISBN 0-7923-9981-1.*
Foon, K.A., Muss, H.B. (eds): *Biological and Hormonal Therapies of Cancer. 1998.* *ISBN 0-7923-9997-8.*
Ozols, R.F. (ed.): *Gynecologic Oncology. 1998.* *ISBN 0-7923-8070-3.*
Noskin, G.A. (ed.): *Management of Infectious Complications in Cancer Patients. 1998.* *ISBN 0-7923-8150-5.*
Bennett, C.L. (ed.): *Cancer Policy. 1998.* *ISBN 0-7923-8203-X.*
Benson, A.B. (ed.): *Gastrointestinal Oncology. 1998.* *ISBN 0-7923-8205-6.*
Tallman, M.S., Gordon, L.I. (eds): *Diagnostic and Therapeutic Advances in Hematologic Malignancies. 1998.* *ISBN 0-7923-8206-4.*
von Gunten, C.F. (ed.): *Palliative Care and Rehabilitation of Cancer Patients. 1999.* *ISBN 0-7923-8525-X.*
Burt, R.K., Brush, M.M. (eds): *Advances in Allogeneic Hematopoietic Stem Cell Transplantation. 1999.* *ISBN 0-7923-7714-1.*
Angelos, P. (ed.): *Ethical Issues in Cancer Patient Care 2000.* *ISBN 0-7923-7726-5.*
Gradishar, W.J., Wood, W.C. (eds): *Advances in Breast Cancer Management. 2000.* *ISBN 0-7923-7890-3.*
Sparano, J.A. (ed.): *HIV & HTLV-I Associated Malignancies. 2001.* *ISBN 0-7923-7220-4.*
Ettinger, D.S. (ed.): *Thoracic Oncology. 2001.* *ISBN 0-7923-7248-4.*
Bergan, R.C. (ed.): *Cancer Chemoprevention. 2001.* *ISBN 0-7923-7259-X.*
Raza, A., Mundle, S.D. (eds): *Myelodysplastic Syndromes & Secondary Acute Myelogenous Leukemia 2001.* *ISBN: 0-7923-7396.*
Talamonti, M.S. (ed.): *Liver Directed Therapy for Primary and Metastatic Liver Tumors. 2001.* *ISBN 0-7923-7523-8.*
Stack, M.S., Fishman, D.A. (eds): *Ovarian Cancer. 2001.* *ISBN 0-7923-7530-0.*
Bashey, A., Ball, E.D. (eds): *Non-Myeloablative Allogeneic Transplantation. 2002.* *ISBN 0-7923-7646-3.*
Leong, S.P.L. (ed.): *Atlas of Selective Sentinel Lymphadenectomy for Melanoma, Breast Cancer and Colon Cancer. 2002.* *ISBN 1-4020-7013-6.*
Andersson, B., Murray, D. (eds): *Clinically Relevant Resistance in Cancer Chemotherapy. 2002.* *ISBN 1-4020-7200-7.*
Beam, C. (ed.): *Biostatistical Applications in Cancer Research. 2002.* *ISBN 1-4020-7226-0.*
Brockstein, B., Masters, G. (eds): *Head and Neck Cancer. 2003.* *ISBN 1-4020-7336-4.*
Frank, D.A. (ed.): *Signal Transduction in Cancer. 2003.* *ISBN 1-4020-7340-2.*

(continued after index)

Radiation Oncology Advances

Edited by

Søren M. Bentzen, Ph.D., D.Sc.
Professor
Department of Human Oncology
University of Wisconsin School of Medicine
Madison, Wisconsin, USA

Paul M. Harari, M.D.
Jack Fowler Professor and Chairman
Department of Human Oncology
University of Wisconsin School of Medicine
Madison, Wisconsin, USA

Wolfgang A. Tomé, M.D., Ph.D
Associate Professor
Department of Human Oncology
University of Wisconsin School of Medicine
Madison, Wisconsin, USA

Minesh P. Mehta, M.D.
Professor
Department of Human Oncology
University of Wisconsin School of Medicine
Madison, Wisconsin, USA

Springer

Søren M. Bentzen, PhD
Paul M. Harari, MD
Wolfgang A. Tomé, PhD
Minesh P. Mehta, MD

University of Wisconsin
Department of Human Oncology
600 Highland Avenue, K4/310
Madison, WI 53792
USA

Series Editor:
Steven T. Rosen
Robert H. Lurie Comprehensive Cancer Center
Northwestern University
Chicago, IL
USA

ISBN-13: 978-1-4419-4221-0 e-ISBN-13: 978-0-387-36744-6

Printed on acid-free paper.

9 8 7 6 5 4 3 2 1

springer.com

Contents

Contributors

Igor Astsaturov, MD
Department of Medical Oncology
Division of Medical Science
Fox Chase Cancer Center
Philadelphia, PA, USA

Søren M. Bentzen, PhD, DSc
Department of Human Oncology and Department of Medical Physics
University of Wisconsin School of Medicine and Public Health
Madison, WI, USA

Robert G. Bristow, MD, PhD, FRCPC
Department of Radiation Oncology
Princess Margaret Hospital – University Health Network
Toronto, ON, Canada M5G 2M9

Kevin Camphausen, MD
Radiation Oncology Branch
National Cancer Institute
Bethesda, MD, USA

Arnab Chakravarti, MD
Laboratory of Cellular and Molecular Neuro-Radiation Oncology
Department of Radiation Oncology
Massachusetts General Hospital/Harvard Medical School
Boston, MA, USA

Deborah Citrin, MD
Radiation Oncology Branch
National Cancer Institute
Bethesda, MD, USA

Roger B. Cohen, MD
Department of Medical Oncology
Division of Medical Science
Fox Chase Cancer Center
Philadelphia, PA, USA

Joseph O. Deasy, PhD
Department of Radiation Oncology
Division of Bioinformatics and Outcomes Research
Washington University School of Medicine
St. Louis, MO, USA

Issam El Naqa, PhD
Department of Radiation Oncology
Division of Bioinformatics and Outcomes Research
Washington University School of Medicine
St. Louis, MO, USA

Oluwatoyosi A. Fatunase, BA
Department of Radiation Oncology
Duke University Medical Center
Durham, NC, USA

John D. Fenwick, PhD
Medical Physics
Clatterbridge Centre for Oncology
Bebington, Wirral, UK

Paul M. Harari, MD
Department of Human Oncology
University of Wisconsin School of Medicine and Public Health
Madison, WI, USA

Robert Jeraj, PhD
Department of Medical Physics
University of Wisconsin School of Medicine and Public Health
Madison, WI, USA

Yusung Kim, PhD
Department of Human Oncology and Department of Medical Physics
University of Wisconsin School of Medicine and Public Health
Madison, WI, USA

Thomas Rockwell Mackie, PhD
Department of Human Oncology and Department of Medical Physics
University of Wisconsin School of Medicine and Public Health
Madison, WI, USA
and
TomoTherapy, Inc.
Madison, WI, USA

Jingfang Mao, MD
Department of Radiation Oncology
Duke University Medical Center
Durham, NC, USA
and
Department of Radiation Oncology
Cancer Hospital, Fudan University
Shanghai, People's Republic of China

Lawrence B. Marks, MD
Department of Radiation Oncology
Duke University Medical Center
Durham, NC, USA

Minesh P. Mehta, MD
Department of Human Oncology
University of Wisconsin School of Medicine and Public Health
Madison, WI, USA

M. Elizabeth Meyerand, PhD
Department of Medical Physics
University of Wisconsin School of Medicine and Public Health
Madison, WI, USA

Kamalakannan Palanichamy, PhD
Department of Radiation Oncology
Massachusetts General Hospital
Boston, MA, USA

Stephen W. Riley, MSc
Medical Physics
Clatterbridge Centre for Oncology
Bebington, Wirral, UK

Mark A. Ritter, MD, PhD
Department of Human Oncology
University of Wisconsin School of Medicine and Public Health
Madison, WI, USA

Jann N. Sarkaria, MD
Mayo Clinic
Department of Radiation Oncology
Rochester, MN, USA

Alison J. D. Scott, MSc
Medical Physics
Clatterbridge Centre for Oncology
Bebington, Wirral, UK

Wolfgang A. Tomé, PhD
Department of Human Oncology and Department of Medical Physics
University of Wisconsin School of Medicine and Public Health
Madison, WI, USA

Gordon Wong, MD
Department of Human Oncology
University of Wisconsin School of Medicine and Public Health
Madison, WI, USA

1
Radiation Oncology Advances: An Introduction

Søren M. Bentzen, Paul M. Harari, Wolfgang A. Tomé, and Minesh P. Mehta

Radiation therapy remains a mainstay of cancer treatment: it is estimated that around half of all cancer patients in Europe, in the US probably close to two-thirds, receive radiation therapy as part of their initial therapy, for salvage or for palliation. There are good reasons to expect the role of radiation therapy in the management of cancer to expand in the next decade. This is partly because of changing demographics: the aging of the population means that an increasing fraction of cancer patients will be elderly and may present with comorbidities making nonsurgical management of their disease an attractive option. At the same time, more widespread implementation of cancer screening programs in the coming years means that more patients will present with early disease where persistent tumor control with organ and functional preservation are realistic treatment aims. But most of all, the role of radiation therapy is likely to expand as a result of a number of recent technological and biological advances that are rapidly changing the way we prescribe, plan and deliver radiation therapy alone or in combination with other modalities and these could potentially widen the indications for combination therapies involving ionizing radiation as one component. These advances are the topic of the current volume. Naturally, a volume like the current one can only highlight some selected areas of progress and we have chosen to organize these thematically under four broad, partly overlapping headings: Imaging and Theragnostic Radiation Oncology, Molecular Biology and Targeted Therapies, Treatment Delivery and Planning, and finally, Clinical Advances.

Advances in Imaging and Theragnostic Radiation Oncology

Ionizing radiation is a unique anticancer agent because it can be precisely modulated in space and time. This anatomical or geometrical targeting is so fundamental to delivering therapeutic radiation that we often do not even think about it; but very few solid malignancies could be controlled by radiation therapy if we had to deliver this systemically, i.e., by total body irradiation. The overall principle of trying to exclude normal tissues and structures from the irradiated volume means on the other hand, that the selection and delineation of target volumes, the prescription of

M.P. Mehta et al. (eds.), *Radiation Oncology Advances.*

a given biologically equivalent dose to these targets and the subsequent verification that the dose is delivered as intended are integral components of high-precision radiation therapy.

Image Guided Radiotherapy (IGRT) is the use of imaging in the treatment room to improve the spatial precision of delivering radiation therapy and these technologies, reviewed by Mackie and Tomé in Chap. 2, are rapidly being introduced in centers all-over the world [1, 2] Some IGRT techniques allow the recording or at least the estimation of the delivered dose distribution which in turn may be used to adapt the dose distribution delivered in subsequent fractions in order to approach the initially prescribed distribution as closely as possible.

Theragnostics, a term formed from the Greek words for medical treatment and knowledge [3] refers to strategies for personalizing therapy based on individual-patient level biological images or biomarkers. Theragnostic imaging for radiation oncology is the use of molecular and functional imaging as a rational basis for delivering biologically targeted external beam radiation therapy. This represents a major extension of the role of imaging in radiation therapy. The ultimate realization of this principle is Dose Painting by Numbers, i.e., the voxel-based prescription of a nonuniform dose distribution estimated to optimize the efficacy:toxicity ratio in an individual patient. This novel treatment paradigm is discussed in Chap. 3 by Bentzen. Theragnostic imaging is becoming a realistic research aim thanks to the rapid advances in functional and molecular imaging, mainly Positron Emission Tomography (PET) and Magnetic Resonance Imaging (MRI), reviewed in some detail by Jeraj and Meyerand in Chap. 4. While these imaging modalities are of great value in traditional anatomical imaging, the current excitement stems from the fact that they can map molecular and phenotypical characteristics with a spatial resolution of a few millimeters. This is a relevant spatial scale for what can be reliably resolved when delivering a nonuniform dose distribution in radiation therapy.

Chapter 5 by Ritter reviews prognostic and predictive markers in prostate cancer. Again, rapid progress in this area may eventually lead to personalized prescriptions of dose fractionation or optimize the use of multiple modalities in managing individual cases. The chapter focuses on immunohistochemical markers in pre-treatment biopsies, where most published data are available, but an increasing number of studies are concerned with high-throughput assays in basic and clinical radiation research.

Advances in Molecular Biology and Targeted Therapies

Recent advances in our understanding of the molecular responses induced in cells by ionizing radiation are expertly reviewed by Sarkaria and Bristow (Chap. 6). Many of these pathways constitute drugable targets for inhibitors that might enhance the efficacy of radiation therapy. Enthusiasm for such strategies is fuelled by the first randomized controlled trial demonstrating a significant clinical benefit from combining radiation with a molecular targeted agent – namely cetuximab, a recombinant mouse/human chimeric monoclonal antibody against the Epidermal Growth Factor (EGF) receptor [4]

Astsaturov, Cohen and Harari present a more indepth review of the biology of the EGF Receptor and its signaling pathway in Chap. 7 as a potential target in combination with fractionated radiotherapy for head and neck squamous cell carcinoma (HNSCC). A flurry of agents are under development for targeting EGFR and in March 2006, the US Food and Drugs Administration approved cetuximab combined with radiation as a primary treatment option for patients with loco-regionally advanced HNSCC in whom chemoradiation therapy is deemed not to be an option.

While blocking the EGF pathway during fractionated radiotherapy may seem an obvious strategy [5], the rationale for combining antiangiogenic and antivascular targeting agents with radiation may be less intuitive. However, recent research shows that there are several reasons why this could result in a therapeutic gain in practice. Chapter 8 is a review of this rapidly expanding field by Citrin and Camphausen.

Targeted agents combined with radiation may offer new opportunities in the treatment of central nervous system malignancies, a tumor type where the outlook remains poor despite some recent progress [6]. Current attempts to overcome radiation resistance in these tumors on the basis of an improved understanding of their molecular biology are the topic of Chap. 9 by Chakravarti and Palanichamy.

Advances in Treatment Delivery and Planning

Advances in radiation oncology have always resulted from successful combinations of technological progress combined with improved biological understanding. The dramatic increase in computer power, and the associated drop in the cost of computing, has already had a major impact of the planning and delivery of radiation therapy. Fenwick, Riley, and Scott (Chap. 10) review the latest developments in Intensity Modulated Radiotherapy (IMRT) using conventional linear accelerators with multileaf collimators and provide an overview of three innovative IMRT planning and delivery systems: tomotherapy, robotic linear accelerators, and conventional linear accelerators modulated by their jaws alone. IMRT delivery typically gives rise to highly nonuniform dose distributions in the surrounding normal tissues and organs. Mathematical models have been introduced and are continually refined for the estimation of normal-tissue complication probabilities arising from nonuniform irradiation and this is the topic of the comprehensive review by Deasy and El-Naqa (Chap. 11). Just around the corner is the use of biologically based objective functions that combine tumor control probability and the risk of normal-tissue complications into a composite score function that form the basis for risk-adaptive optimization, a topic discussed in Chap. 12 by Kim and Tomé.

Clinical Advances

All of the above advances are in various stages of clinical or preclinical development and many of these are already becoming integrated into clinical practice. When looking at the current growth areas of clinical radiation research, we have chosen to highlight two additional topics. One is the advances in combining cytotoxic chemotherapy with radiation in many of the most common solid malignancies, a topic reviewed by Wong and Mehta in Chap. 13. While most current strategies for combining drugs with radiation have been developed empirically, improved understanding of the exploitable mechanisms in combining drugs with fractionated radiotherapy provides a framework for rational progress in this field [7]. The other area is the less established, but potentially very promising, use of drugs for normal tissue protection [8]. The most clinically advanced o f these drugs is amifostine, a free-radical scavenger with potential as a cytoprotector, and the experience with this compound is reviewed here by Mao, Fatunase and Marks (Chap. 14). The technological and conceptual advances presented in this book are likely to improve the efficacy:toxicity ratio of radiation therapy for a number of indications and will almost certainly revolutionize the practice of radiation oncology in the next decade. They represent the future of radiation therapy in the era of molecular oncology.

References

1. Mackie TR, Kapatoes J, Ruchala K, Lu W, Wu C, Olivera G, Forrest L, Tome W, Welsh J, Jeraj R, Harari P, Reckwerdt P, Paliwal B, Ritter M, Keller H, Fowler J, Mehta M. Image guidance for precise conformal radiotherapy. Int J Radiat Oncol Biol Phys 2003; 56:89–105.
2. Jaffray DA. Emergent technologies for 3-dimensional image-guided radiation delivery. Semin Radiat Oncol 2005; 15:208–216.
3. Bentzen SM. Theragnostic imaging for radiation oncology: dose-painting by numbers. Lancet Oncol 2005; 6:112–117.
4. Bonner JA, Harari PM, Giralt J, Azarnia N, Shin DM, Cohen RB, Jones CU, Sur R, Raben D, Jassem J, Ove R, Kies MS, Baselga J, Youssoufian H, Amellal N, Rowinsky EK, Ang KK. Radiotherapy plus cetuximab for squamous-cell carcinoma of the head and neck. N Engl J Med 2006; 354:567–578.
5. Harari PM, Huang SM. Epidermal growth factor receptor modulation of radiation response: preclinical and clinical development. Semin Radiat Oncol 2002; 12:21–26.
6. Stupp R, Mason WP, van den Bent MJ, Weller M, Fisher B, Taphoorn MJ, Belanger K, Brandes AA, Marosi C, Bogdahn U, Curschmann J, Janzer RC, Ludwin SK, Gorlia T, Allgeier A, Lacombe D, Cairncross JG, Eisenhauer E, Mirimanoff RO. Radiotherapy plus concomitant and adjuvant temozolomide for glioblastoma. N Engl J Med 2005; 352:987–996.
7. Bentzen SM, Harari PM, Bernier J. Exploitable mechanisms for combining drugs with radiation: concepts, achievements and future directions. Nat Clin Pract Oncol 2007; 4:172–180.
8. Bentzen SM. Preventing or reducing late side effects of radiation therapy: radiobiology meets molecular pathology. Nat Rev Cancer 2006; 6:702–713.

Section I
Advances in Imaging and Biologically-Based Treatment Planning

2
Advanced Image-Guided External Beam Radiotherapy

Thomas Rockwell Mackie and Wolfgang Tomé

Introduction

In 2003, Schultz and Kagan speculated that even with a perfect ability to deliver the ideal radiation dose distribution, it would be unlikely that outcomes would be improved. They imagined a perfect radiation treatment machine, which they called the "Infinitron," that could deliver a dose distribution with any dose level and a zero dose outside of the target volume. They proposed that the Infinitron might not be preferable to surgery except for the reduced morbidity that would accompany its use. Schultz and Kagan were overly pessimistic as their argument that better radiation technology would not affect cure was easily countered by Keall and Williamson (2003) who provided several examples to the contrary. However, Schultz and Kagan (2003) were correct on one point; without the knowledge of where the disease is and where it is not present, the Infinitron could not guarantee a cure. As more and better treatment systems to deliver radiation come into existence, the key to their use will be to identify the target volume more exactly and to ensure that the targeted region is treated as prescribed.

Radiation therapy treatment planning was the first application to use quantitative imaging in medicine to determine an accurate representation of the patient including the tumor volume. Other allied fields such as radiology and surgery traditionally used images in a qualitative sense. Images have long been used to determine the position and extent of the tumor. In modern radiation therapy, CT images are routinely used to obtain density and tissue type information in order to determine tissue attenuation accurately. More recently, images are used not just to determine physical quantities but are also increasingly being used to incorporate biological information into the treatment planning process [1–4].

The goal of radiation therapy research and development is to increase the chance of tumor control and/or reduce the chance of causing harm to normal tissues. 3D imaging modalities can pinpoint the location of many anatomical structures within the body, and their function can be mapped with reasonable precision. Intensity-modulated radiotherapy (IMRT) can deliver radiation to target volumes of complex shape (ASTRO/AAPM 2001) [5–8] and so it is now possible to improve the delivery of radiation to those regions that are truly afflicted and to avoid better those areas that

M.P. Mehta et al. (eds.), *Radiation Oncology Advances*.

are at risk of radiation injury. With IMRT, it is possible to increase the magnitude of the gradient between the target and normal tissue, which places more demand on imaging as a verification tool for this form of radiation delivery.

Until the advent of 3D imaging systems, the extent of the diseased volume was uncertain unless surgery was performed. This is because the exclusive use of 2D images presupposes an underlying shape in order to deduce volumes. For example, the tradition of staging tumor size based on lineal measurements in orthogonal planes is from an earlier era when 2D imaging was dominant. 3D CRT planning systems can augment the poor image quality of planar radiographs and improve their comparability with CT by the construction of digital reconstructed radiographs (DRRs) from CT [9, 10] or even MR [11] image sets in the same treatment setup and beam position as the radiographs. However, when mismatches occur between DRRs and planar radiographs, the reasons are usually not readily obvious or easily determined. Radio-opaque markers can be placed in certain structures such as the prostate to assist in its localization with EPIDs [12–14] but this is a highly invasive procedure and does not have universal applicability.

The International Committee of Radiation Units and Measurements (ICRU) have developed nomenclature and procedures for defining tumor and normal tissue structures in radiotherapy [15, 16]. 3D imaging modalities such as computed tomography (CT), magnetic resonance imaging (MRI), and positron emission tomography (PET) have enabled ever more precise localization of the gross tumor volume (GTV) for many sites and most sensitive structures. The location of microscopic extensions of the tumor around the GTV remains uncertain because tumor extension or tumorlets visible close to the GTV have to consist of millions of cells to be visible on a PET scan, typically the most sensitive (not necessarily the most specific) imaging system for cancer. The concept of clinical target volume (CTV) surrounding the GTV with a margin for invasion undetectable by current imaging systems is used to define the region of presumed spread that is inferred occasionally by evidence from pathology but usually only by clinical experience [15, 16]. A margin around the CTV defining a volume called the planning target volume (PTV) takes into account uncertainties affecting the precise treatment of the target volume. The uncertainty arises because the target volumes cannot be set up precisely from day to day, the organ shape and position may vary due to organ filling (or voiding), the patient may have lost (or gained) weight, the tumor may have shrunk (or grown), or the organ could be in periodic motion. In modern radiotherapy, the dose given to the GTV is typically higher than the dose applied to the CTV. If the dose difference is substantial, a PTV margin should also surround the GTV to ensure that it is getting adequate dose. Figure 1 illustrates the concepts of GTV, CTV, and PTV [15, 16].

In-room image guidance is also not a new topic. 2D image guidance using portal imaging systems has been used for decades. The current state of the art for curative radiotherapy is to produce a portal image once a week, which is an image of the beam exiting the patient [17–19]. This may be acquired with radiographic film but increasingly electronic portal imaging detector (EPID) systems are used. EPIDs are an improvement over film because they are less sensitive to over- or underexposure and there is an opportunity for image enhancement [20–23]. EPIDs have been used to automatically correct patient setup, for example, using a "tilt and roll" couch

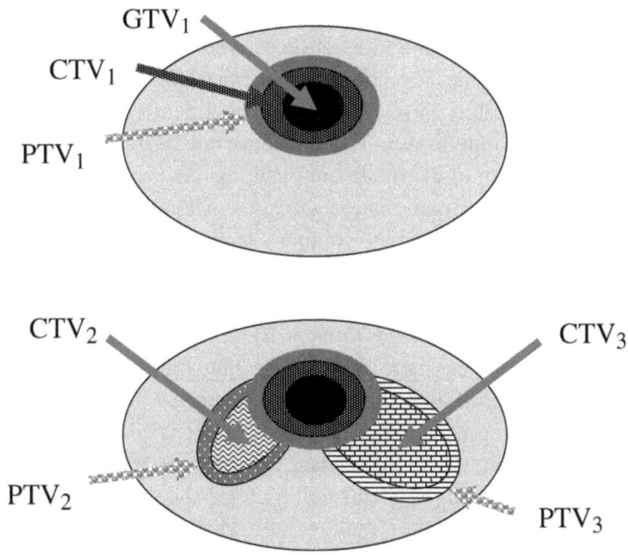

Fig. 1 Illustration of the use of the concepts of gross tumor volume (GTV), clinical target volume (CTV), and planning target volume (PTV). In the *upper figure*, a CTV (CTV_1) is the margin for microscopic tumor extension surrounding GTV_1. The dose prescription is assigned to the PTV (PTV_1) which is the extension to account for setup variation and organ motion. In the *lower figure*, in addition to CTV_1, there are clinical target volumes (CTV_2 and CTV_3) that are the regional extensions of the disease. Correspondingly, the planning target volumes account for setup variability and organ motion. The dose prescriptions for PTV_1, PTV_2, and PTV_3 could be all different

[24]. Many investigators have shown that it is possible to collect the "exit dose" from the EPID signal [25–30]. This exit dosimetry information could be compared to the exit dose calculated from the treatment plan and employed as the basis to halt the treatment.

Even the best portal images will be inferior to typical diagnostic X-ray planar radiographs because of the smaller focal spot size in X-ray tubes and higher bony contrast of diagnostic X-rays. Planar radiographs are difficult to interpret because they are not in reference to 3D CT image sets and out-of-plane rotations of the patient are not as readily evident as translations [31–33].

Image Guidance for Defining Target Volumes

Of all likely uncertainties in radiotherapy, position and extent of the contoured volumes have the greatest uncertainty. The CTV margin is almost never satisfied by a simple constant distance extension around the GTV. Many studies have shown that the accuracy of the definition of the CTV is not accurate to even 10s of percent in the lung [34–36], esophagus [37], breast [38], bladder [39, 40], and cervix [41].

A major goal of future radiotherapy procedures and systems will be to reduce the uncertainty in tumor extent and location as well as to reduce the uncertainties related to treatment delivery. The conventional fractionation paradigm of radiation therapy has been predicated on relatively large treatment volumes, which irradiate a large volume of normal tissue. The conventional 2 Gy per fraction has been established during the era of 2D treatment planning. As target volumes are reduced due to improved imaging, fractionation schedules should be re-evaluated. Recent evidence indicates that many target volume sites are likely to respond to higher doses per fraction [42] without impacting normal tissue tolerance. The α/β ratio for prostate carcinoma is likely to be low [43–48] as compared to other treatment sites, with estimates as low as 1.5 instead of the 8–10 typical for early responding tissues and tumors. In lung cancer, there is evidence that the dose per fraction should be increased and the overall time should be shortened [49, 50] to avoid wasted dose because of accelerated repopulation of the tumor. IMRT is enabling a higher dose per fraction to be more safely delivered because the dose per fraction to normal tissues is not significantly increased [51]. This will increase the importance of image guidance because a higher dose per fraction will decrease the number of fractions treated; hence the increased effort of image guidance is justifiable. All of these strategies taken together will reduce the margins around the GTV and reduce the amount of integral dose that needs to be deposited in the patient.

There are two types of CTV. The first type takes into account that an occult microscopic disease exists around the visible tumor extent defined to be the GTV. If there are no highly sensitive normal tissue structures close to the GTV, a CTV accounting for the microscopic extension typically receives a dose close to or equal to that received by the GTV. This use of CTV is illustrated in the upper panel of Fig. 1.

Reducing the uncertainty of the microscopic extension of the tumor is a difficult task. The CTV margin for some sites like breast might be too generous (hence the interest in partial breast radiotherapy) whereas for other sites like glioblastoma multiforme it might encompass most of the brain. What is needed is a three-pronged research attack on the problem:

1. High-sensitivity and potentially high-specificity imaging systems, such as PET, correlated with image-registered pathological specimens should be used to help delineate disease extent from normal tissue at the tumor periphery so that knowledge of the probability of spread can be determined. This approach attempts to make occult disease visible, in effect, turning CTVs into GTVs.
2. Outcome analysis has to be precisely quantified so that it can be determined whether or not patients are failing at the margin or within the tumor. This will be a tremendous complement to dose escalation trials because even extremely high doses will not be sufficient to eradicate high probability tumors that are routinely missed [52].
3. Begin treating patients with a conformal avoidance methodology in addition to conformal radiotherapy; this allows for the use of modestly large CTV margins while still sparing critical normal structures.

Radiation therapy treatment planning requires sufficient sensitivity and specificity to be able to delineate tumor and normal tissues with confidence. CT, alone or fused with other imaging modalities [53], is still the predominant imaging modality on which the delineation of most tissue structures is based. Improved CT contrast agents have led to improved definition of tumor boundaries. CT simulation with 3D treatment planning is now conventional practice in all radiotherapy centers and the need for conventional simulators in radiotherapy departments has been called into question [54]. Even with dedicated 3D imaging systems common in the clinic and a generation of radiation oncologists trained in their use, there is considerable variation of the GTV for many sites [55].

MRI is gaining in importance in radiation therapy. Usually, the MRI scans are fused with CT scans and the MRI is used to aid in delineation of tumor volumes and normal structures. Dedicated MRI simulation that eliminates the need for fusion is being investigated for sites, like prostate, for which tissue heterogeneity dose calculation algorithms are not necessary [56]. MRI is now the preferred way by which most central nervous system malignancies are delineated [57, 58]. Even though its resolution is not comparable with conventional MR images, magnetic resonance spectroscopy (MRS) is being used to determine the location of the most active disease site within the prostate, in effect, identifying the GTV within the prostate CTV volume [59–62]. Selective boosting of active disease will require excellent tumor and target localization at the time of treatment [cf. 52].

The best MRI or contrast CT imaging today is capable of defining tumors with a clonogen density of about 10^6 or 10^7 tumor cells per square centimeter as compared to 10^9 cells/cm^3 (range from 10^8 to 10^{10} cells/cm^3) for normal tissue. Tumorlets which have fewer than 10^6 cells extending over a cubic centimeter will not be visible.

The role of PET will be greatly enhanced by the new generation of PET/CT scanners from which fully correlated PET and CT images emerge. PET/CT simulators will augment or even replace CT simulators during this decade. Using PET images, one will be able to delineate the extent of the GTV and the CTV with much more precision. PET will begin to enable a probabilistic formulation for the GTV and CTV whereby the GTV is that region where the probability of the occupancy by tumor approaches 100% and the CTV is at the boundary where that probability approaches zero. The PET successors to Prostascint scans might identify minimally involved lymph nodes in prostate cancer. Radiopharmaceuticals to complement ^{18}FDG, a good marker of proliferative metabolic activity in many cases, are emerging [63]. Labeling of proliferation, hypoxia, perfusion, even the status of the P53 gene in the tumor, will be possible [37, 64, 65].

The best PET imaging today is capable of improved sensitivity as compared to MRI or contrast-enhanced CT. That means that it may be possible to detect tumors with a density as low as 10^5 cells/cm^3. This could be improved in a number of ways. The efficiency of tumor uptake could be improved. With faster PET detector electronics, the absolute activity of the isotope could be increased for patients undergoing radiotherapy. The scan times could be increased. Each of these factors would only increase the contrast by the square root of the counts detected and so all of these approaches may be necessary for a significant improvement. Decreasing the background of the isotope in normal tissues would improve the detectability in a linear fashion but this requires new imaging compounds that have lower uptake and/or faster clearance in normal tissue.

Only detailed examination of pathological specimens can reveal information about the margin around the GTV necessary to ensure that the tumor is completely within the treatment field [66, 67]. Image guidance should be carried into the microscopic realm. Systems that automate the screening of pathological samples and correlate this information with imaging studies need to be developed in order to gather information on nodal disease spread on individual patients and populations of patients so that rational margins around the GTVs can be established [68].

The other major reason for defining a CTV is to define the volume of regional spread of the disease (see the lower panel of Fig. 1). Often this CTV is prescribed a dose that is lower than that of the GTV. The regional spread can never be defined with the use of a simple margin around the GTV but rather on anatomical grounds defining the volume of likely spread. The ability of radiation oncologists to define the extent of the tumor needs to be improved. At the present time, the inconsistency of contouring the CTV to define the regional spread makes the interpretation of clinical trials difficult; therefore, if accuracy is not possible then at least consistency should be improved. Better training of radiation oncologists in visualizing tissue structures and the routes of likely spread of disease is necessary to improve the accuracy of the CTV. Education will likely have the biggest cost/benefit of any approach to improve the CTV definition.

Conformal avoidance is the complement to conformal therapy [69, 70] and it is used if the CTV extent is uncertain. The strategy of conformal avoidance is to treat the tumor with generous treatment volumes but to "carve out" dose-limiting regions around sensitive structures where there is no possibility of tumor extensions. Conformal therapy should be used when the GTV is well delineated and the CTV extension is small. Conformal avoidance should be used when the GTV is not well delineated or the CTV is large. This strategy was not possible prior to the advent of IMRT because it was extremely difficult to produce arbitrarily shaped treatment volumes with standard uniform field irradiation. Examples of conformal avoidance include sparing uninvolved parotid glands, auditory apparatus, mucosa and larynx in head and neck radiotherapy. In advanced prostate, the paraprostatic nodes are the ones at the highest risk of involvement. A treatment envelope could cover the nodes but avoid the rectum and the lower bladder [cf. 71].

Conformal avoidance radiotherapy requires image-guided delivery. Carving out regions around sensitive structures will result in placing high gradients near the sensitive structures. In order to have confidence in this strategy, the second major objective for precise delivery of radiotherapy, the reduction of setup uncertainty and organ motion and confirmation of accurate dose delivery, has to be met.

Radiation therapy has not routinely gathered highly accurate information on distributions of failure in and near the treatment volume and that information is needed even more now [72]. As CTV margins around disease sites are reduced and doses are escalated, there must be careful monitoring to determine whether the patterns of failure are changing. Smaller margins will result in more motion blurring of the dose inside the target volume [73]. There is plenty of data on failure from autopsy series; the problem is that the fine structure of local failure is blurred by overgrowth of the recurrence. Without image-based follow-up correlated to the treatment plan to provide in vivo recurrence detection, failures could masquerade as a consequence of inadequate dose instead of inadequate margin. Shrinking the margins for the sake of shrinking the margins, when there is no critical sensitive tissue to spare, might lead to a decreased therapeutic ratio.

Margins blur the radius of curvature of GTV contours to a value no less than the margin width. Today's large margins moderate the demand for high-resolution planning, delivery, and verification systems. As margins shrink, there will be a need for tighter resolution requirements of image-guidance systems.

Image Guidance at the Time of Delivery

Image guidance at the time of treatment delivery is useful to prevent setup variations and when the patient representation varies from day-to-day. Interfractional variations are patient variations due to weight loss or tumor shrinkage and can be detected by imaging the patient. Variations in the patient representation happening on a timescale comparable with the time to perform a treatment are called intrafractional variations. Table 1 summarizes techniques used to ensure that the patient is set up correctly. Figure 2 illustrates the timescales for intrafractional and interfractional variations.

The day-to-day movement of the prostate has been well established mainly due to differential filling of the rectum with fecal matter or gas [74]. The predominant translational displacement of the prostate is in the anterior–posterior direction with an accompanying pitch along a lateral axis. This movement may be accounted with

Table 1 Methodologies to effect precision radiation delivery

	Translation + Rotation	Organ Deformation	Organ Motion
Immobilization	√	X	X
Planar imaging			
Film	Depends on Contrast	X	X
EPID	Improvement from Film	X	X
DDR	Improves use of EPID	X	X
Stationary X-ray	OK when used with markers	X	√
Ultrasound Imaging	Good where applicable	Possibly in Prostate	X
CT imaging			
KVCT	√	√	X
MVCT	√	√	X

X Indicates lack of effectiveness
√ Indicates effectiveness

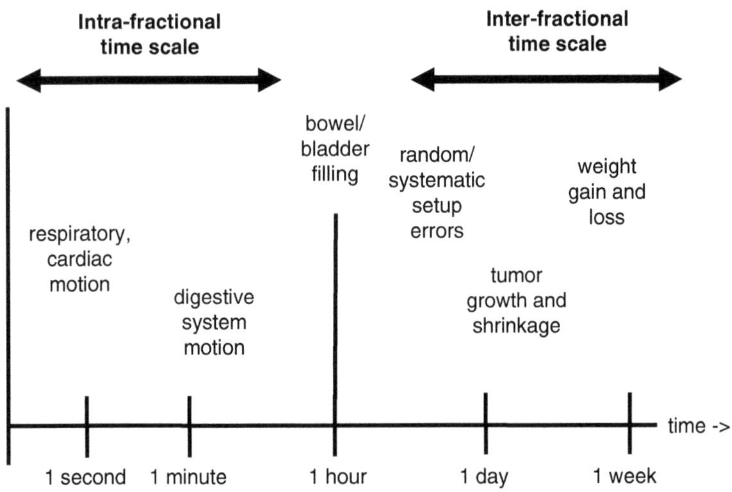

Fig. 2 Illustration of intrafraction and interfraction timescales and their corresponding geometrical errors

a sufficient PTV margin. If the margin is too large, the rectum and bladder will get significant unwanted dose. A balloon inserted into the rectum may improve the setup and reduce the margins [75–78]; however, most radiation oncologists worry that the balloon will not be well tolerated and do not use it.

Image-guided delivery is required for precise conformal therapy or conformal avoidance therapy for many treatment sites. There are examples of radiation therapy today for which setup uncertainty or organ motion is not an issue. In stereotactic radiosurgery, the use of imaging to localize the disease with pin-point precision is justified because the brain is held relatively fixed within the cranium and the cranium is fixed to rigid external devices or implanted markers [79–82]. When it can be guaranteed that the representation of the patient at the time of delivery is the same as at the time of imaging, and the tumor volume is small, one or a few high doses of radiation can be delivered to the tumor. However, even in stereotactic radiosurgery, imaging can be used to verify that the fiducial frame position did not become altered between planning and delivery [83].

Optical Guidance

Optically guided radiation therapy systems have played an important role in improving the precision of patient treatment. Since these systems allow one to accurately position internal targets relative to the isocenter of a treatment machine and also allow one to track patients in real time, they theoretically enable one to reduce PTV margins to include only uncertainties due to imaging and contouring, and therefore allow one to limit the amount of normal tissue included in the irradiated volume. Moreover, optical guidance, both alone and in conjunction with imaging systems such as ultrasound or digital X-ray imaging, can be used for localization of extracranial targets. In what follows, we describe the process of optical tracking, discuss patient localization systems that exploit optically guided techniques to improve patient setup for radiotherapy, as well as their clinical utilization.

Optical Tracking Systems

Tracking is the process of measuring the location of instruments, anatomical structures, and/or landmarks in 3D space and in relationship to each other in real time. Various technologies have been tested for determining an object's location, including mechanical, magnetic, acoustic, inertial, and optical position sensors. Most of these technologies have been tested for medical use in either image-guided surgery or image-guided tracking in radiation therapy. In what follows, only optical tracking techniques are considered and the reader is referred to Allen et al. [84] for a description of more general tracking systems.

Infrared light is employed in optical tracking to determine the position of an object. The object might consist of either an active or a passive marker. The most commonly used active markers are infrared light emitting diodes (IRLED). Passive markers are generally spheres or disks coated with a highly reflective surface that reflects the infrared light emitted from an external source. A variety of detectors can be used to determine the positions of either active or passive optical markers; however, charged couple device (CCD) cameras are the detector system used most often. CCD cameras consist of a collection of light sensitive pixels, and these pixels can be arranged either in a linear or a planar geometry. When light strikes a CCD pixel, the number of electrons produced in the pixel is proportional to the intensity of the incident light. The charge collected per pixel yields a pixel luminance value; a planar CCD array therefore provides a 2D digital "image" of the target in terms of intensity values, where brighter pixels correspond to higher light intensity and darker pixels correspond to lower light intensity. This digital image can then be analyzed to determine the pixel with the highest intensity. Each camera in a planar CCD array determines a 3D ray in space. When an optical system uses two planar CCD cameras, the intersection of the 3D rays from the cameras determines a line in space while if it uses three planar CCD cameras, the intersection of the rays from the cameras determines a single point in space.

Several optical tracking systems have been developed for use in radiation therapy [cf. 85–91]. All of these systems function similarly, namely infrared markers (passive or active) that are either attached to the patient or are correlated to the patients position are optically tracked and are used to determine the patient's position relative to the treatment machine isocenter. This real-time feedback can be used to position the patient and gate the radiation beam during delivery.

Optical Tracking in Fractionated Stereotactic Radiotherapy, Intracranial, and Head and Neck IMRT

The first commercially available optical tracking system for radiation therapy was developed at the University of Florida [92–97] and is commercially available under the trade name FreeTrack™ (Varian, Inc., Ashland, MA). It can be employed for fractionated stereotactic radiotherapy, intracranial and Head and Neck IMRT [95, 96]. This system employs a hybrid Polaris position sensor unit (Northern Digital, Inc., Waterloo, Ontario), which is an array of two planar CCD cameras surrounded by a ring of infrared light-emitting diodes, to optically track the position of either active or passive infrared markers arranged in an array to form a fixed rigid body. For the Free Track system, the CCD camera is permanently mounted to the ceiling at a distance of approximately 1.8 m from the isocenter of the treatment machine (cf. Fig. 3). Therefore, the origin of the optical tracking system is located at the ceiling of the treatment room and the axes of its coordinate system are dependent upon the camera's orientation. The most logical origin for clinical use in radiotherapy is of course the treatment machine isocenter, with the coordinate axes

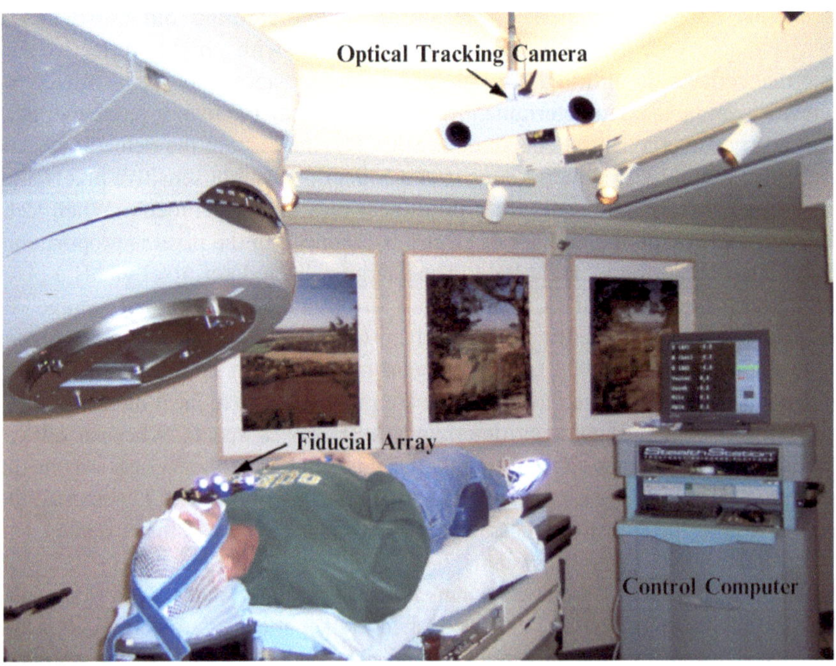

Fig. 3 A patient undergoing optical-guided head and neck radiotherapy. A camera system monitors the translations and rotations of a set of markers that are rigidly fixed to a special bite block

located parallel to the vertical, lateral, and longitudinal motions of the treatment couch. Using a calibration procedure, the native coordinate system of the optical tracking system is transformed to that of the treatment machine that has the isocenter of the treatment machine as its origin.

Patient localization is accomplished through detection of an optical fiducial array containing four passive markers. This fiducial array is attached to a custom bite plate that links to the maxillary dentition of the patient to form a rigid system. The patient position (determined using optical guidance) is then compared to the desired patient position (determined during treatment planning). During CT simulation, the bite plate fiducial array complex is kept in place, and the image coordinates of the reflective markers are determined as part of treatment planning (cf. Fig. 4). During treatment planning, the desired target, or isocenter, coordinates

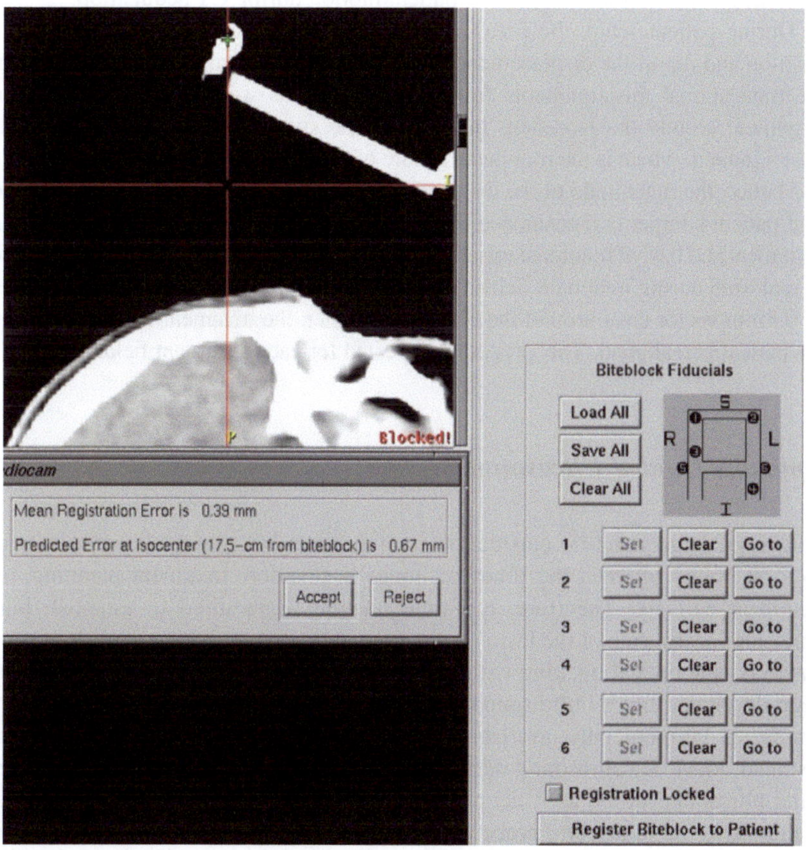

Fig. 4 The mean registration error is a quality assurance allowing the assessment of the quality of the registration of the fiducal array bite block complex to the patient. The predicted error at Isocenter at a given distance from the bite block allows assessment of the expected error in target localization, which in this particular case is 0.67 mm

are determined in CT space. The centers of the spherical fiducial markers in the optical reference array are also localized in CT space, thus determining their positions relative to the treatment isocenter and defining a stereotactic coordinate system. After selecting the fiducials from the scan, the best fit between the image-defined coordinates of the reference array and the known geometry of the reference array is determined. The residual error between the image localization of the markers and the known geometry after the best fit is obtained is called the mean registration error, and is calculated for each patient. The mean registration error provides quality assurance measure for frameless localization, as it ensures integrity of both the fiducial array and image data set [94]. In phantom, it has consistently been shown that the mean registration error is approximately 0.3 mm, which is governed entirely by the finite size of the CT voxels. For most clinical situations, the mean registration error can be maintained below 0.5 mm. For a given image set, values larger than this are indicative of either spatial CT inaccuracies, mechanical inaccuracy of the fiduicial array, or patient motion during CT acquisition.

During patient setup, the FreeTrack™ system is used to determine the patient's position and report the displacement from isocenter in real time. The system reports the translational misalignments from the isocenter as well as the rotational misalignment around the Isocenter. In addition, the system reports overall the vector misalignment, which is the root mean square of the three translational misalignments, and hence, the magnitude of the displacement vector of the target from the isocenter. The patient's target is repositioned to the desired position within 0.3 mm vector misalignment and 0.3° of rotational misalignment about each axis. The patient is monitored in real time during treatment delivery. If a patient moves out of the tolerance sphere of 0.5 mm vector error around the planned isocenter, the treatment is interrupted and the patient is realigned. This process is repeated for each treatment field.

Optically Guided Ultrasound

Soft-tissue targets that lie outside the cranial region can move relative to external fixation points between the times of image acquisition, treatment planning, and treatment delivery. Therefore, real-time imaging is required to establish high-precision localization of the lesion at the time of treatment. To accomplish this, one has to couple optical tracking with a real-time imaging system; such a system has been developed for 3D ultrasound guidance for target localization [98–103]. This system is commercially available under the trade name SonArray™ (Varian, Ashland, MA). 3D ultrasound data sets are generated by optically tracking a free-hand ultrasound probe as it acquires 2D ultrasound image planes. The operator manipulates the ultrasound probe over the anatomical region of interest to acquire real time planar ultrasound image data of the region of interest. The acquired raw image planes are then transferred to a computer workstation via video link. The position and angulation of the ultrasound probe in any arbitrary orientation is determined using an active array containing four IRLEDs that is attached to the probe.

Just as is the case for intracranial optical tracking, the hybrid Polaris optical tracking system is used to determine the positions of the active probe attached to the ultrasound probe, and this information is used in the construction of a full 3D Ultrasound volume. Using the optical tracking data, the position of each ultrasound voxel can therefore be determined and a 3D ultrasound volume can be reconstructed by linking the position information of the 2D Ultrasound probe with the raw ultrasound data (see Fig. 5).

In addition to constructing a true 3D Ultrasound image volume, optical guidance is used to determine the absolute position of this 3D ultrasound volume in the treatment room. Since the relative positions of the ultrasound volume and the ultrasound probe are fixed, the knowledge of the probe position in the treatment room coordinate system at the time of data acquisition is sufficient to determine the position of the image volume relative to the treatment machine isocenter. The determination of the relative position of the image and probe corresponds to a calibration step that has to be performed prior to use of the system and the validity of this calibration is checked daily prior to clinical use of the system [98].

Ultrasound localization has been employed for target localization in conformal and intensity-modulated radiotherapy of prostate cancer [78], in the localization of the bladder base in the conformal and intensity-modulated therapy in the post prostatectomy setting [104], and for target localization for patients undergoing extracranial radiosurgery for a variety of abdominal, paraspinal, and pelvic lesions [100, 102]. Clinically, the system is used as follows: first, a CT is acquired with the patient immobilized in the intended treatment position in order to maintain a

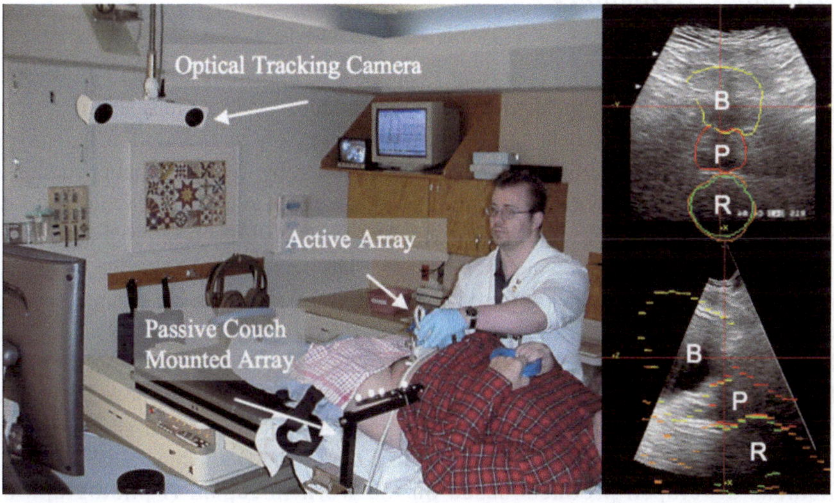

Fig. 5 Free hand ultrasound target localization using optical guided 3D ultrasound for the treatment of a patient with intact prostate. As shown in the axial and sagittal ultrasound image panel on the right, the prostate is the target structure of interest. The labels B, P, and R refer to the bladder, the prostate, and the rectal balloon, respectively

consistent position of the mobile anatomy as far as possible. The CT image data set is then transferred to the treatment planning system where target and normal tissue volumes are defined and a treatment plan is generated. The CT data set together with the generated treatment plan is then transferred to SonArray™ (Varian, Inc., Ashland, MA) control computer. On the day of the treatment, the patient is positioned in treatment position based on the skin marks placed at the time of CT simulation using in-room lasers, this defines the boney anatomy. The setup based on boney anatomy is then verified using portal images and necessary adjustments to the patient's position are made. To localize the internal target, a 3D ultrasound volume of the volume interest is then acquired and reconstructed. The outlines of target volume and critical structures that have been delineated on the CT data set at the time of treatment planning are then overlaid on the acquired ultrasound volume in relation to treatment machine isocenter. These contours are then manipulated until they align with the anatomic structures seen on the ultrasound images. The amount of movement required to align the contours with the ultrasound images determines the magnitude of the target misalignment with isocenter based on the conventional setup technique. The target is then placed at the isocenter by tracking an infrared array attached to the treatment couch which allows precise translation in the submillimeter range from the position determined using portal imaging to the 3D ultrasound determined position. Before treatment commences, a verification Ultrasound scan can be acquired to confirm that the target is now at isocenter. Once this set is complete, treatment proceeds as planned.

In-Room CT Guidance

The CT scanner is the most important imaging modality used in radiation therapy. 3D radiation therapy is typically planned with patient representations acquired from CT scanners. Its geometrical precision is not based on its calibration but on its geometry. This is in contrast to an MRI scanner whereby the positional encoding is not based on its geometry but its calibration, which can lead to geometric distortions. First and foremost, verification of the treatment setup requires positional accuracy.

There are three ways in which CT guidance has been brought into the treatment room. The first approach, pioneered in Japan, was to put a CT scanner in the treatment room and to use the patient support couch for both the CT scanner and the treatment unit [105]. The patient was first set up and then CT scanned. While the CT scan was being reconstructed and analyzed, the couch was moved from the CT scanner to the treatment unit. The operators would determine what shifts to make and the couch position would be altered before treatment. Both General Electric and Siemens developed products based on the work in Japan. A photograph of the Siemens version called the Somotom is shown in Fig. 6.

Helical tomotherapy is the marriage of a linac with a helical CT scanner [69, 106–109]. This system uses a fan-beam CT system like a conventional CT but uses the treatment linac to produce a scan at megavoltage energies [110, 111]. During

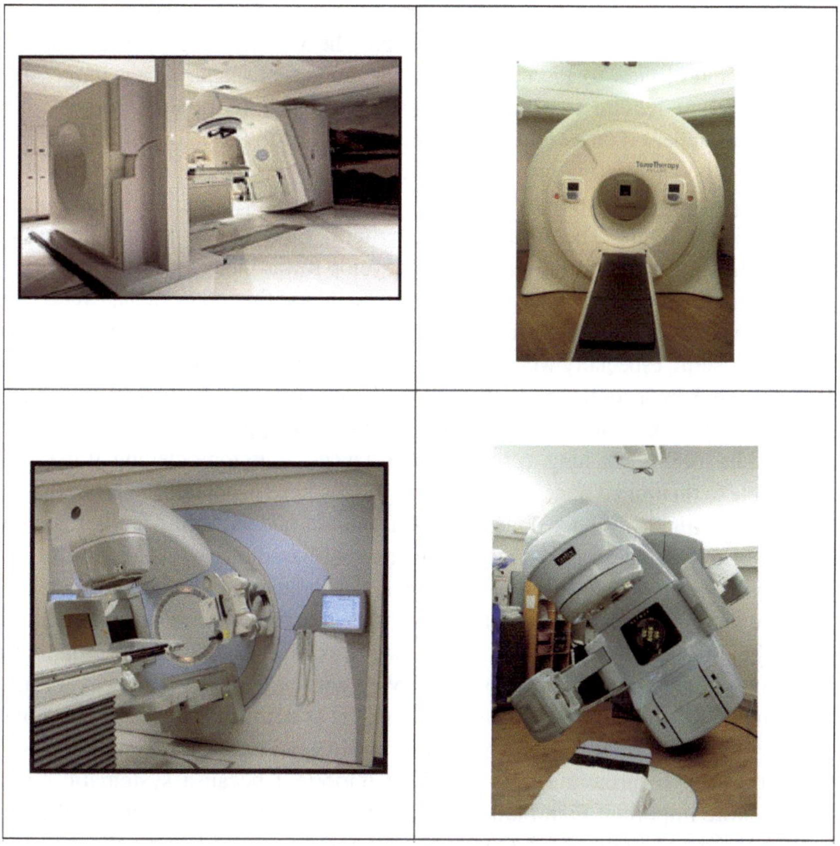

Fig. 6 In-room CT guidance. The *upper left panel* is a Siemens Primatom™ in-room CT system. The *upper right panel* is the TomoTherapy Hi-Art™ helical tomotherapy unit. The *lower left panel* is the Elekta Synergy™ system with a cone-beam CT system. The *lower right panel* is the Varian Trilogy™ system also with an on-board cone-beam CT system

treatment, a dedicated binary MLC modulates the same fan beam to provide rotational IMRT. The collimator is binary in the sense that it leaves rapid transition between open (leaf-retracted) and closed (leaf-blocking) states [106, 112] to provide the modulation. When operating as an MVCT system, the leaves are fully retracted to the open state. Figure 6 shows a photograph of one of the helical tomotherapy units installed at the University of Wisconsin.

It is also feasible to put a CT scanner onto a conventional C-arm linac gantry [113, 114]). Cone-beam CT using flat panel detectors can acquire many slices with one rotation. There are two radiation sources used: a megavoltage beam produced by the linac as is done with the Siemens Oncol™ product and kilovoltage beams produced by a separate X-ray tube as done with both the Elekta Synergy™ and Varian Trilogy™ linacs. Cone-beam CT on conventional accelerators requires correcting for gantry sag [115]. The correction can be accomplished by calibration using a phantom. Scatter on a kilovoltage cone-beam scanner is considerable if the longitudinal field of view is large. For example, the Varian Trilogy™ cone-beam CT limits the field of view to 17 cm to control the amount of scatter. Scans longer than 17 cm therefore require two separate rotation acquisitions of the Trilogy™. The gantry rotation period on a conventional linac is limited to 60 s. To move faster, they will have to be enclosed in covers to prevent collisions with patients or staff. Both tomotherapy and conventional linacs may be equipped with multirow kilovoltage detectors in the future. Therefore, in the long term, there will be technical pressure for tomotherapy and conventional units to develop toward the same solutions.

Putting a linear accelerator into a ring gantry means that noncoplanar treatments for certain sites in the body are not possible. There are times when noncoplanar beams are useful, especially when the tumor is surrounded by a parallel normal tissue structure and the noncoplanar distances through the normal tissue is less than or equal to those for the coplanar directions. This is most often applicable to the brain but it may also be true for the lung in some circumstances. With tomotherapy, it may still be possible to do limited noncoplanar delivery to the head using the natural capability of the head to tilt as was once done before CT gantries had the ability to tilt. Recently, Kamino et al. [116] described a large diameter ring-based linear accelerator that had the capability of tilting and panning the linear accelerator and rotating the couch.

There are a number of verification processes that are possible with a CT scanner on board. One of the first proposed uses was to only use CT information to determine the margins to apply to the CTV to get the PTV [117]. It was felt that only a few CT scans were needed to eliminate the systematic error inherent in only using a single CT image set for planning but it would not eliminate day-to-day random errors. In principle, this could be important because systematic errors may be more important than random errors in setting the PTV margin [118].

With the introduction of CT scanners in the room, it was felt that patients would be CT scanned on a weekly basis much as had been done with portal imaging systems. Daily image guidance with CT scanning is becoming the norm rather than the exception. Immediately after the scan, the image set can be fused with a planning CT image set to determine if the patient is set up correctly. This eliminates both the systematic and random setup error. The fusion process must be done carefully enough to be accurate but fast enough so that the patient's setup does not change. A combination of automated [119, 120] and manual fusion techniques is essential as the operator must be able to override the automated procedure, if necessary. Is daily CT guidance necessary? A recent paper by Zeidan et al. [121] showed that weekly image guidance results in more 50% of the head and neck patients having setup errors greater than 3 mm and this is reduced to about a 25% chance if the CT guidance is done every second day. The probability of setup errors greater than 5 mm occurs about 30% of the time for weekly and about 15% for imaging every second day.

Daily imaging for lung cases is especially important for dose escalation procedures like stereotactic body radiosurgery. CT scanning of lung tumors does not require contrast agents. Doing daily CT scans for lung cancer can also be used to determine the treatment response, as in many patients it is possible to observe the tumor shrinking during the course of treatment [122, 123]. Figure 7 is an example

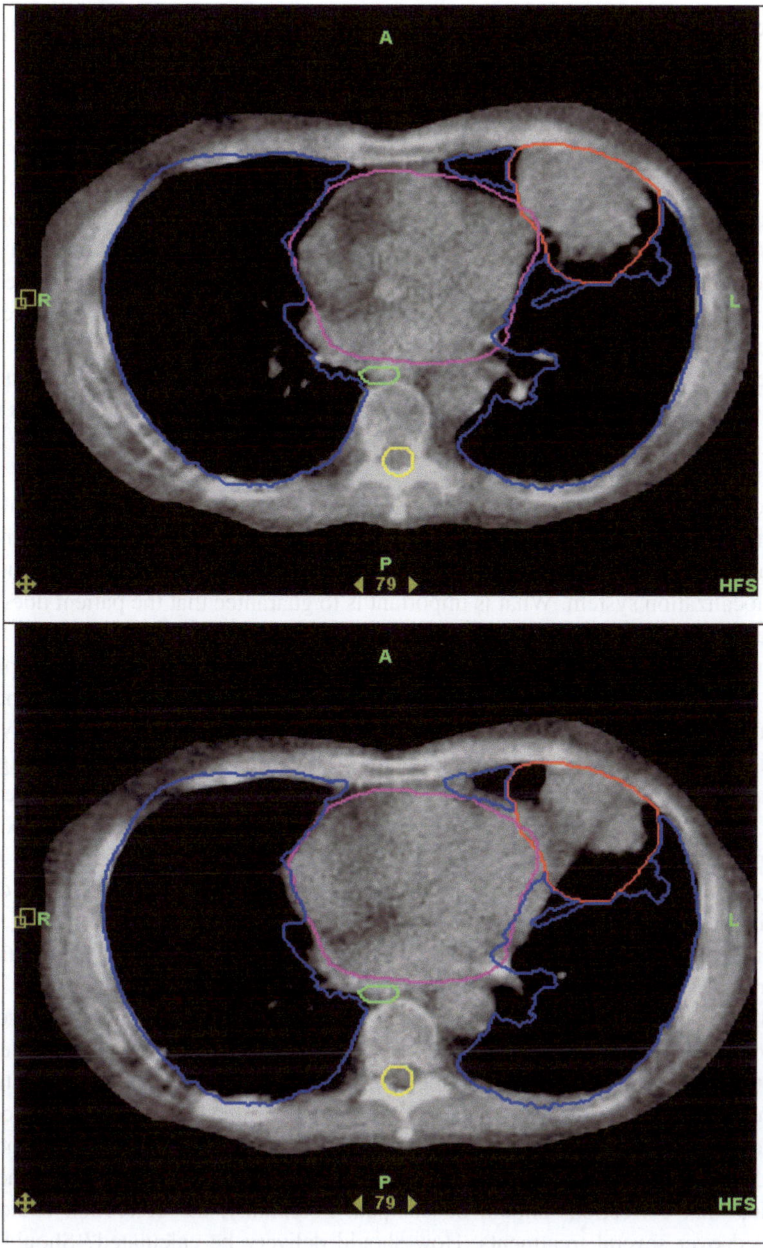

Fig. 7 Example of visualization of tumor shrinkage. The *upper panel* was taken on the second treatment day and the *lower panel* was taken on the 18th treatment day. Both images were acquired on the TomoTherapy Hi-Art™ helical tomotherapy unit

of the change in a lung tumor during treatment as imaged on a MVCT scan at the time of treatment.

The capabilities of having a CT image at the time of treatment will not be fulfilled without image analysis software. 3D treatment planning analysis requires segmentation of relevant structures. The most time-consuming aspect of 3D treatment planning is the segmentation of the planning image. It is unreasonable to expect physicians to repeat their segmentation tasks routinely. Automated tools to segment the relevant volumes on treatment CT images are more practical in this application because the planning CT will have been segmented and can be used as a template for autosegmentation. Computers cannot be expected to automatically render contour volumes in an unsupervised manner. Physicians, or those well trained in anatomy, will be required to approve the automated procedures and to correct mistakes. Similar to automated processing of scanned paper documents into text, the utility of these systems will depend on their error rate and how easy it is to correct them.

Acquiring a CT scan immediately before treatment puts less emphasis on patient localization devices, such as stereotactic coordinate frames, and more emphasis on patient immobilization. The CT representation at the time of treatment forms its own localization system. What is important is to guarantee that the patient does not move during the treatment.

One complicating factor is that the patient representation in the original planning CT might be significantly deformed from the representation at the time of treatment. Deformable registration of the two patient representations may be required to accurately associate features in the two image sets [124, 125]. Figure 8 is a deformable registration example. Here two kVCT scans taken on different days have been registered together. As proof of the registration technique, the second image was deformed so that it appeared to be nearly identical to the first image. Once the mapping from one image set to another is determined, the dose distribution can be mapped using the same transformation. Like automated contouring, physicians or trained anatomists will have to approve the results of deformable registration.

The process of applying feedback to the image-guided radiotherapy processes is called adaptive radiotherapy. The best way in which this feedback can be applied is under active research [126, 127]. Is there an optimal way to estimate the corrections when the verification results are uncertain? Methods from statistical signal processing can be applied to find, in a statistical sense, the most likely position of an organ based on an uncertain setup verification measurement [128]. Basic control theory predicts that corrections should be damped. Potentially, the correction could be effected over several treatments. How should delivery be calculated? Should the original prescription be modified? These questions will be answered as experience is gained.

Figure 9 is a head and neck radiotherapy example of what is currently possible for adaptive modification of the treatment. In this case, patient weight loss changed the contour of their neck, and their parotid glands were entering the field. Deformable registration was used to determine how the contours had changed and

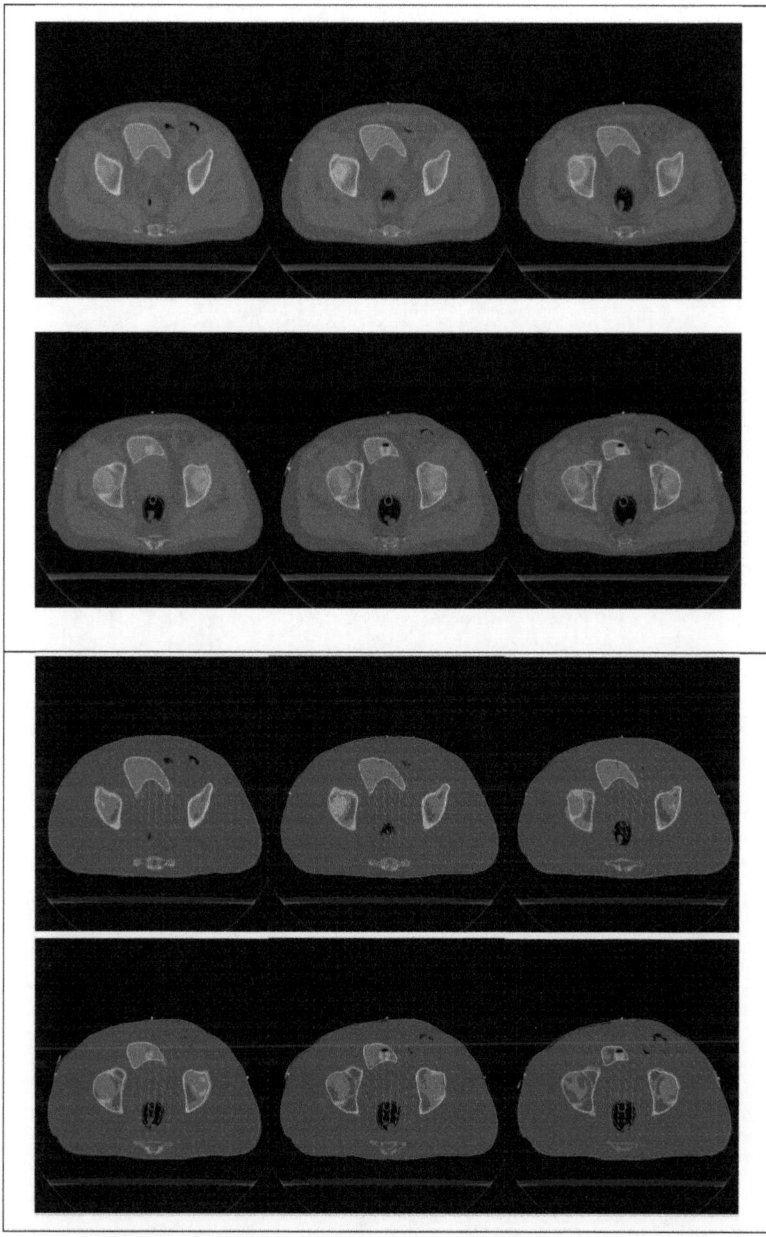

Fig. 8 Deformable registration example. In the *upper panel* of six images the contours are the bladder, prostate and rectum delineated by a physician. The *lower panels* are the contours which have been autocontoured using deformable registration on an image set taken on a different day. It can be seen that the image contents of the rectum were much different on these 2 days. A vector display of the mapping from one image set to the other is also shown. Figure courtesy of Dr. Weiguo Lu, TomoTherapy Inc. (Madison WI).

a)

b)

c)

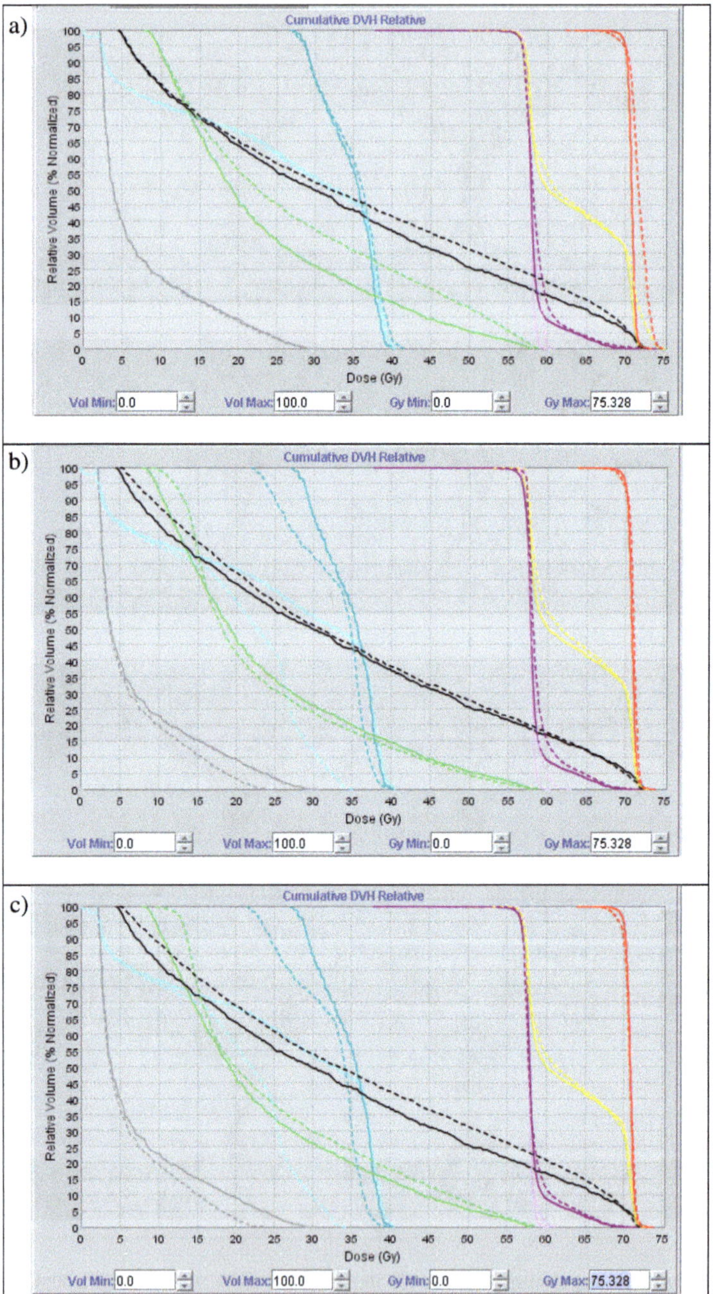

Fig. 9 Dose–volume histograms documenting adaptive radiotherapy applied to a head and neck case. (**a**) A DVH comparing the original plan with the forecast of what would be the outcome if nothing is changed. The *solid lines* are from the original plan and the *dashed line* is the forecast at the end of the treatment if the plan is not altered and the patient remains as they are at Day 17.

the dose delivered on each fraction was deformably registered and summed and then the patient replanned. Reoptimization was performed after the 17th fraction was delivered. Figure 9a shows a comparison between the original planned distribution and the dose that would be delivered at the end of the 35 fraction treatment if the patient does not change from fraction 18 to 35 and the original plan is continued to be delivered. Clearly, the right parotid would receive too much dose and the left parotid dose would be somewhat elevated. Figure 9b shows the dose that could be delivered with a reoptimized plan again presuming the patient does not change subsequent to fraction 17. Notice that the reoptimization was able to reduce the planned dose to the cord as well as the parotids. Not surprisingly, the patient anatomy continued to change but now more due to tumor shrinkage than weight loss. Figure 9c shows what was actually achieved at the end of the 35 fractions as compared to the original plan. The parotid dose is higher than originally desired but less than what was seen at the end of fraction 17. The cord dose is actually lower than the original plan and the dose to the target volume was acceptable. In this case a midcourse correction enables the rest of the treatments to be planned on a more correct patient representation and the original intent is more correctly carried out than it would have been had nothing been done. It is obvious in this example that having even more reoptimization could make the dose even more accurately delivered throughout the treatment course. As computers become faster, the adaptive radiotherapy processes will become potentially more powerful enabling full reoptimization of dose distributions before each treatment and even adapting to organ motion while it occurs.

Image Guidance and Organ Motion

For conventional conformal radiotherapy, intrafraction organ motion is accounted for by placing an internal target volume (ITV), a component of the PTV boundary around the CTV [15, 16]. However, intrafraction organ motion may limit the accuracy of IMRT delivery [129, 130] even with image guidance just prior to or immediately before treatment. Adding an ITV margin has been shown to guarantee that the CTV is receiving adequate dose for some types of IMRT delivery using conventional MLCs. For dynamic MLC (moving window) and static MLC (step and shoot) styles of delivery, it is possible for hot and cold spots to develop in the intensity profile from a beam direction. For tomotherapy delivery this is less of a problem. That is because the fan beams overlap for tomotherapy effectively "repainting" the same area many times. However, like conventional conformal

Fig. 9 (continued) (**b**) A DVH comparing the original plan (*solid lines*) and the *dashed lines* are the new planned forecast at the end of the treatment if a reoptimization is done. (**c**) A DVH comparing the original plan with the actual result at the end of 35 fractions after plan had been changed beginning on Day 18. The final result is better than it would have been had the plan not been altered. Figure courtesy of Dr. Katja Langen, M.D. Anderson Cancer Center, (Orlanda FL).

radiotherapy, tomotherapy will still result in blurring of the dose distribution at the edge of the field and so an ITV margin is required [131].

The uncertainty of the delivery depends a great deal on the typical size of the aperture, the amplitude of motion, the periodicity of organ motion (e.g., regular vs. irregular breathing), the rate of motion, and the number of treatment fractions or the degree of repainting [120, 129, 131]. The greatest excursions for organ motion are in the thorax where respiration can sometimes move lungs and liver appreciably [132]. Many other thoracic structures are less mobile [133]. The prostate of some patients in the prone position appears to have a larger range of motion due to breathing than patients in the supine position [134].

The visualization is usually accomplished by placing fiducial markers in the tumor and performing repeat X-ray imaging from two or more directions in order to determine the position of the markers [135, 136]. A new type of implanted electronic localization marker system developed by Calypso Medical enables markers to be tracked within 1.5 mm without the use of X-rays [137]. These methods of tumor tracking implicitly assume that the tumor is a rigid body and ignore the changing shape of the normal tissue. Kamino et al. [116] described a combination CT scanner and treatment unit from Mitsubishi Heavy Industries that was capable of acquiring a CT scan, not just before the radiation was delivered, but simultaneously with delivery. It accomplishes this by having two separate kilovoltage X-ray systems irradiating their own flat-panel image detectors. The gimbal on the system enables the linac to be tilted and panned to enable arbitrary tracking of a tumor with typical excursions. The degree of organ motion should always be judged on a case-by-case basis using fluoroscopy with an implanted marker or 4D CT scans. Siemens announced a product called the Artiste™ which has a flat panel in the path of the therapy beam for verification of the entrance beam [138]. The same panel can be used as a detector for X-rays from a tube mounted on the exit side of the patient. This system can in principle be used to acquire images of the patient during treatment or be a cone-beam CT scanner for pretreatment verification.

There have been four approaches to mitigate the effect of organ motion so that an ITV margin expansion is not necessary: gating, maximum breath hold, active breathing control (ABC), and tumor tracking [139]. Gated delivery applies the radiation only when the organ is in preselected breathing phase [140] typically at maximum inspiration or maximum expiration. Gated delivery is easiest for conventional uniform field delivery although it may also be possible with simpler forms of IMRT such as static MLC (step and shoot) IMRT techniques. If the patient can tolerate breath-holding for a reasonable period, a second method that can be pursued is maximum breath-hold delivery. During normal breathing, the lung is in the maximum expiration for the longest fraction of the time [141]; however, when asked to hold their breath people typically inspire deeply. During maximum inspiration, the lung is fully inflated so that normal lung tissue is maximally displaced from the high-dose regions. One problem with maximum inspiration is that the lung position is not as certain as it is for maximum expiration. If the patient is in good health, but they are uncooperative, it is possible to use active breathing control (ABC) [141, 142] to control the movement of the lung. In order to deliver IMRT using gating or breath-holding, the beam delivery has to be suspended after only a part of the volume has been treated in order to allow the patient to "catch" their breath.

Tumor tracking continuously moves the patient into the beam or moves the beam to the patient. The tracking is accomplished by anticipating the motion of the tumor, visualization of the tumor in real time, and continuously adjusting the motion. The Accuray CyberKnife™ uses two ceiling-mounted X-ray systems and two flat panel detector systems to monitor the motion of the patient [143]. It does this by automatically comparing digital reconstructed radiographs of the patient with the X-ray images. The CyberKnife™ robotic deliver system can adjust the beam delivery to take into account the motion of the patient in real time. The motion of the tumor demonstrates hysteresis in that the trajectory of the tumor during inspiration might not be the reverse of the trajectory during expiration. In dynamic MLC IMRT, it is possible to move the leaves to track the beam to the patient [144]. On the helical tomotherapy unit, the independent pair of jaws defining the field width could track in the superior–inferior direction corresponding to the majority of the respiratory motion and still account for residual lateral movement using the fast moving binary collimator. This would allow tumor motion to be tracked without oscillatory movements of the patient. The simplest approach to tracking is to move the patient couch to realign the patient to the beam. This could be done with a robotic couch on any treatment delivery system but periodic breathing could result in the patient developing motion sickness.

Rather than assuming that the tumor is rigidly moving, it is possible to determine a 4D model of the patient including deformation of the tumor, lung, diaphragm, and liver. Both 4D CT and 4D MRI are possible [136]. These 4D representations are obtained by encoding each of the slices acquired with a breathing phase and reordering the slices if necessary. A treatment plan can be computed using the 4D representation but the patient has to be not only registered in space but also in time. This means that there has to be coordination of the breathing phase with the delivery [145].

Image Guidance for Follow-Up Imaging and Retreatments

Radiotherapy is ultimately limited by the ability of visualization systems to detect small tumor masses. Chemotherapy is limited by its effectiveness against larger tumor sizes. Chemotherapy agents are effective when the cell density is less than 10^3 cell/cm^3. It may be that targeted agents like Bexxar or Zevalin are more effective. This means that there is a "visualization gap" extending through two or three orders of magnitude from the largest tumor density effective for a targeted agent and the smallest tumor density visualizable with PET. The concept of the visualization gap is shown in the number line in Fig. 10.

The importance of the visualization gap as shown in Fig. 10 may be profound. If the gap could be closed by either improving the effectiveness of systemic agents

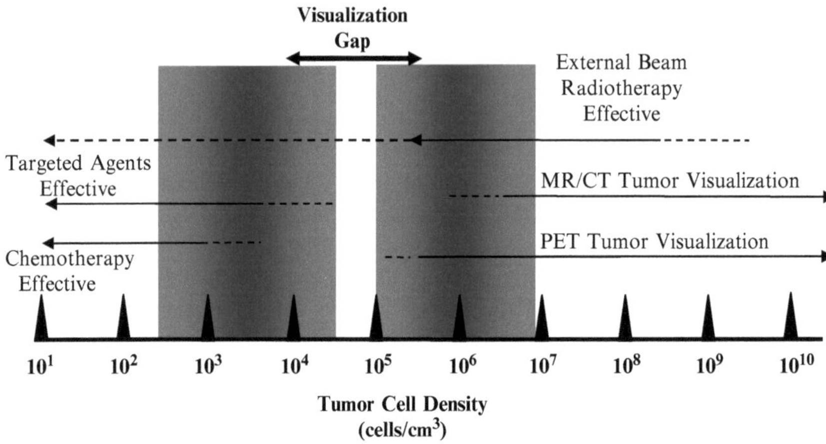

Fig. 10 Illustration of the visualization gap. PET imaging is capable of visualizing tumors that have a clonogen cell density of about 10^5 cells/cm^3. MRI or CT can visualize to about the about one million per cubic centimeter. Chemotherapy is effective up to a cell density of 10^3–10^4 cells/cm^3 and targeted agents may able to do better. There is little expectation that systemic therapy agents will be effective at the limits of detectability of modern imaging systems. A gap of visibility extends from the upper threshold of the effectiveness of systemic agents to the lower limit of detectability of modern imaging that is a prerequisite for effective radiotherapy

or by improving the visualization of PET, cancer has the real possibility of being treated as a chronic disease by the combined role of systemic agents and radiotherapy for the treatment of systemic disease. There is at least one agent that has the possibility of closing the visualization gap from both directions. NM404 is a phosolipid ether compound that is preferentially taken up by all tumor cells thus far tested but rejected from normal tissues [146]. It may be easily labeled with iodine. It has been called a "diapeutic" agent because it may have a role as both a diagnostic and a therapeutic agent. When labeled with I-125 or I-131, it has the potential to be a powerful targeted agent that could push the lower boundary of the visualization gap to the right. When labeled with a PET emitting isotope like I-124, it has the potential to push the upper boundary to the left enabling the visualization so that surgery or radiotherapy could treat the smaller tumorlets.

What would be the role of external beam radiotherapy? In repeat follow-up visits, if small tumorlets were visible, they could be treated with focused radiosurgery or fractionated stereotactic radiotherapy so long as the number of focal areas was not too large but as the size of the region to treat shrinks the number of such sites that may be safely treated could increase. External beam radiotherapy would likely be able to treat many more focal regions than either surgery or brachytherapy. The treatment of multiple focal metastatic lesions has been termed the treatment of oligometastases. Such a treatment regime will only be effective if the location of, and dose delivered by, the treatments are well documented so that long term radiation complications would not ensue. In order for the number of focal areas to not increase, chemotherapy or targeted agents would be most effective when used when the scan was negative so that the number of occult tumorlets could be reduced in number before they could grow into visible tumors later on. A corollary to the concept of visualization gap is the realization that the use of chemotherapy when a tumorlet is visible will not be effective at complete tumor eradication but will only reduce the tumor bulk and provide palliation but buys the patient additional life. The role of chemotherapy and radiotherapy when viewed in this way is analogous to the control of weeds in a garden. Systemic agents are most effective against small or preemergent weeds. The radiotherapy treatment of oligo-metastases is like "weeding" the garden and as such it is important to find and eradicate the tumorlets before more metastases are seeded. Of course, the authors realize that practice of the use of chemotherapy or targeted agents when imaging systems present no evidence of disease, and its more limited role when there is imaging evidence of disease, is radical and unproven, and is only presented here as a conceptual hypothesis.

Summary

The goal of radiation therapy is to eradicate tumor stem cells while sparing healthy tissue. Therefore, the first aim must be to delineate tumor from healthy tissue. Advanced imaging techniques will enable one to reduce the uncertainty of microscopic extension of disease. Ultimately, advanced functional imaging systems correlated with image-registered pathological specimens will allow one to delineate disease extent from normal tissue at the tumor periphery. When it is not possible to determine the CTV margin with reasonable certainty, the margins must remain generous and conformal avoidance methodology could and should be deployed to spare critical normal structures.

Of equal importance to defining the CTV is the need to guarantee that this target is indeed treated. For this purpose, image guidance using a variety of systems including portal images, ultrasound devices, and CT scanners at the time of treatment has been implemented. Some image-guided methods, portal images for instance, are more amenable for use with rigid structures such as encountered in the sinus whereas others like ultrasound or CT scanners are able to account for nonrigid setup variations. Several strategies for preventing organ motion from degrading the precision that radiotherapy offers have been described.

In particular, a CT scan at the time of treatment delivery can also be used as the basis to reconstruct the dose received by the patient [30, 147–152]. Dose reconstruction will allow the dose just delivered to be superimposed on the pretreatment CT scan and will allow one to compare the reconstructed delivered dose distribution with the planned dose distribution to assess discrepancies between these. Furthermore, reconstruction of the delivered dose distributions holds the promise of allowing one to accumulate dose delivered to the tumor and normal structures on a fraction per fraction basis. This will ultimately allow for the determination of treatment-specific tumor control probabilities and normal tissue complication probabilities.

Acknowledgments The authors would like to acknowledge the support of NIH P01 CA088960, and TomoTherapy, Inc. TRM has a financial interest in TomoTherapy, Inc.

References

1. Bentzen SM. Theragnostic imaging for radiation oncology: dose-painting by numbers. Lancet Oncol 2005; 6:112–117.
2. Kim Y, Tomé WA. Risk-Adaptive Optimization: Selective Boosting of high-risk tumor subvolumes. Int J Radiat Oncol Biol Phys 2006; 66:1528–1542.
3. Tomé WA, Fowler JF: Selective boosting of tumor subvolumes. Int J Radiat Oncol Biol Phys 2000; 48(2):593–599.
4. Ling CC, Humm J, Larson S, Amols H, Fuks Z, Leibel S, Koutcher JA. Towards multidimensional radiotherapy (MD-CRT): Biological imaging and biological conformity. Int J Radiat Oncol Biol Phys 2000; 47:551–560.
5. Koper PCM, Stroom JC, van Putten WLJ, et al. Acute morbidity reduction using 3DCRT for prostate carcinoma: a randomized study. Int J Radiat Oncol Biol Phys 1999; 43:727–734.
6. Nutting CM, Convery DJ, Cosgrove VP, et al. Reduction of small and large bowel irradiation using an optimized intensity-modulated pelvic radiotherapy technique in patients with prostate cancer. Int J Radiat Oncol Biol Phys 2000; 48:649–656.
7. Pirzkall A, Carol M, Lohr F, et al. Comparison of intensity-modulated radiotherapy with conventional conformal radiotherapy for complex-shaped tumors. Int J Radiat Oncol Biol Phys 2000; 48:1371–1380.
8. Portelance L, Chao KSC, Grigsby PW, et al. Intensity-modulated radiation therapy (IMRT) reduces small bowel, rectum, and bladder doses in patients with cervical cancer receiving pelvic and para-aortic irradiation. Int J Radiat Oncol Biol Phys 2001; 51:261–266.
9. Goitein M, Abrams M, Rowell D, et al. Multidimensional treatment planning. II. Beam's-eye-view, back projection, and projection through CT sections. Int J Radiat Oncol Biol Phys 1983; 9:789–797.
10. Sherouse G, Novins KL, Chaney EL. Computation of digitally reconstructed radiographs for use in radiotherapy. Int J Radiat Oncol Biol Phys 1990; 18:651–658.
11. Ramsey CR, Arwood D, Scaperoth D, et al. Clinical application of digitally-reconstructed radiographs generated from magnetic resonance imaging for intracranial lesions. Int.J Radiat Oncol Biol Phys 1999; 45:797–802.
12. Vigneault E, Pouliot J, Laverdiere J, et al. Electronic portal imaging device detection of radioopaque markers for the evaluation of prostate position during megavoltage irradiation – A clinical study. Int J Radiat Oncol Biol Phys 1997; 37:205–212.
13. Bergström P, Lofröth P-O, Widmark A. High-precision conformal radiotherapy (HPCRT) of prostate cancer-a new technique for exact positioning of the prostate at the time of treatment. Int J Radiat Oncol Biol Phys 1998; 42:305–311.
14. Pang G, Beachey DJ, O'Brien PF, et al. Imaging of 1.0-mm-diameter radiopaque markers with megavoltage X-rays: an improved online imaging system. Int J Radiat Oncol Biol Phys 2002; 52:532–537.
15. ICRU Report 50, Prescribing, Recording and Reporting Photon Beam Therapy. Bethesda MD, 1993. International Commission on Radiation Units and Measurements (ICRU).
16. ICRU Report 62, Prescribing, Recording, and Reporting Photon Beam Therapy, Supplement to ICRU Report No. 50. Bethesda MD, 1999. International Commission on Radiation Units and Measurements (ICRU).
17. Mubata CD, Bidmead AM, Ellingham LM, et al. Portal imaging protocol for radical dose-escalated radiotherapy treatment of prostate cancer. Int J Radiat Oncol Biol Phys 1998; 40:221–231.

18. Stroom JC, Olofsen-van Acht MJJ, Quint S, et al. On-line setup corrections during radiotherapy of patients with gynecologic tumors. Int J Radiat Oncol Biol Phys 2000; 46:499–506.
19. Alasti H, Petric MP, Catton CN, et al.: Portal imaging for evaluation of daily on-line setup errors and off-line organ motion during conformal irradiation of carcinoma of the prostate. Int J Radiat Oncol Biol Phys 2001; 49:869–884.
20. Leong J. Use of digital fluoroscopy as an on-line verification device in radiation therapy. Phys Med Biol 1986; 31:985–992.
21. Munro P, Rawlinson JA, Fenster A. A digital fluoroscopic imaging device for radiotherapy localization. Proc SPIE 1989; 1090:321–329.
22. Meertens H, Bijold J, Strackee J. A method for the measurement of field placement errors in digital portal images. Phys Med Biol 1990; 35:299–323.
23. Ezz A, Munro P, Porter AT, et al. Daily monitoring and correction of radiation field placement using a video-based portal imaging system: a pilot study. Int J Radiat Oncol Biol Phys 1992; 22:159–165.
24. Hornick DC, Litzenberg DW, Kam KL, et al. A tilt and roll device for automated correction of rotational setup errors. Med Phys 1998; 25:1739–1740.
25. Wong J, Binns R, Cheng A, et al. On-line radiotherapy imaging with an array of fiber-optic image reducers. Int J Radiat Oncol Biol Phys 1990; 18:1477–1484.
26. Essers M, Hoogervoorst BR, van Herk M, et al. Dosimetric characteristics of a liquid-filled electronic portal imaging device. Int J Radiat Oncol Biol Phys 1995; 33:1265–1272.
27. Kirby MC, Williams PC. The use of an electronic portal imaging device for exit dosimetry and quality control measurements. Int J Radiat Oncol Biol Phys 1995; 31:593–603.
28. Zhu Y, Jiang X-Q, Van Dyk J. Portal dosimetry using a liquid ion chamber matrix: Dose response studies. Med. Phys. 1995; 22:1101–1106.
29. Hansen VN, Evans PM, Swindell W: The application of transit dosimetry to precision radiotherapy. Med Phys 1996; 23:713–721.
30. McNutt TR, Mackie TR, Reckwerdt PJ, et al. Modeling dose distributions from portal dose images using the convolution/superposition method. Med Phys 1996; 23:1381–1392.
31. Balter JM, Chen GTY, Pelizzari CA, et al. On-line repositioning during treatment of the prostate: A study of potential limits and gains. Int J Radiat Oncol Biol Phys 1993; 27:137–143.
32. Van de Steene J, Van den Heuvel F, Bel A, et al. Electronic portal imaging with on-line correction of setup error in thoracic irradiation: Clinical evaluation. Int J Radiat Oncol Biol Phys 1998; 40:967–976.
33. Remeijer P, Geerlof E, Ploeger L, et al. 3-D portal image analysis in clinical practice: an evaluation of 2-D and 3-D analysis techniques as applied to 30 prostate cancer patients. Int J Radiat Oncol Biol Phys 2000; 46:1281–1290.
34. Senan S, van Sörnsen de Koste J, Samson M, Tankink H, Jansen P, Nowak PJCM, Krol ADG, Schmitz P, and Lagerwaard FJ. Evaluation of a target contouring protocol for 3D conformal radiotherapy in non-small cell lung cancer. Radiotherapy Oncol 1999; 53:247–255.
35. Giraud P, Elles S, Helfre S, De Rycke Y, Servois V, Carette M, Alzieu C, Bondiau P, Dubray B, Touboul E, Housset M, Rosenwald J, and Cosset J. Conformal radiotherapy for lung cancer: different delineation of the gross tumor volume (GTV) by radiologists and radiation oncologists. Radiat Oncol 2002; 62:27–36.
36. Van de Steene J, Linthout N, de May J, Vinh-Hung V, Claassens C, Noppen M, Bel A, Storme G. Definition of gross tumor volume in lung cancer: inter-observer variability. Radiat Oncol 2002; 62:37–49.
37. Tai P, Van Dyk J, Yu E, et al. Variability of target volume delineation in cervical esophageal cancer. Int J Radiat Oncol Biol Phys 1998; 42:227–288.

38. Hurkmans CW, Boger JH, Pieter BR, Russell NS, Jansen EPM, and Mijnheer BJ. Variability in target volume delineation on CT scans of the breast. Int J Radiat Oncol Biol Phys 2001; 50:1366–1372.
39. Logue JP, Sharrock CL, Cowan RA, Read G, Marrs J, Mott D. Clinical variability in target volume description in conformal radiotherapy planning. Int J Radiat Oncol Biol Phys 1998; 41:929–931.
40. Meijer GJ, Rasch C, Remeijer P, and Lebesque JV. Three-dimensional analysis of delineation errors, setup errors, and organ motion during radiotherapy of bladder cancer. Int J Radiat Oncol Biol Phys 2003; 55: 1277–1287.
41. Weiss E, Richter S, Krauss T, Metzelthin SI, Hille A, Pradier O, Sikmeyer B, Vorwerk H, Hess CF. Conformal radiotherapy planning of cervix carcinoma: Differences in the delineation of the clinical target volume: A comparison between gynaecologic and radiation oncologists. Radiotherapy Oncol 2003; 67:87–95.
42. Fowler J, Chappell R, Ritter M. The prospects for new treatments for prostate cancer. Int J Radiat Oncol Biol Phys 2002; 52:3–5.
43. Brenner DJ, Hall EJ. Fractionation and protraction for radiotherapy of prostate carcinoma. Int J Radiat Oncol Biol Phys 1999; 43:1095–1101.
44. Brenner DJ. Toward optimal external-beam fractionation for prostate cancer. Int J Radiat Oncol Biol Phys 2000; 48:315–316.
45. D'Souza WD, Thames HD. Is the α/β ratio for prostate cancer low? Int J Radiat Oncol Biol Phys 2001; 51:1–3.
46. King CR, Fowler JF. A simple analytic derivation suggests that prostate cancer α/β ratio is low. Int J Radiat Oncol Biol Phys 2001; 51:213–214.
47. Fowler J, Chappell R, Ritter M. Is α/β for prostate tumors really low? Int J Radiat Oncol Biol Phys 2001; 50:1021–1031.
48. Brenner DJ, Martinez AA, Edmundson GK, et al. Direct evidence that prostate tumors show high sensitivity to fractionation (low α/β ratio), similar to late-responding normal tissue. Int J Radiat Oncol Biol Phys 2002; 52:6–13.
49. Mehta M, Scrimger R, Mackie R et al. A new approach to dose escalation in non-small-cell lung cancer. Int J Radiat Oncol Biol Phys 2001; 49:23–33.
50. Fowler JF, Tomé WA, Fenwick JD, Mehta MP. Stereotactic Body radiotherapy: A challenge to conventional radiation oncology. Int J Radiat Oncol Biol Phys 2004; 60(4):1241–1256.
51. Mohan DS, Kupelian PA, Willoughby TR. Short-course intensity-modulated radiotherapy for localized prostate cancer with daily transabdominal ultrasound localization of the prostate gland. Int J Radiat Oncol Biol Phys 2000; 46:575–580.
52. Tomé WA, Fowler JF: On Cold Spots in Tumor Subvolumes. Med Phys 2002; 29:1590–1598.
53. Mutic S, Dempsey JF, Bosch WR, et al. Multimodality image registration quality assurance for conformal three-dimensional treatment planning. Int J Radiat Oncol Biol Phys 2001; 51:255–260.
54. de Boer HCJ, van Sornsen de Koste JR, Senan S, et al. Analysis and reduction of 3D systematic and random setup errors during the simulation and treatment of lung cancer patients with CT-based external beam radiotherapy dose planning. Int J Radiat Oncol Biol Phys 2001; 49:857–868.
55. Valicenti RK, Sweet JW, Hauck WW, et al. Variation of clinical target volume definition in three-dimensional radiation therapy for prostate cancer. Int J Radiat Oncol Biol Phys 1999; 44:931–935.
56. Chen L, Price RA Jr, Wang L, Li J, Qin L, McNeeley S, Ma C-M, Freedman GM, Pollack A. MRI-based treatment planning for radiotherapy: Dosimetry verification for prostate IMRT. Int J Radiat Oncol Biol Phys 2004; 60:636–647.
57. Huber PE, Hawishorst H, Fuss M, et al. Transient enlargement of contrast uptake on MRI after linear accelerator (linac) stereotactic radiosurgery for brain metastases. Int J Radiat Oncol Biol Phys 2001; 49:1339–1349.

58. Aoyama H, Shirato H, Nishioka T, et al. Magnetic resonance imaging system for three-dimensional conformal radiotherapy and its impact on gross tumor volume delineation of central nervous system tumors. Int J Radiat Oncol Biol Phys 2001; 50:821–827.
59. Kurhanewicz J, Dahiya R, Macdonald JM, et al. Citrate alterations in primary and metastatic human prostate adenocarcinoma – 1H magnetic resonance spectroscopy and biochemical study. Magn Reson Med 1993; 29:149–157.
60. Zaider M, Zelefsky MJ, Lee EK, et al. Treatment planning for prostate implants using magnetic-resonance spectroscopy imaging. Int J Radiat Oncol Biol Phys 2000; 47:1085–1096.
61. Menard C, Smith ICP, Somorjai RL, et al. Magnetic resonance spectroscopy of the malignant prostate gland after radiotherapy: a histopathologic study of diagnostic validity. Int J Radiat Oncol Biol Phys 2001; 50:317–323.
62. DiBiase SJ, Hosseinzadeh K, Gullapalli RP, et al. Magnetic resonance spectroscopic imaging-guided brachytherapy for localized prostate cancer. Int J Radiat Oncol Biol Phys 2002; 52:429–438.
63. Gross MW, Weber WA, Feldmann HJ, et al. The value of F-18-fluorodeoxyglucose PET for the 3-D radiation treatment planning of malignant gliomas. Int J Radiat Oncol Biol Phys 1998; 41:989–995.
64. Nuutinen J, Sonninen P, Lehikoinen P, et al. Radiotherapy treatment planning and long-term followup with [11C]methionine PET in patients with low-grade astrocytoma. Int J Radiat Oncol Biol Phys 2000; 48:43–52.
65. Van de Wiele C, Lahorte C, Oyer, W, Boerman O, Goethals I, Siegers G, Bierckx RA, Nuclear medicine imaging to predict response to radiotherapy: a review. Int J Radiat Oncol Biol Phys 2003; 55:5–15.
66. Ellis RJ, Kim EY, Conant R, et al. Radioimmunoguided imaging of prostate cancer foci with histopathological correlation. Int J Radiat Oncol Biol Phys 2001; 49:1281–1286.
67. Epstein JJ, Walsh PC, Carmichael M, et al. Pathological and clinical findings to predict tumor extent of nonpalpable (stage T1c) prostate cancer. JAMA 1994; 271:368–374.
68. Mackie TR, Kapatoes J, Ruchala K, Lu W, Wu C, Olivera G, Forrest L, Tome W, Welsh J, Jeraj R, Harari P, Reckwerdt P, Paliwal B, Ritter M, Keller H, Fowler J, Mehta M. Image-guidance for precise conformal radiotherapy. Int J Radiat Oncol Biol Phys 2003; 56:89–105.
69. Mackie TR. CT in Radiotherapy and Tomotherapy. In: Goldman LW, Fowlkes JB, editors. Medical CT & Ultrasound: Current Technology and Applications. Madison, WI: 1995. Advanced Medical Publishing.
70. Aldridge JS: Tomographic patient registration and conformal avoidance tomotherapy. In Dept. of Medical Physics; 1999. Madison: University of Wisconsin.
71. Hong TS, Tomé WA, Jaradat HA, Raisbeck BM, Ritter MA. Pelvic Nodal Dose Escalation with Prostate Hypofractionation Using Conformal Avoidance Defined (H-CAD) Intensity Modulated Radiation Therapy, Acta Oncologica 2006; 45:717–727.
72. Pameijer FA, Hermans R, Mancuso AA, et al. Pre- and post-radiotherapy computed tomography in laryngeal cancer: Imaging-based prediction of local failure. Int J Radiat Oncol Biol Phys 1999; 45:359–366.
73. Levitt SH, Khan FM. The rush to judgment: does the evidence support the enthusiasm over three-dimensional conformal radiation therapy and dose escalation in the treatment of prostate cancer? Int J Radiat Oncol Biol Phys 2001; 51:871–879.\
74. Yan D, Xu B, Lockman D, Kota K, Brabbins DS, Wong J, Martinez AA. The influence of interpatient and intrapatient rectum variation on external beam treatment of prostate cancer. Int J Radiat Oncol Biol Phys 2001; 51:1111–1119.
75. Teh, BS Woo SY, Butler EB, et al. Intensity modulated radiation therapy – A new promising technology in radiation oncology. The Oncologist 1999; 4:433–442.
76. Teh BS, Mai W-Y, Uhl BM, et al. Intensity-modulated radiation therapy (IMRT) for prostate cancer with the use of a rectal balloon for prostate immobilization: acute toxicity and dose–volume analysis. Int J Radiat Oncol Biol Phys 2001; 49:705–712.

77. D'Amico AV, Manola J, Loffredo M, et al. A practical method to achieve prostate gland immobilization and target verification for daily treatment. Int J Radiat Oncol Biol Phys 2001; 51:1431–1436.
78. Patel RR, Orton NP, Tomé WA, Chappell R, Ritter MA, Rectal dose-sparing with a balloon catheter and ultrasound localization in conformal radiation therapy for prostate cancer. Radiotherapy and Oncology 2003; 67(3):285–294.
79. Petereit D, Mehta M, Turski P, et al. Treatment of arteriovenous malformations with stereotactic radiosurgery employing both magnetic resonance angiography and standard angiography as a database. Int J Radiat Oncol Biol Phys 1993; 25:309–313.
80. Bednarz G, Downes B, Werner-Wasik M, et al. Combined stereotactic angiography and 3D time-of-flight magnetic resonance angiography in treatment planning for arteriovenous malformation radiosurgery. Int J Radiat Oncol Biol Phys 2000; 46:1149–1154.
81. Salter BJ, Fuss M, Vollmer DG, et al. The Talon removable head frame system for stereotactic radiosurgery/radiotherapy: measurement of the repositioning accuracy. Int J Radiat Oncol Biol Phys 2001; 51:555–562.
82. Ebert MA, Zavgorodni SF, Kendrick LA, et al. Multi-isocenter stereotactic radiosurgery: implications for target dose distributions of systematic and random localization errors. Int J Radiat Oncol Biol Phys 2001; 51:545–554.
83. Otto K, Fallone G. Frame slippage verification in stereotactic radiosurgery. Int J Radiat Oncol Biol Phys 1998; 41:199–205.
84. Allen BD, Bishop G, Welch G. Tracking: Beyond 15 min of thought. Course 11, SIGGRAPH 2001.
85. Baroni G, Ferrigno G, Pedotti A, Implementation and application of real-time motion analysis based on passive markers. Med Biol Eng Comput 1998; 36:693–703.
86. Cardinale RM, Benedict SH, Bump EA, et al. Automated target positioning for extracranial radiosurgery. Int J Radiat Oncol Biol Phys 1999, S45:206.
87. Kai J, Shiomi H, Sasama T, Sato Y. Optical high-precision three-dimensional position measurement system suitable for head motion tracking in frameless stereotactic radiosurgery. Comput Aided Surg 1998; 3:257–263.
88. Kubo HD, Len PM, Minohara S, Mostafavi. Breathing-synchronized radiotherapy program at the University of California Davis Cancer Center. Med Phys 2000;27:346–353.
89. Menke M, Hirschfeld F, Mack T, et al. Photogrammetric accuracy measurements of head holder systems used for fractionated radiotherapy. Int J Radiat Oncol Biol Phys 1994; 29:1147–1155.
90. Rogus RD, Stern RL, Kubo HD. Accuracy of a photogrammetry-based patient positioning and monitoring system for radiation therapy. Med Phys 1999; 26:721–728.
91. Wang T, Solberg T, Medin P, Boone R. Infrared patient positioning for stereotactic radiosurgery of extracranial tumors. Comput Biol Med 2001; 31:101–111.
92. Bova FJ, Buatti JM, Friedman WA, et al. The University of Florida frameless high-precision stereotactic radiotherapy system. Int J Radiat Oncol Biol Phys 1997; 38:875–882.
93. Buatti JM, Bova FJ, Friedman WA, et al.: Preliminary experience with frameless stereotactic radiotherapy. Int J Radiat Oncol Biol Phys 1998; 42:591–599.
94. Meeks SL, Bova FJ, Wagner TH, et al. Image localization for frameless stereotactic radiotherapy. Int J Radiat Oncol Biol Phys 2000; 46:1291–1299.
95. Tomé WA, Meeks SL, Buatti JM, et al. A high-precision system for conformal intracranial radiotherapy. Int J Radiat Oncol Biol Phys 2000; 47:1137–1143.
96. Tomé WA, Meeks SL, McNutt TR, et al. Optically guided intensity modulated radiotherapy. Radiother Oncol 2001; 61:33–44.
97. Ryken TC, Meeks SL, Pennington EC, et al. Initial experience with frameless stereotactic radiosurgery. Int J Radiat Oncol Biol Phys 2001a; 51(4):1152–1158.
98. Bouchet LG, Meeks SL, Goodchild G, et al. Calibration of three-dimensional ultrasound images for image-guided radiation therapy. Phys Med Biol 2001;46:559–577.
99. Bouchet LG, Meeks SL, Bova FJ, et al. 3D ultrasound image guidance for high precision extracranial radiosurgery and radiotherapy. Radiosurgery, 2002; 4:262–278.

100. Ryken TC, Meeks SL, Buatti JM, et al. Ultrasonic guidance for spinal extracranial radiosurgery: technique and application for metastatic spinal lesions. Neurosurgical Focus 2001b; 11(6):8.
101. Tomé WA, Meeks SL, Orton NP, et al. Commissioning and quality assurance of an optically guided 3D ultrasound target localization system for radiotherapy. Med Phys 2002; 29(8):1781–1788.
102. Meeks SL, Buatti JM, Bouchet LG, et al. Ultrasound guided extracranial radiosurgery: technique and application. Int J Radiat Oncol Biol Phys 2003; 55(4):1092–1101.
103. Orton NP, Jaradat HA, Tomé WA. Clinical Assessment of three-dimensional ultrasound prostate localization for external beam radiotherapy. Med Phys 2006; 33:4710–4717.
104. Chinnaiyan P, Tomé WA, Patel R, Chappell R, Ritter MA: Feasibility of Ultrasound-Guidance of Radiation Therapy in the Post-prostatectomy Setting. Technol Cancer Res Treat 2003; 2(5):455–458.
105. Uematsu M, Shioda A, Suda A, et al. Intrafractional tumor position stability during computed tomography (CT)-guided frameless stereotactic radiation therapy for lung or liver cancers with a fusion of CT and linear accelerator (FOCAL) unit. Int J Radiat Oncol Biol Phys 2000; 48:443–448.
106. Mackie TR, Holmes T, Swerdloff S, et al. Tomotherapy: A new concept for the delivery of dynamic conformal radiotherapy. Med Phys 1993; 20:1709–1719.
107. Mackie TR. Tomotherapy. In Leavitt DD, Starkshall G, editors. XII International Conference on the Use of Computers in Radiation Therapy. Salt Lake City, UT, USA: Medical Physics Publishing, 1997, pp. 9–11.
108. Mackie TR, Balog J, Ruchala K, et al. Tomotherapy. Sem Radiat Oncol 1999; 9:108–117.
109. Olivera GH, Shepard DM, Ruchala K, et al. Tomotherapy. In Modern Technology of Radiation Oncology. Van Dyk J, editor. Madison: 1999. Medical Physics Publishing.
110. Ruchala KJ, Olivera GH, Kapatoes JM, et al. Megavoltage CT image reconstruction during tomotherapy treatments. Phys Med Biol 2000; 45:3545–3562.
111. Forrest LJ, Mackie TR, Ruchala K, Turek M, Kapatoes J, Jaradat H, Hui S, Balog J, Vail DM, Mehta MP. The utility of megavoltage computed tomography images from a helical tomotherapy system for setup verification purposes. Int J Rad Oncol Biol Phys 2004; 60:1639–1644.
112. Carol M. A system for planning and rotational delivery of intensity-modulated fields. Int J Imaging Syst Tech 1995; 6:56–61.
113. Jaffray DA, Drake DG, Moreau M, et al. A radiographic and tomographic imaging system integrated into a medical linear accelerator for localization of bone and soft-tissue targets. Int J Radiat Oncol Biol Phys 1999; 45:773–789.
114. Siewerdsen JH, Jaffray DA. Cone-beam computed tomography with a flat-panel imager: Magnitude and effects of X-ray scatter. Med Phys 2001; 28:220–231.
115. Pouliot J, Bani-Hashemi A, Svatos M, Ghelmansarai F, Mitschke M, Aubin M, Xia P, Morin O, Bucci K, Roach III M. Low-dose megavoltage cone-beam CT for radiation therapy. Int J Radiat Oncol Bio Phys 2005; 61:552–560.
116. Kamino Y, Takayama K, Kokubo M, Narita Y, Hirai E, Kawawda N, Mizowaki T, Nagata Y, Nishidai T, Hiraoka M. Development of a four-dimensional image-guided radiotherapy system with a gimbaled X-ray head. Int J Radiat Oncol Biol Phys 2006; 66:271–278.
117. Yan D, Wong J. Adaptive modification of treatment planning to minimize the deleterious effects of treatment setup errors. Int J Radiat Oncol Biol Phys 1997; 38:197–206.
118. van Herk M, Remeijer P, Rasch C, et al. The probability of correct target dosage: Dose-population histograms for deriving treatment margins in radiotherapy. Int J Radiat Oncol Biol Phys 2000; 47:1121–1135.
119. Ardekani BA, Braun M, Hutton BF, et al. A fully automatic multimodality image registration algorithm. J Comput Assist Tomogr 1995; 19:615–623.
120. Alexander ME, Somojai RL. The registration of MR images using multiscale robust methods. Mag Reson Imaging 1996; 14:453–468.

121. Zeidan OA, Langen KM, Meeks SL, Manon RR, Wagner TH, Willoughby TR, Jenkins DW, Kupelian PA. Evaluation of image-guidance protocols in the treatment of head and neck cancer. Int J Radiat Oncol Biol Phys 2007; 67:670–677.
122. Kupelian P, Ramsey C, Meeks S, Willoughby T, Forbes A, Wagner T, Langen K Serial megavoltage CT imaging during external beam radiotherapy for non-small-cell lung cancer: Observations on tumor regression during treatment. Int J Radiat Oncol Biol Phys 2005; 63:1024–1028.
123. Siker M, Tomé W, Mehta M. Tumor volume changes on serial imaging with megavoltage CT for non-small-cell lung cancer during intensity-modulated radiotherapy: How reliable, consistent, and meaningful is the effect? Int J Radiat Oncol Biol Phys 2006; 66:135–141.
124. Blake A, Isard M. Active Contours. Berlin: Springer-Verlag; 1998.
125. Lu W, Chen M-L, Olivera G, Ruchala K, Mackie TR. Fast free-form deformable registration via calculus of variations. Phys Med Biol 2004; 49:3067–3087.
126. Wu C, Jeraj R, Olivera GH, Mackie TR. Re-optimization in adaptive radiotherapy. Phys Med Biol 2002; 47:3181–3195.
127. Keller H, Ritter MA, and Mackie TR. Optimal stochastic correction strategies for rigid-body target motion. Int J Radiat Oncol Biol Phys 2003; 55:261–270.
128. Keller H, Tomé WA, Ritter MA, Mackie TR: Design of adaptive treatment margins for non-neglible measurement uncertainty: application to ultrasound-guided prostate radiation therapy. Phys Med Biol 2004; 49:69–86.
129. Yu CX, Jaffray DA, Wong JW. The effects of intra-fraction organ motion on the delivery of dynamic intensity modulation. Phys Med Biol 1998; 43:91–104.
130. Yang JN, Mackie TR, Reckwerdt P, Deasy JO, Thomadsen BR. Investigation of tomotherapy beam delivery. Med Phys 1997; 24:425–436.
131. Kissick MW, Boswell SW, Jeraj R, and Mackie TR. Confirmation, refinement, and extension of a study in intrafraction motion interplay with sliding jaw motion. Med Phys 2005; 32:2346–3250.
132. Balter JM, Ten Haken RK, Lawrence TS et al. Uncertainties in CT-based radiation therapy treatment planning associated with patient breathing. Int J Radiat Oncol Biol Phys 1996; 36:167–174.
133. Samson MJ, van Sornsen de Koste JR, de Boer HCJ, et al. An analysis of anatomic landmark mobility and setup deviations in radiotherapy for lung cancer. Int J Radiat Oncol Biol Phys 1999; 43:827–832.
134. Dawson LA, Litzenberg DW, Brock KK, et al. A comparison of ventilatory prostate movement in four treatment position. Int J Radiat Oncol Biol Phys 2000; 48:319–323.
135. Shirato H, Shimizu S, Kitamura K, et al. Four-dimensional treatment planning and fluoroscopic real-time tumor tracking radiotherapy for moving tumor. Int J Radiat Oncol Biol Phys 2000; 48:435–442.
136. Shimizu S, Shirato H, Aoyama H, et al. High-speed magnetic resonance imaging for four-dimensional treatment planning of conformal radiotherapy of moving body tumors. Int J Radiat Oncol Biol Phys 2000; 48:471–474.
137. Willoughby TR, Kupelian PA, Pouliot J, Shinobara K, Aubin M, Roach M 3rd, Skrumeda LL, Balter JM, Litzenberg DW, Hadley SW, Wei JT, Sandler HM. Int J Radiat Oncol Biol Phys 2006; 65:434–528.
138. Oelfke U, Tücking T, Nill S, Seeber A, Hesse B, Huber P, Thilmann C. Linac-integrated kV-cone beam CT: Technical features and first applications. Med Dos 2006; 31:62–70.
139. Vedem SS, Keall PJ, Kini VR, Mohan R. Determining parameters for respiration-gated radiotherapy. Med Phys 2001; 28:2139–2146.
140. Kubo HD, Hill BC. Respiration gated radiotherapy treatment: A technical study. Phys Med Biol 1996; 41:83–91.
141. Wong JW, Sharpe MB, Jaffray DA, et al. The use of active breathing control (ABC) to reduce margin for breathing motion. Int J Radiat Oncol Biol Phys 1999; 44:911–919.
142. Balter JM, Brock KK, Litzenberg DW, et al. Daily targeting of intrahepatic tumors for radiotherapy. Int J Radiat Oncol Biol Phys 2002; 52:266–271.

143. Adler JR, Chang SD, Murphy MJ, Doty J, Geis P, Hancock SL. The Cyberknife: a frameless robotic system for radiosurgery. Stereotact Funct Neurosurg 1997; 69:124–128.
144. Keall PJ, Kini VR, Vedam SS, Mohan R. Motion adaptive X-ray therapy: a feasibility study. Phys Med Biol 2001; 46:1–10.
145. Zhang T, Jeraj R, Keller H, Lu W, Olivera G, McNutt T, Mackie TR, Paliwal B. Treatment plan optimization incorporating respiratory motion. Med Phys 2004; 1576–1586.
146. Counsell RE, Longino MA, Pinchuk AN, Rampy MA, Weichert MA. Radioiodinated phospholipid ether analogs and methods of using the same. US Patent #6,255,519 (2001).
147. Kapatoes JM. Olivera GH. Ruchala KJ. et al. A feasible method for clinical delivery verification and dose reconstruction in tomotherapy. Med Phys 2001a; 28:528–542.
148. Kapatoes JM. Olivera GH. Balog JP, et al. On the accuracy and effectiveness of dose reconstruction for tomotherapy. Phys Med Biol 2001b; 46:943–966.
149. Kapatoes JM, Olivera GH, Reckwerdt PJ, Fitchard EE, Schloesser EA, Mackie TR. Delivery verification in sequential and helical tomotherapy. Phys Med Biol 1999; 44:1815–1841.
150. Yan, D, Jaffray D.A., Wong, J.W. A model to accumulate fractionated dose in a deforming organ. Int J Radiat Oncol Biol Phys 1999; 44:665–675.
151. Pasma KL, Kroonwijk M, Quint S, Visser AG, Heijman BJ. Transit dosimetry with an electronic portal imaging device (EPID) for 115 prostate cancer patients. Int J Radiat Oncol Biol Phys 1999; 45:1297–1303.
152. Partridge M, Ebert M, Hesse B–H. IMRT verification by three-dimensional dose reconstruction from portal beam measurements. Med Phys 2002; 29:1847–1858.

3
Dose Painting and Theragnostic Imaging: Towards the Prescription, Planning and Delivery of Biologically Targeted Dose Distributions in External Beam Radiation Oncology

Søren M. Bentzen

Radiation Theragnostics

Theragnostics (from Greek *therapeia:* to treat and *gnosis:* knowledge) is the use of individual patient-level biological information in deciding the optimal therapy for that individual. Thus, theragnostic radiation therapy aims to go from a population-based, typically uniform, dose prescription to a personalized prescription of a, generally nonuniform, dose distribution [1]. The two main research fields are:

- *Theragnostic imaging*, i.e., the use of functional or molecular imaging data for prescribing radiation dose distributions, which is of particular interest in RT due to our ability to modulate and titrate biological effective dose in space and time. The ultimate goal is *dose painting by numbers*, i.e., direct prescription of a voxel-based biologically targeted 4D dose distribution based on 3D maps of validated imaging surrogates reflecting local radioresistance/radiosensitivity. The main imaging modalities under investigation are positron emission tomography (PET) and magnetic resonance imaging (MRI), see also Chap. 4 by Jeraj and Meyerand in this book.
- *Molecular radiation theragnostics*, which is the use of molecular biomarkers for "molecular phenotyping" of an individual tumor to optimize the radiation therapy delivered as a single modality or in combination with systemic therapies [2, 3]. Much of the research in this area is based on immunohistochemical detection of candidate proteins in tumor biopsies (see Chap. 5 by Ritter in this book) but there are also an increasing number of studies using high-throughput assays [4–6].

Clearly, these two approaches are potentially complementary although little systematic work has been done on combining them. In this chapter, the focus is on theragnostic imaging and the potential clinical gain from delivery of a biologically targeted rather than a uniform radiation dose distribution. An overview is presented of this emerging research field and the technological and biological challenges in prescription, planning and delivery of biologically targeted dose distributions will be briefly discussed.

M.P. Mehta et al. (eds.), *Radiation Oncology Advances*.

From Anatomical to Biological Targeting in Radiation Therapy

Among the nonsurgical agents for treating cancer, radiation is unique because it can be precisely modulated in space and time. The vast majority of cancer patients receiving radiation therapy will have a relatively limited tissue volume irradiated to the prescribed target dose, typically not more than a few percent of their body volume. As side effects of radiation therapy are generally confined to the irradiated tissues, this geometrical exclusion of healthy normal tissues is such a fundamental aspect of radiation therapy that we often do not even think about it.

A brief look at the evolution of radiation therapy targeting over the last 30 years or so, may form an interesting background for what we discuss here. Due to the limited ability of X-rays and fluoroscopy to visualize the anatomical spread of malignant disease, most definitions of target volumes before 1980 were based on the normal X-ray anatomy. This was "looking for the keys under the lamppost" but was rationalized by noting that specific anatomical regions were "at high risk of microscopic spread," thereby justifying the application of a curative dose to more than the actual macroscopic malignant tumor. With the event of whole-body computed tomography around 1980, and the parallel development of CT-based dose-planning systems, anatomical targeting became increasingly based on the visual (morphological) extent of tumor on CT scans at times supported by biopsies from suspicious tissues: we may call this, patho-anatomical targeting. The prescribed radiation dose distribution became a uniform dose distribution with high geometrical conformality to the clinical target volume, so-called 3D conformal radiation therapy. In some cases more than one dose level was prescribed to separate target volumes depending on the estimated risk of tumor recurrence.

When moving from wide-field to 3D conformal radiotherapy, selection and delineation of the target volume become critical. Several studies have demonstrated large interoperator variability in traditional target volume delineation in a variety of anatomical sites including brain [7], prostate [8], esophagus [9], breast [10], and uterine cervix [11]. This has created a push for multimodality imaging as a means of improving the sensitivity and specificity of target selection and reducing variabililty in target delineation among operators. The use of functional and molecular imaging in diagnosis and staging has been called anato-molecular imaging (Richard Wahl).

Biologically targeted radiotherapy was the goal of research into the therapeutic administration of internal emitters combined with a biologically selective vehicle. Typical examples are radioimmunotherapy [12, 13] or the use of bone-seeking radiopharmaceuticals [14, 15]. This field has shown some progress over the last couple of decades [16–18] but is still not widely used for the treatment of solid tumors. There are several reasons for this, but part of the explanation is that with internal emitters the biological targeting is achieved at the expense of anatomical targeting. This means in practice that it is difficult to deliver a very high radiation dose to localized tumors without unacceptable normal-tissue toxicity. On the other hand, the systemic application of internal emitters does entail a potential advantage in patients with disseminated disease, e.g., nonfocal bone metastases.

Biologically targeted external beam radiation therapy (bio-EBRT) is emerging as a theoretically attractive alternative to conventional uniform dose delivery and biological targeting using internal emitters [1]. Bio-EBRT combines the fundamental advantage of geometrical targeting offered by conventional EBRT with the theoretical advantage of delivering higher dose to potentially resistant tumor subvolumes. With the technological advances in treatment planning and delivery, most notably the conceptual development of inverse treatment planning and the technological development of intensity modulated (IMRT) and image guided (IGRT) radiation therapy [19], bio-EBRT is gradually becoming a realistic treatment paradigm.

From Target Selection and Delineation to 4D Dose Prescription

Medical imaging is an integral component of planning, delivery, and follow-up of modern radiation therapy (Fig. 1). Imaging, typically CT or MRI, is used in diagnosis and staging of malignant disease. Once the indication for radiation therapy is established for a given case, planning CT scans with or without additional imaging information from PET or MRI are used for selecting and delineating the target.

In-room imaging refers to imaging in the radiation treatment room conducted to verify the position of the patient, the tumor or target volume or critical normal structures: so-called image-guided radiation therapy or IGRT [20]. A number of new technologies are in clinical use or under development [19, 21], including electronic portal imaging devices, cone-beam CT, megavoltage CT, and optical tracking devices as well as more elaborate schemes such as CT on rails, where the

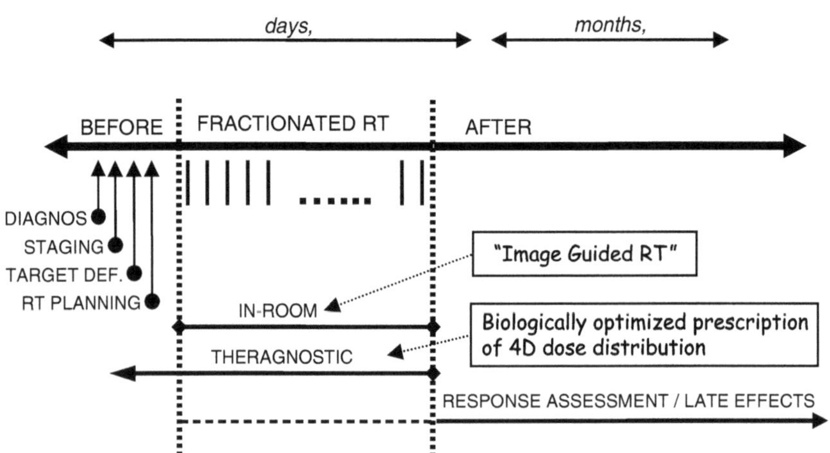

Fig. 1 The many roles of imaging in modern radiation theraphy. Theragnostic imaging is the use of molecular or functional imaging as a basis for prescribing a 4D dose distribution that is estimated to optimize the efficacy:toxicity ratio.

patient is translated, while lying in treatment position on the couch, from the treatment machine to a CT scanner in the treatment room.

Imaging is also applied in the monitoring of tumor response, traditionally in the form of volume regression assessed from CT scans or X-rays. However, the utility of PET/CT is being studied in this context [22], leading to the assessment of metabolic response rather than clinical (volume) response. In addition, a number of novel PET tracers are under evaluation for response assessment [23]. The hope is that molecular imaging of specific surrogates of biological properties will improve the sensitivity and decrease the time interval for establishing a potential significant response. Also, functional MRI is of major interest in this context [24]. One obvious field of application is with molecular targeted agents, where the imaging surrogate may directly reflect target inhibition, but it is also likely that some imaging markers could reliably map response to cytotoxic chemotherapy or radiation.

Theragnostic imaging represents the logical next frontier in the integration of imaging and radiation oncology: the goal is to prescribe the full 4D radiation dose distribution for a specific individual patient based on a functional or molecular imaging map of a biological characteristics or a cellular phenotype [1]. Imaging theragnostics is the topic of this chapter.

The Case for Nonuniform Theragnostic Dose Distributions

Under quite general assumptions it can be shown that for a given integral dose to a tumor with uniform radiation sensitivity, a uniform dose distribution maximizes the tumor control probability [25–27]. However, for a tumor with a spatial variation in radiosensitivity, a uniform dose distribution is no longer optimal as demonstrated theoretically 20 years ago in a mathematical modeling paper by Brahme and Ågren [28]. Intuitively, it is clear that spending more of the dose on irradiating the most resistant areas will improve the overall probability of controlling the tumor. With the event of functional and molecular imaging, many authors suggested that this could form the basis for selective boosting of tumor subvolumes with potentially resistant cells [29–33]. Numerous modeling studies provide support for this concept [28, 34–38] and in these, admittedly often highly idealized, studies gains in tumor control probability of 50% or more have been estimated.

Some basic features of biotargeted EBRT are revealed by a simple “caricature model” of a tumor containing a radiosensitive and a radioresistant compartment of cells, see Fig. 2. The two compartments are assumed not to interact, in other words, the probability of controlling both compartments, and thereby achieving tumor control of the whole tumor, is simply the product of the tumor control probabilities (TCP) for each compartment. Tumor control in these compartments are assumed to follow a logistic dose–response curve with a γ_{50}-value of 2, the typical shape and steepness of clinical dose–control curves [39, 40]. The position of the dose–response curve is quantified by the dose required for 50% tumor control, the TCD_{50} [39]. The comparison is made against a homogenous tumor consisting of two equal-sized

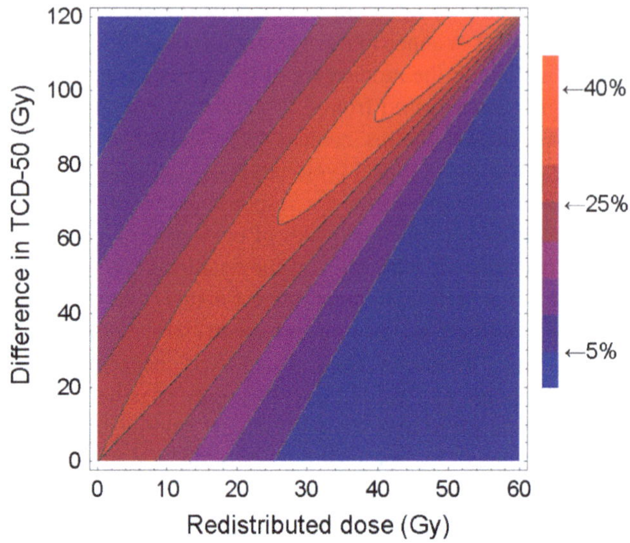

Fig. 2 Contour plot of the tumor control probability (scale on the left) as a function of the difference in the position of the dose–response curves for the sensitive and resistant compartments in a two-compartment tumor model. Giving a uniform 70-Gy dose to the whole tumor is associated with a decrease in TCP with increasing difference in the position of the two curves (moving along the y-axis). Similarly, redistributing too high a dose is associated with a poor outcome (lower right corner of graph). For more details, see text

subvolumes with a TCD_{50} of 70 Gy and treated with a uniform dose of 70 Gy in 2-Gy fractions. This tumor will have a TCP of 25%. For simplicity, we assume that in the heterogeneous case, the two tumor control curves are symmetrically shifted by subtracting and adding the same dose, ΔTCD_{50}, from the two TCD_{50}'s. There are an infinite number of potential strategies for treating the heterogeneous tumor with some measure of dose intensification to the more resistant compartment. Again, it may be instructive to study just one such strategy, called dose redistribution [35], whereby the integral tumor dose is kept constant. We assume that this two-level prescribed dose distribution can be delivered such that 100% of the two compartmental volumes receive the prescribed dose. Figure 2 shows how TCP varies as the difference in the two TCD_{50}'s increases: if no dose redistribution is implemented, the TCP of the tumor tends to zero. Clearly, if the two radiosensitivities, quantified here by the TCD_{50} of the corresponding dose–response curves, could be reliably assessed, there would be an optimal-redistributed dose that would maximize TCP. As we "borrow" dose from the sensitive and deliver this to the resistant compartment, the TCP of a heterogeneous tumor may in fact exceed that of a homogenous tumor receiving the same integral dose; the intuitive reason for this being that the hypothetical existence of a sensitive subpopulation of effectively over-treated cells represents an opportunity to escalate the dose to the more resistant cells.

Figure 3 illustrates some of the above strategies in a plot of the dose–control curves for a two-compartment tumor with a 60-Gy difference between the two TCD_{50}'s. Delivering a 70-Gy uniform dose to this tumor yields an 8% TCP. A simple optimization shows that TCP can be maximized for the same integral tumor dose by redistributing 24.4 Gy from the sensitive to the resistant compartment: this gives rise to a 29% TCP.

In practice, it may seem risky to lower the dose to any part of the target volume, and a simple alternative strategy may be to keep the dose at 70 Gy for the sensitive compartment and escalate the dose to the resistant compartment by 24.4 Gy, corresponding to arrows A and D in Fig. 2. This increases the TCP to 39%, considerably better than if the same integral dose, i.e., a dose of 82.2 Gy was delivered to the whole tumor, producing a calculated TCP of 19%. Although the boosting *without* dose redistribution is clearly a safe strategy, it should be noted, for the sake of argument, that this way of spending the integral tumor dose is still not optimal: optimal dose redistribution in case of a uniform integral dose of 82.2 Gy to the whole tumor would further increase the calculated TCP to 48%.

Three slightly different implementations of biologically targeted EBRT are under investigation. *Dose painting* was the term coined by Cliff Ling and colleagues [33] and refers to the identification of a discrete tumor subvolume with potential radioresistance and then prescribing an additional boost dose to this region. This approach was used in a proof-of-principle planning study by Chao and colleagues [32].

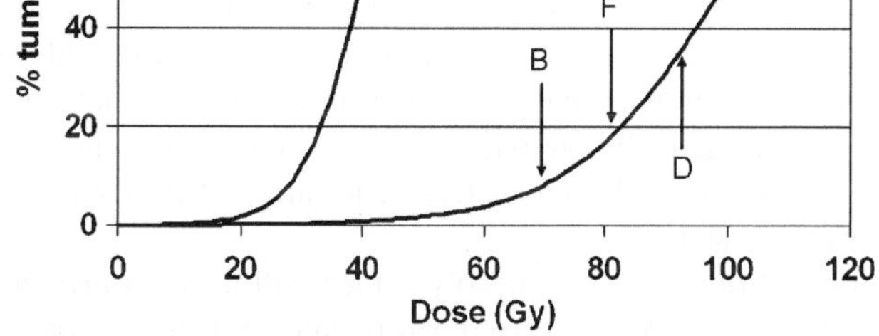

Fig. 3 A two-compartment tumor comprising equal-sized volumes of sensitive and resistant cells. The doses required for 50% tumor control probability, the TCD-50s, are 40 Gy and 100 Gy, i.e., a 60-Gy difference, for the two compartments. A 70 Gy uniform dose (A and B) produces an 8.3% TCP. Keeping the integral tumor dose at 70 Gy but redistributing dose from the sensitive to the resistant compartments (C and D) increases TCP to 29.4%. The optimal-redistributed dose turns out to be 24.4 Gy. Keeping the 70 Gy to the sensitive cells (A) and boosting the resistant cells by the 24.4 Gy (D) produces a 39% TCP. In contrast, a 12.2 Gy uniform boost (E and F) will produce a TCP of 19%.

The alternative approach has been called *dose painting by numbers* [1] whereby a full 3D or more generally 4D dose distribution is prescribed and presented to the treatment plan optimization software on a voxel-by-voxel basis. The link between image intensity and radiation dose is called the *prescription function*, see below. The technical feasibility of *planning* such a distribution has been shown by several groups [41–43]. *Delivering* this kind of dose distribution is yet another matter, and this has not been systematically investigated for biologically realistic prescription maps. A hybrid between these two strategies is *multilevel dose painting* where several, typically 3 or 4, dose levels are prescribed in discrete regions defined by the average regional image intensity [35], see also Chap. 12 by Kim and Tomé in this book. These implementations are all means to the same end and their relative merits have not been rigorously compared yet.

Two planning studies have demonstrated the clinical feasibility of dose painting according to ^{18}F-FDG intensity: Das et al. [42] scanned and planned two lung cancer patients and Vanderstraeten et al. [34] performed a planning study comprising 15 cases with HNSCC. While the biological basis for boosting FDG avid regions remains to be established, these studies are valuable contributions to the conceptual and technical development of dose painting in radiotherapy.

Precision Requirements

As mentioned above: unless a spatial variation in radioresponsiveness can be precisely mapped and dose painted, the patient would be better off in terms of tumor control by receiving a uniform dose distribution. So, what are the requirements for taking this forward in the clinic?

Sufficient predictive power of the imaging surrogate for local tumor radioresponsiveness is a sine qua non. Much of the current research aims to identify adequate imaging surrogates for the clinically established biological mechanisms behind locoregional failure: hypoxia and rapid tumor cell proliferation. As radiobiologically relevant hypoxia and cell proliferation are not directly quantifiable, most studies on validation of imaging surrogates resort to showing correlation between the image intensity on one hand and a (locally) measurable tumor characteristic on the other. This characteristic in turn is then assumed to correlate with clinical radioresistance.

Spatiotemporal stability of the phenotype map will decide *when* and *how often* that patient would have to be rescanned and replanned. It is necessary to evaluate both the short- and the longterm stability during fractionated radiotherapy. Test–retest reliability is an important aspect of an imaging modality used directly in clinical decision making or treatment planning.

Estimating the dose prescription function is the next logical step. After establishing the correlation between the local intensity of a molecular imaging agent and the local outcome of radiation therapy, the challenge is to estimate the dose of radiation required to offset this level of local radioresistance.

Planning the dose painted distribution can be achieved using standard commercial software in the case of single- or multilevel dose painting whereas dose painting by numbers requires research optimization software that is currently not on the market. Optimization of the prescribed dose plan must be conducted under appropriate normal-tissue dose–volume constraints.

Delivery and verification of the painted dose plan is not principally different from the delivery and verification of any other IMRT plan, only harder! The long-established way to incorporate setup accuracy for a uniform dose plan is to add margins to expand the clinical target volume, CTV, to a planning target volume, PTV. Ideally, this can be achieved rationally using a margin recipe derived from empirical data [44]. This approach breaks down when the goal is accurate delivery of a prescribed nonuniform dose distribution. While margins can be added around a single hot area to be dose painted with a defined dose, this is not practical in case of dose painting by numbers. A special issue arises with involuntary motion of the target volume for example the movement of thoracic tumors close to the diaphragm as a function of phase in the breathing cycle where verification of the accuracy of patient setup will be the first step only. On top of this, it is necessary to use gated or breathing synchronized dose delivery.

Clinical testing represents the ultimate validation of dose painting as a therapeutic interventional strategy. Early clinical trials are in progress aimed at proving feasibility, optimizing imaging protocols and correlating imaging parameters with outcome. Phase III randomized controlled trials, comparing biologically targeted with standard EBRT are likely to be initiated within the next 5–7 years, depending on the outcome of the early trials.

Targeting Hypoxia Using EBRT: Are We Ready for Dose Painting by Numbers?

At the time of writing the most advanced research area in theragnostic imaging for radiation oncology is hypoxia targeting and it may be instructive to review the current state of the research with respect to the various components listed above.

Hypoxia as a Cause of Clinical Failure of Radiation Therapy

In vitro irradiation of cells under hypoxia or anoxia has long been known to produce a higher surviving fraction after a specific dose than if the same cells had been given the same dose under normal oxygen conditions [45]. Traditionally this has been explained by the damage-fixation hypothesis: that free radicals produced in DNA can be repaired under hypoxic conditions but will be "fixed" in the presence of oxygen. A clear demonstration of the oxygen effect in vivo is obtained when irradiating transplantable tumors on the leg of mice where clamps can be used to restrict blood flow and thereby induce hypoxia: the dose required to control 50% of the tumors increases dramatically when irradiating tumors under clamp hypoxia [46–48]. Transplantable mouse tumors implanted in inbred experimental animals show increasing heterogeneity in oxygenation status assessed by microelectrode pO_2 measurements with increasing tumor volume and they follow a more shallow radiation dose–response curve consistent with this intertumor heterogeneity [48]. This suggests that tumor oxygenation is not only associated with radioresistance but is a major source of variability even in the response of well-stratified experimental tumors to radiation therapy.

More than 50 years ago, Thomlinson and Gray [49] demonstrated in a study of histological sections from patients with lung cancer that some solid human tumors contain hypoxic cells. Since then, numerous assays have been developed and applied in the detection and quantification of hypoxia in human tumors including direct physical measurement of the partial oxygen tension by means of polarographic microelectrodes, detection of extrinsic markers such as pimonidazole or endogenous hypoxia markers such as HIF-1α, HIF-2α, or CAIX in tumor biopsies and more recently noninvasive functional and molecular imaging.

Significant association between tumor oxygenation status and the outcome of radiotherapy has been most convincingly demonstrated in squamous cell carcinoma of the head and neck (HNSCC). Physical measurement of partial oxygen tension by means of polarographic microelectrodes [50] has been shown to correlate with outcome after definitive radiation therapy in a joint analysis of a large series of 397 tumors from seven institutions [51]. There is also evidence from studies of endogenous hypoxia markers detected by immunohistochemistry in tumor biopsies that tumors expressing these markers have a relatively poor outcome after radiation therapy [52].

A number of randomized controlled clinical trials have tested hypoxic modification in patients receiving radiotherapy, for example by treating patients in hyperbaric oxygen chambers or by administering oxygen-mimetic hypoxic cell sensitizers. A meta-analysis identified 91 published or unpublished trials with more than 11,000 patients [53] and found a significant benefit of combining hypoxic modification with radiation therapy, especially on locoregional control in head and neck cancer, 46% versus 39% for radiotherapy alone. As hypoxic cell sensitization affects the locoregional effect of radiation therapy only, the fact that these strategies are associated with an improved outcome lends indirect support to the idea that local treatment intensification in hypoxic regions could be advantageous.

On the other hand, the overall effect of hypoxic modification has not been all that great and there is probably an important lesson there too. Hypoxia is a strong driver of malignant progression [54] and it is now evident that the prognostic impact of tumor hypoxia is not solely the result of classic hypoxic radioresistance as explained by the damage-fixation hypothesis. Support for this assertion comes partly from a study showing that in carcinoma of the uterine cervix hypoxic tumors as assessed by microelectrode measurement do worse than well-oxygenated tumors after definitive surgery as well as after radiation therapy [55] and partly from studies showing an increased rate of metastases in patients harboring hypoxic soft tissue sarcoma [56] or HNSCC [52]. This is also consistent with recent data from prostate cancer biopsies showing a correlation between strong staining with the intrinsic hypoxia marker pimonidazole and increasing Gleason score [57]. Also, the mechanism underlying hypoxia as a factor modulating radiation response seems to be more complex than suggested by the damage-fixation hypothesis. Recent studies have shown that HIF-1 plays an active role in mediating hypoxia induced radiation resistance [58]. Williams et al. [59] found no difference in the in vitro radiation response of wild type and HIF-1 deficient mouse hepatoma cell lines. However, when these cell lines were grown in nude mice, the HIF-1 deficient tumors were considerably more radiosensitive than wild type tumors. Microelectrode measurements of pO_2 and assessment of the binding of an extrinsic hypoxia marker in tumor biopsies showed no difference in oxygenation status. These experiments suggest that activation of the hypoxia response pathways produce a survival advantage for cells after irradiation. Indirect support for this picture comes from a large clinical study using immunohistochemistry on diagnostic biopsies to quantify two hypoxia-responsive proteins, HIF-2α and CAIX [52]. Again, rather than just being endogenous markers of a low chemical oxygen concentration, activation of these two hypoxia response pathways appears to have an independent negative impact on prognosis after definitive radiotherapy.

The above observations, together with a large body of experimental data, suggest a more active biological view on hypoxia whereby hypoxia is a cause as well as a consequence of malignant progression. If tumor cells in a hypoxic environment have already activated multiple hypoxia-inducible survival pathways, then attempts to restore the local radiosensitizing effect of oxygen may not be that effective. This is the rationale for radiation dose escalation to hypoxic areas: cells in these areas are in part protected by the direct DNA damage from radiation, but are also likely to have acquired biological strategies that make them more aggressive and less susceptible to cytotoxic therapy. The logical therapeutic approach would therefore seem to be a combined systemic and locoregional intensification, combining cytotoxic or molecular targeted therapies with biological targeted radiation dose distributions.

Hypoxia Imaging

Quite a number of imaging surrogates for hypoxia are in various stages of preclinical and clinical development, see also Chap. 4 by Jeraj and Meyerand in this volume. The present chapter will be limited to hypoxia imaging using PET.

The pioneering study in this field was conducted by Janet Rasey and colleagues from the University of Washington, Seattle more than 10 years ago [60]. These authors published on ^{18}F-labeled fluoromisonidazole (FMISO) PET scans in 37 patients with various tumor types: 21 nonsmall cell lung cancer patients, seven head and neck cancer patients, four prostate cancer patients, and five patients with other histologies. Defining the fractional hypoxic volume (FHV) as the proportion of pixels in the imaged tumor volume with a tissue-to-blood (T/B) ^{18}F activity ratio $\geq$1.4 at 2–2.5 h after the injection, Rasey and colleagues found an FHV>0 in all except one (97%) of the 37 tumors. Rischin et al. [61] used a qualitative scale for grading hypoxia based on FMISO PET scans in 45 patients with HNSCC, 32 of whom (71%) were classified as having hypoxic tumors at baseline. A similar estimate is obtained from the large HNSCC study from Seattle [62] where 58/73 (79%) showed "significant hypoxia," defined as tumor regions with a T/B ≥ 1.4. The proportion of PET-hypoxic tumors depends, of course, on the exact definition of hypoxia – and the above prevalence estimates are therefore to some extend circular. Unfortunately, there is still no consensus on the most appropriate definition of PET hypoxia. The general impression from the published studies, however, is that PET-detected hypoxia is a frequent characteristic of solid malignancies.

PET Tracers for Imaging Hypoxia

Clinical PET studies have used tracers belonging to one of two broad classes of compounds. The most widely used of these are the radiofluorinated nitroimidazoles in particular FMISO [60–68] but also fluoroerythronitroimidazole (FETNIM) has been used in human studies [69, 70]. Several more compounds of this type are under preclinical development (see Chap. 4 by Jeraj and Meyerand). These tracers are derived from compounds originally developed as oxygen-mimetic hypoxic cell radiosensitizers with a high electron affinity. Under low oxygen tension they are reduced and bind covalently to intra- or extracellular molecules. Thus, the nitroimidazole-based tracers may reflect the physicochemical presence of oxygen quite directly. The other tracer that has been used in several clinical studies [32, 71, 72] is Cu(II)-diacetyl-bis(N4-methylthiosemicarbazone) (Cu-ATSM), a chelated Cu compound, that has also been shown to be retained in cells under hypoxia [73–76]. The reduction of Cu-ATSM predominantly takes place in the microsome/cytosol rather than in the mitochondria and reflects the activity of bioreductive enzymes such as NADH-cytochrome b5 reductase and NADPH-cytochrome P450 reductase [76]. The level of these enzymes are increased several fold, especially in chronic hypoxic areas and it may therefore be that such areas are particularly well visualized in Cu-ATSM images. The retention of Cu-ATSM is therefore more dependent on the biological consequences of hypoxia, rather than oxygen concentration per se. It remains to be seen whether this theoretical advantage – from the perspective of hypoxia as an active biological process – converts into a stronger predictive and prognostic power in clinical applications.

The two lead tracers, FMISO and Cu-ATSM, each has its proponents and opponents – and at the time of writing their clinical performance has not been directly compared. It is possible that hypoxic regions in human tumors would be correctly identified in scans using either of the two tracers. In terms of imaging properties, Cu-ATSM is rapidly washed out from norm-oxic cells and tissues and therefore provides images with a high signal-to-background ratio, i.e., high image contrast. FMISO images suffer from a lower signal-to-background ratio partly due to a relatively low binding of FMISO in hypoxic regions and partly due to the lipophilicity and slower clearance of this compound [77]. Tracer concentration is often quantified by the T/B or tumor-to-muscle (T/M) ratio. Chapman et al. [30] have suggested that the ideal surrogate tracer for hypoxia imaging would preferentially bind in the same range of oxygen concentrations where radiobiological hypoxia is seen. However, the relevance of this criterion is debatable in view of the current more active biological view of hypoxia. Even under the "old" hypothesis regarding the radiobiological effect of hypoxia, modeling studies have suggested that it may be cells at moderate levels of hypoxia that will contribute most to hypoxia-related failure of fractionated radiotherapy [78]. Also, Rajendran and Krohn [77] have argued that due to the difference in tracer kinetics and binding mechanism, FMISO may be more sensitive to rapid changes in oxygenation status than Cu-ATSM. Again, it can be argued that if the main effect of hypoxia is the biological response to this factor, then tracking the actual oxygen tension may be relatively less important than thought under the traditional radiobiological paradigm. Nevertheless, FMISO is currently the tracer that has been used in the majority of clinical studies. More clinical and preclinical studies are needed to fully characterize the relative merits of these tracers for PET hypoxia imaging.

Perhaps it is worth mentioning that ^{18}F-FDG does not appear to be a good imaging surrogate for hypoxia. In vitro, several cell lines do show a hypoxia-dependent increase in FDG uptake [79, 80]. In vivo studies in rodent tumors [81, 82] have also shown increased FDG uptake in regions with marked immunohistochemical staining for pimonidazole, an extrinsic immunohistochemical marker of hypoxia. However, the correlation between FMISO and FDG PET seems to be low. Cherk et al. [83] found no significant correlation between tumor FMISO SUV_{max} and FDG SUV_{max} in 21 patients with NSCLC, $r = 0.26$. In an interesting study, Zimny et al. [84] compared FDG PET, FMISO PET, and pO_2 microelectrode measurements in 24 patients with HNSCC. Both PET scans and the pO_2 measurements were obtained within 1 week. A moderate correlation, $r = 0.53$, was found between the T/B ratio of FMISO at 2 h and the FDG SUV_{max}. However, the FDG uptake was not correlated with the pO_2 measurements, in contrast to the retention of FMISO that *did* show such a correlation (see below). Finally, the large series published by Rajendran and colleagues [85] provides important information also in this regard. Forty-nine patients with a mix of tumor histologies (26 HNSCC, 11 soft tissue sarcoma, seven breast cancer, and five glioblastoma multiforme) had both FMISO and FDG PET scans and the pixel-by-pixel correlation between FMISO and FDG uptake was estimated for each patient. The mean correlation coefficients were 0.62 for HNSCC, 0.47 for breast cancer, 0.38 for glioblastoma multiforme, and 0.32 for soft tissue sarcoma. However, the correlation between the overall tumor FDG SUV_{max} and the hypoxic volume estimated from FMISO PET scans was low with a Spearman's rank correlation coefficient, $r_S = 0.24$.

Validation of Hypoxia PET Imaging

The hypoxia targeting PET tracers that are currently in clinical trials have all been validated in preclinical in vitro and in vivo models. Direct clinical validation, however, is more of a challenge, in part because of the difficulty in manipulating human tumor oxygenation and demonstrating sensitivity of the tracers to pick up these changes, and in part, for the simple reason that there is no accepted gold standard for quantifying biologically relevant tumor hypoxia in patients. Correlations have been shown between Eppendorf microelectrode measurements of physical oxygen tension and FMISO PET scans by Zimny et al. [84], who found that FMISO retention was significantly higher in hypoxic tumors than in normoxic tumors (T/M ratios at 2h of 1.8 ± 0.4 versus 1.4 ± 0.1, $p<0.05$). Furthermore, FMISO T/M showed good correlation with the proportion of microelectrode readings with $pO_2 \leq 5$ mmHg ($r=0.80$, $p<0.001$).

At the time of writing, the most convincing, and ultimately also the most relevant, support for the value of current PET hypoxia imaging techniques comes from studies testing a direct association between PET hypoxia and clinical outcome. Table 1 summarizes the results of nine studies addressing this issue, six of them in head and neck cancer and one each in nonsmall cell lung cancer, cervix cancer, and glioblastoma. Two-thirds of these studies have used FMISO PET and two have used Cu-ATSM. A variety of PET hypoxia descriptors have been used and the clinical endpoints as well as the actual study designs vary considerably across studies. Most studies published to date have been exploratory or hypothesis-generating, as opposed to hypothesis-testing, and the significant *p*-values should be taken with a pinch of salt. Still, the overall picture is encouraging: PET hypoxia invariably shows some association with clinical outcome.

Spatiotemporal Stability of the PET Hypoxia Map

Very few studies have investigated the spatial dynamics of the hypoxia map *before* the start of radiation therapy and the spatiotemporal evolution of the map *during* fractionated radiotherapy. Note that even if the pretherapy hypoxia map eventually is found to correlate only weakly with maps assessed during therapy, it is still possible that boosting the areas that were hypoxic before the start of radiation therapy could be therapeutically advantageous. Lee et al. [89] have published, in abstract form, an analysis of repeat FMISO scans recorded 2 days apart before therapy in a single patient with HNSCC. They concluded that the distribution of FMISO in the gross tumor volume was "heterogeneous but reproducible" between the two scans. A scatter plot of pairs of pixel intensities of the two coregistered FMISO scans showed some correlation between the intensities but the correlation coefficient was not given in the abstract. Paulsen et al. [67] performed FMISO scans at baseline and after reaching 30–40 Gy in eight patients with locally advanced HNSCC. A "clear shrinkage of hypoxic areas" was seen and the authors noted that in "some patients" residual hypoxic regions remained after 30+ Gy. According to the authors, these regions of residual hypoxia correlated well with the regions showing high uptake at baseline.

Reoxygenation at the whole tumor rather than regional level has been monitored in a few studies. In the study by Rischin et al. [61], of the 32 HNSCC tumors

Table 1 Studies looking at the possible correlation between hypoxia PET imaging and clinical outcome

Imaging agent	Tumor site	Sample size, N	Hypoxi a descriptor	Clinical endpoint	Significance of association	Comment	References
FMISO	HNSCC	73	Max T/B, FHV	Survival	T/B: $p = 0.006$ FHV: $p = 0.001$	p-Values are from a multivariate model adjusting for nodal stage	[62]
FMISO	HNSCC	12	Max SUV	Local relapse	$p = 0.045$	Same patients as in the study below (?)	[86]
FMISO	HNSCC	13[a]	SUV at 2 and 4 h	Clinical response	2 h: $p = 0.16$ 4 h: $p=0.04$	Exploratory data analysis looking at multiple hypoxic descriptors; T/M ratios claimed to discriminate better but no formal test stated in paper	[66]
FMISO	HNSCC	45	Qualitative consensus score by two blinded observers	Clinical response after chemoradiation therapy ± the bioreductive drug tirapazamine	Significant interaction between hypoxic status and response to tirapazamine $p < 0.05$		[61]
FMISO	NSCLC	8[a]	SUV at 2 and 4 h	Clinical response	2 and 4 h: $p =$ NS	T/M ratios claimed to produce better discrimination but no formal test stated in paper	[66]
FMISO	gliomas	14	"FMISO uptake" (yes/no)	Survival	$p = 0.03$	p-Value calculated from data in original paper (Fisher's Exact test)	[87]

(continued)

Table 1 (continued)

Imaging agent	Tumor site	Sample size, N	Hypoxia descriptor	Clinical endpoint	Significance of association	Comment	References
FETNIM	HNSCC	21	FHV	Survival	$p = 0.04$		[70]
Cu-ATSM	NSCLC	14	Mean T/M	Clinical response	$p = 0.002$		[72]
Cu-ATSM	Uterine cervix	14	T/M > 3.5	Progression-free (PFS) and overall survival (OS)	PFS: $p = 0.0005$ OS: $p = 0.015$		[88]

FHV fractional hypoxic volume, *T/B* tumor-to-blood ratio, *T/M* tumor-to-muscle ratio, *FMISO* [^{18}F]fluoromisonidazole, *FETNIM* [18F]fluoroerythronitroimidazole, *Cu-ATSM* [^{60}Cu]Cu-diacetyl-bis(N4-methylthiosemicarbazone

[a]Patients with both valid hypoxia imaging and clinical outcome data

(out of 45) judged to be hypoxic at baseline, 29 had a repeat FMISO scan in weeks 4 or 5 and six of these patients (21%) had residual hypoxia at that time. No attempt was made to correlate the spatial distribution of PET hypoxia during therapy and at baseline. Also the Seattle group [90] performed serial FMISO scans during radiotherapy in seven patients with locally advanced nonsmall cell lung cancer. Again, no attempt was made to correlate the spatial distribution of FMISO intensity before and during radiation therapy. Also these authors concluded that reoxygenation takes place in some tumors but that there was considerable variability among individual cases and there was no obvious way to predict this process.

The above observations are in broad agreement with preliminary data from studies in progress at the University of Wisconsin – Madison, showing relative spatial stability of the hypoxia map, but this is clearly an area where more research is needed.

Dose Painting by Numbers

Assuming that local hypoxia can be reliably mapped using functional or molecular imaging, the next challenge is to select the additional ("boost") dose to be delivered to these regions. As discussed above, there are several strategies for doing this; here, only the voxel-based dose painting by numbers will be considered. The key step is to define the *prescription function* that is the mathematical link between the image contrast parameter and the prescribed dose to that specific voxel.

In the absence of an evidence-based prescription function derived from clinical data sets, the simplest reasonable prescription function is probably a linear interpolation between a minimum desirable tumor dose, D_{min}, and a maximum safe dose, D_{max}, according to the pixel intensity, I [34, 42]

$$D(I) = D_{min} + \frac{I - I_{min}}{I_{max} - I_{min}}(D_{max} - D_{min}).$$

In other words, as I increases from the minimum (I_{min}) to the maximum (I_{max}) intensity value observed in the tumor volume, the prescribed dose will increase from D_{min} to D_{max}. It is likely that the optimal prescription function will be a nonlinear function of the image intensity, I. On the other hand, there are good reasons to believe that $D(I)$ is a monotonic function, and the simple linear formula may turn out to be a good first approximation.

More elaborate prescription functions, some of them estimated from clinical observations, are being studied and the possible advantage of using these relative to the simple form above is being quantified using mathematical bioeffect models.

Dose Delivery and Expected Change in Outcome

As mentioned above, there is no principal difference between delivering a uniform versus a nonuniform dose distribution, but the required precision in dose planning as well as in the treatment room may effectively limit the clinical gain from theragnostic dose distributions. The truth is that a reasonable assessment of the precision requirements cannot be made before a more thorough understanding of the temperospatial aspects of the dose prescription map has been established through clinical research.

How effective will hypoxia targeted EBRT be? Again, this is currently an open question. Bioeffect modeling, partly based on clinical empirical data on the prognostic impact of hypoxia, suggests that very large improvements in tumor control probability could be achievable. However, the estimated gain depends on a long string of assumptions, many of which have been summarized above. The estimated gain will depend on tumor type and may likely vary from patient to patient. The ultimate treatment goal is to improve the life expectancy and/or the quality of life for the patient. How improved local control will contribute to this, depends again on the natural history of the disease. It has been estimated from a meta-analysis of clinical trials, that for squamous cell carcinoma of the head and neck, a 10% point improvement in locoregional control converts into a 6–7% point improvement in 5-year survival [91]. Obviously, this ratio will be less favorable for other tumor histologies. Unless, that is, competing risks models will allow us in the future to select patients for dose painting who have a high risk of locoregional compared with systemic relapse [3].

Conclusion

More research is needed – and is currently underway – on both the biological and technical feasibility of dose painting by numbers. There are many technical and biological challenges and only future research will allow an evidence-based definition of the indication for theragnostic radiation dose distributions and an estimation of the potential benefit to individual patients as well as at the population level. On the other hand, dose painting by numbers as a therapeutic strategy is at the very heart of what makes external beam radiation therapy a unique cancer therapy modality. With advances in predictive oncology and with a rapidly increasing number of cytotoxic and molecular targeted agents at our disposal, the dream of personalized cancer medicine, optimizing the individual efficacy:toxicity ratio for locoregional as well as for systemic therapy, is finally within reach. Theragnostic radiation oncology is likely to be a major component of the personalized therapeutic package we will be offering patients 5–10 years from now.

References

1. Bentzen SM. Theragnostic imaging for radiation oncology: dose-painting by numbers. Lancet Oncol 2005; 6(2):112–117.
2. Buffa FM, Bentzen SM, Daley FM, Dische S, Saunders MI, Richman PI, et al. Molecular marker profiles predict locoregional control of head and neck squamous cell carcinoma in a randomized trial of continuous hyperfractionated accelerated radiotherapy. Clin Cancer Res 2004; 10(11):3745–3754.
3. Ataman OU, Bentzen SM, Wilson GD, Daley FM, Richman PI, Saunders MI, et al. Molecular biomarkers and site of first recurrence after radiotherapy for head and neck cancer. Eur J Cancer 2004; 40(18):2734–2741.
4. Ghadimi BM, Grade M, Difilippantonio MJ, Varma S, Simon R, Montagna C, et al. Effectiveness of gene expression profiling for response prediction of rectal adenocarcinomas to preoperative chemoradiotherapy. J Clin Oncol 2005; 23(9):1826–1838.
5. Wong YF, Selvanayagam ZE, Wei N, Porter J, Vittal R, Hu R, et al. Expression genomics of cervical cancer: molecular classification and prediction of radiotherapy response by DNA microarray. Clin Cancer Res 2003; 9(15):5486–5492.
6. Torres-Roca JF, Eschrich S, Zhao H, Bloom G, Sung J, McCarthy S, et al. Prediction of radiation sensitivity using a gene expression classifier. Cancer Res 2005; 65(16):7169–7176.
7. Leunens G, Menten J, Verstraete J, van der Schueren E. Quality assessment of medical decision making in radiation oncology: variability in target volume delineation for brain tumours. Radiother Oncol 1993; 29:169–175.
8. Logue JP, Sharrock CL, Cowan RA, Read G, Marrs J, Mott D. Clinical variability of target volume description in conformal radiotherapy planning. Int J Radiat Oncol Biol Phys 1998; 41(4):929–931.
9. Tai P, Van Dyk J, Yu E, Battista J, Stitt L, Coad T. Variability of target volume delineation in cervical esophageal cancer. Int J Radiat Oncol Biol Phys 1998; 42(2):277–288.
10. Hurkmans CW, Borger JH, Pieters BR, Russell NS, Jansen EP, Mijnheer BJ. Variability in target volume delineation on CT scans of the breast. Int J Radiat Oncol Biol Phys 2001; 50(5):1366–1372.
11. Weiss E, Richter S, Krauss T, Metzelthin SI, Hille A, Pradier O, et al. Conformal radiotherapy planning of cervix carcinoma: differences in the delineation of the clinical target volume. A comparison between gynaecologic and radiation oncologists. Radiother Oncol 2003; 67(1):87–95.
12. Hernandez MC, Knox SJ. Radiobiology of radioimmunotherapy with 90Y ibritumomab tiuxetan (Zevalin). Semin Oncol 2003; 30(6 Suppl 17):6–10.
13. Macklis RM. Clinical Radioimmunotherapy and Systemic Targeted Radiopharmaceutical Therapy (STaRT) programs in a radiation oncology environment. Am J Clin Oncol 2006; 29(6):543–547.
14. Bruland OS, Nilsson S, Fisher DR, Larsen RH. High-linear energy transfer irradiation targeted to skeletal metastases by the alpha-emitter 223Ra: adjuvant or alternative to conventional modalities? Clin Cancer Res 2006; 12(20 Pt 2):6250s–6257s.
15. Lewington VJ. Bone-seeking radionuclides for therapy. J Nucl Med 2005; 46(Suppl 1):38S–47S.
16. Witzig TE, Gordon LI, Cabanillas F, Czuczman MS, Emmanouilides C, Joyce R, et al. Randomized controlled trial of yttrium-90-labeled ibritumomab tiuxetan radioimmunotherapy versus rituximab immunotherapy for patients with relapsed or refractory low-grade, follicular, or transformed B-cell non-Hodgkin's lymphoma. J Clin Oncol 2002; 20(10):2453–2463.
17. Fisher RI, Kaminski MS, Wahl RL, Knox SJ, Zelenetz AD, Vose JM, et al. Tositumomab and iodine-131 tositumomab produces durable complete remissions in a subset of heavily pretreated patients with low-grade and transformed non-Hodgkin's lymphomas. J Clin Oncol 2005; 23(30):7565–7573.

18. Kaminski MS, Zelenetz AD, Press OW, Saleh M, Leonard J, Fehrenbacher L, et al. Pivotal study of iodine I 131 tositumomab for chemotherapy-refractory low-grade or transformed low-grade B-cell non-Hodgkin's lymphomas. J Clin Oncol 2001; 19(19):3918–3928.
19. Bentzen SM. Radiation therapy: intensity modulated, image guided, biologically optimized and evidence based. Radiother Oncol 2005; 77(3):227–230.
20. Mackie TR, Kapatoes J, Ruchala K, Lu W, Wu C, Olivera G, et al. Image guidance for precise conformal radiotherapy. Int J Radiat Oncol Biol Phys 2003; 56(1):89–105.
21. Jaffray DA. Emergent technologies for 3-dimensional image-guided radiation delivery. Semin Radiat Oncol 2005; 15(3):208–216.
22. Weber WA, Figlin R. Monitoring cancer treatment with PET/CT: does it make a difference? J Nucl Med 2007; 48(Suppl 1):36S–44S.
23. Neves AA, Brindle KM. Assessing responses to cancer therapy using molecular imaging. Biochim Biophys Acta 2006; 1766(2):242–261.
24. Galbraith SM, Lodge MA, Taylor NJ, Rustin GJ, Bentzen S, Stirling JJ, et al. Reproducibility of dynamic contrast-enhanced MRI in human muscle and tumours: comparison of quantitative and semi-quantitative analysis. NMR Biomed 2002; 15(2):132–142.
25. Webb S, Nahum AE. A model for calculating tumour control probability in radiotherapy including the effects of inhomogeneous distributions of dose and clonogenic cell density. Phys Med Biol 1993; 38(6):653–666.
26. Webb S, Evans PM, Swindell W, Deasy JO. A proof that uniform dose gives the greatest TCP for fixed integral dose in the planning target volume. Phys Med Biol 1994; 39(11):2091–2098.
27. Levin-Plotnik D, Hamilton RJ. Optimization of tumour control probability for heterogeneous tumours in fractionated radiotherapy treatment protocols. Phys Med Biol 2004; 49(3):407–424.
28. Brahme A, Agren AK. Optimal dose distribution for eradication of heterogeneous tumours. Acta Oncol 1987; 26(5):377–385.
29. Tome WA, Fowler JF. Selective boosting of tumor subvolumes. Int J Radiat Oncol Biol Phys 2000; 48(2):593–599.
30. Chapman JD, Schneider RF, Urbain JL, Hanks GE. Single-photon emission computed tomography and positron-emission tomography assays for tissue oxygenation. Semin Radiat Oncol 2001; 11(1):47–57.
31. Rosenman J. Incorporating functional imaging information into radiation treatment. Semin Radiat Oncol 2001; 11(1):83–92.
32. Chao KS, Bosch WR, Mutic S, Lewis JS, Dehdashti F, Mintun MA, et al. A novel approach to overcome hypoxic tumor resistance: Cu-ATSM-guided intensity-modulated radiation therapy. Int J Radiat Oncol Biol Phys 2001; 49(4):1171–1182.
33. Ling CC, Humm J, Larson S, Amols H, Fuks Z, Leibel S, et al. Towards multidimensional radiotherapy (MD-CRT): biological imaging and biological conformality. Int J Radiat Oncol Biol Phys 2000; 47(3):551–560.
34. Vanderstraeten B, Duthoy W, De GW, De NW, Thierens H. [18F]fluoro-deoxy-glucose positron emission tomography ([18F]FDG-PET) voxel intensity-based intensity-modulated radiation therapy (IMRT) for head and neck cancer. Radiother Oncol 2006; 79(3): 249–258.
35. Sovik A, Malinen E, Bruland OS, Bentzen SM, Olsen DR. Optimization of tumour control probability in hypoxic tumours by radiation dose redistribution: a modelling study. Phys Med Biol 2007; 52(2):499–513.
36. Stavreva NA, Stavrev PV, Round WH. A mathematical approach to optimizing the radiation dose distribution in heterogeneous tumours. Acta Oncol 1996; 35(6):727–732.
37. Brahme A. Biologically optimized 3-dimensional in vivo predictive assay-based radiation therapy using positron emission tomography-computerized tomography imaging. Acta Oncol 2003; 42(2):123–136.
38. Popple RA, Ove R, Shen S. Tumor control probability for selective boosting of hypoxic subvolumes, including the effect of reoxygenation. Int J Radiat Oncol Biol Phys 2002; 54(3):921–927.

39. Bentzen SM, Tucker SL. Quantifying the position and steepness of radiation dose–response curves [see comments]. Int J Radiat Biol 1997; 71(5):531–542.
40. Bentzen SM. Radiobiological considerations in the design of clinical trials. Radiother Oncol 1994; 32:1–11.
41. Alber M, Paulsen F, Eschmann SM, Machulla HJ. On biologically conformal boost dose optimization. Phys Med Biol 2003; 48(2):N31–N35.
42. Das SK, Miften MM, Zhou S, Bell M, Munley MT, Whiddon CS, et al. Feasibility of optimizing the dose distribution in lung tumors using fluorine-18-fluorodeoxyglucose positron emission tomography and single photon emission computed tomography guided dose prescriptions. Med Phys 2004; 31(6):1452–1461.
43. Vanderstraeten B, De GW, Duthoy W, De NW, Thierens H. Implementation of biologically conformal radiation therapy (BCRT) in an algorithmic segmentation-based inverse planning approach. Phys Med Biol 2006; 51(16):N277–N286.
44. Van Herk M. Errors and margins in radiotherapy. Semin Radiat Oncol 2004; 14(1):52–64.
45. Gray LH, Conger AD, Ebert M, Hornsey S, Scott OC. The concentration of oxygen dissolved in tissues at the time of irradiation as a factor in radiotherapy. Br J Radiol 1953; 26(312):638–648.
46. Howes AE. An estimation of changes in the proportions and absolute values of hypoxic cells after irradiation of transplanted C3H mouse mammary tumours. Br J Radiol 1969; 42:441–447.
47. Bentzen SM, Grau C. Direct estimation of the fraction of hypoxic cells from tumour-control data obtained under aerobic and clamped conditions. Int J Radiat Biol 1991; 59:1435–1440.
48. Khalil AA, Bentzen SM, Overgaard J. Steepness of the dose–response curve as a function of volume in an experimental tumor irradiated under ambient or hypoxic conditions [see comments]. Int J Radiat Oncol Biol Phys 1997; 39(4):797–802.
49. Thomlinson RH, Gray LH. The histological structure of some human lung cancers and the possible implications for radiotherapy. Br J Cancer 1955; 9(4):539–549.
50. Nordsmark M, Bentzen SM, Overgaard J. Measurement of human tumour oxygenation status by a polarographic needle electrode. An analysis of inter- and intratumour heterogeneity. Acta Oncol 1994; 33(4):383–389.
51. Nordsmark M, Bentzen SM, Rudat V, Brizel D, Lartigau E, Stadler P, et al. Prognostic value of tumor oxygenation in 397 head and neck tumors after primary radiation therapy. An international multi-center study. Radiother Oncol 2005; 77(1):18–24.
52. Koukourakis MI, Bentzen SM, Giatromanolaki A, Wilson GD, Daley FM, Saunders MI, et al. Endogenous markers of two separate hypoxia response pathways (hypoxia inducible factor 2 alpha and carbonic anhydrase 9) are associated with radiotherapy failure in head and neck cancer patients recruited in the CHART randomized trial. J Clin Oncol 2006; 24(5):727–735.
53. Horsman MR, Overgaard J. Overcoming tumour radioresistance resulting from hypoxia. In: Steel GG, editor. Basic Clinical Radiobiology. 3 ed. London: Arnold; 2002. p. 169–181.
54. Harris AL. Hypoxia – a key regulatory factor in tumour growth. Nat Rev Cancer 2002; 2(1):38–47.
55. Hockel M, Schlenger K, Aral B, Mitze M, Schaffer U, Vaupel P. Association between tumor hypoxia and malignant progression in advanced cancer of the uterine cervix. Cancer Res 1996; 56(19):4509–4515.
56. Brizel DM, Scully SP, Harrelson JM, Layfield LJ, Bean JM, Prosnitz LR, et al. Tumor oxygenation predicts for the likelihood of distant metastases in human soft tissue sarcoma. Cancer Res 1996; 56(5):941–943.
57. Carnell DM, Smith RE, Daley FM, Saunders MI, Bentzen SM, Hoskin PJ. An immunohistochemical assessment of hypoxia in prostate carcinoma using pimonidazole: implications for radioresistance. Int J Radiat Oncol Biol Phys 2006; 65(1):91–99.
58. Moeller BJ, Dewhirst MW. HIF-1 and tumour radiosensitivity. Br J Cancer 2006; 95(1):1–5.
59. Williams KJ, Telfer BA, Xenaki D, Sheridan MR, Desbaillets I, Peters HJ, et al. Enhanced response to radiotherapy in tumours deficient in the function of hypoxia-inducible factor-1. Radiother Oncol 2005; 75(1):89–98.

60. Rasey JS, Koh WJ, Evans ML, Peterson LM, Lewellen TK, Graham MM, et al. Quantifying regional hypoxia in human tumors with positron emission tomography of [18F]fluoromisonidazole: a pretherapy study of 37 patients. Int J Radiat Oncol Biol Phys 1996; 36(2):417–428.
61. Rischin D, Hicks RJ, Fisher R, Binns D, Corry J, Porceddu S, et al. Prognostic significance of [18F]-misonidazole positron emission tomography-detected tumor hypoxia in patients with advanced head and neck cancer randomly assigned to chemoradiation with or without tirapazamine: a substudy of Trans-Tasman Radiation Oncology Group Study 98.02. J Clin Oncol 2006; 24(13):2098–2104.
62. Rajendran JG, Schwartz DL, O'Sullivan J, Peterson LM, Ng P, Scharnhorst J, et al. Tumor hypoxia imaging with [F-18] fluoromisonidazole positron emission tomography in head and neck cancer. Clin Cancer Res 2006; 12(18):5435–5441.
63. Koh WJ, Rasey JS, Evans ML, Grierson JR, Lewellen TK, Graham MM, et al. Imaging of hypoxia in human tumors with [F-18]fluoromisonidazole. Int J Radiat Oncol Biol Phys 1992; 22(1):199–212.
64. Koh WJ, Bergman KS, Rasey JS, Peterson LM, Evans ML, Graham MM, et al. Evaluation of oxygenation status during fractionated radiotherapy in human nonsmall cell lung cancers using [F-18]fluoromisonidazole positron emission tomography. Int J Radiat Oncol Biol Phys 1995; 33(2):391–398.
65. Schwartz DL, Ford EC, Rajendran J, Yueh B, Coltrera MD, Virgin J, et al. FDG-PET/CT-guided intensity modulated head and neck radiotherapy: a pilot investigation. Head Neck 2005; 27(6):478–487.
66. Eschmann SM, Paulsen F, Reimold M, Dittmann H, Welz S, Reischl G, et al. Prognostic impact of hypoxia imaging with 18F-misonidazole PET in non-small cell lung cancer and head and neck cancer before radiotherapy. J Nucl Med 2005; 46(2):253–260.
67. Paulsen F, Eschmann SM, Alber M, Buck D, Machulla HJ, Bares R, et al. Time course of hypoxia in head and neck cancer patients treated by radiotherapy. Int J Radiat Oncol Biol Phys 2003; 57(Suppl 2):S406.
68. Hicks RJ, Rischin D, Fisher R, Binns D, Scott AM, Peters LJ. Utility of FMISO PET in advanced head and neck cancer treated with chemoradiation incorporating a hypoxia-targeting chemotherapy agent. Eur J Nucl Med Mol Imaging 2005; 32(12):1384–1391.
69. Lehtio K, Oikonen V, Gronroos T, Eskola O, Kalliokoski K, Bergman J, et al. Imaging of blood flow and hypoxia in head and neck cancer: initial evaluation with [(15)O]H(2)O and [(18)F]fluoroerythronitroimidazole PET. J Nucl Med 2001; 42(11):1643–1652.
70. Lehtio K, Eskola O, Viljanen T, Oikonen V, Gronroos T, Sillanmaki L, et al. Imaging perfusion and hypoxia with PET to predict radiotherapy response in head-and-neck cancer. Int J Radiat Oncol Biol Phys 2004; 59(4):971–982.
71. Takahashi N, Fujibayashi Y, Yonekura Y, Welch MJ, Waki A, Tsuchida T, et al. Evaluation of 62Cu labeled diacetyl-bis(N4-methylthiosemicarbazone) as a hypoxic tissue tracer in patients with lung cancer. Ann Nucl Med 2000; 14(5):323–328.
72. Dehdashti F, Grigsby PW, Mintun MA, Lewis JS, Siegel BA, Welch MJ. Assessing tumor hypoxia in cervical cancer by positron emission tomography with 60Cu-ATSM: relationship to therapeutic response-a preliminary report. Int J Radiat Oncol Biol Phys 2003; 55(5):1233–1238.
73. Lewis J, Laforest R, Buettner T, Song S, Fujibayashi Y, Connett J, et al. Copper-64-diacetyl-bis(N4-methylthiosemicarbazone): an agent for radiotherapy. Proc Natl Acad Sci USA 2001; 98(3):1206–1211.
74. Lewis JS, Sharp TL, Laforest R, Fujibayashi Y, Welch MJ. Tumor uptake of copper-diacetyl-bis(N(4)-methylthiosemicarbazone): effect of changes in tissue oxygenation. J Nucl Med 2001; 42(4):655–661.
75. Lewis JS, McCarthy DW, McCarthy TJ, Fujibayashi Y, Welch MJ. Evaluation of 64Cu-ATSM in vitro and in vivo in a hypoxic tumor model. J Nucl Med 1999; 40(1):177–183.
76. Obata A, Yoshimi E, Waki A, Lewis JS, Oyama N, Welch MJ, et al. Retention mechanism of hypoxia selective nuclear imaging/radiotherapeutic agent cu-diacetyl-bis(N4-methylthiosemicarbazone) (Cu-ATSM) in tumor cells. Ann Nucl Med 2001; 15(6):499–504.

77. Rajendran JG, Krohn KA. Imaging hypoxia and angiogenesis in tumors. Radiol Clin North Am 2005; 43(1):169–187.
78. Wouters BG, Brown JM. Cells at intermediate oxygen levels can be more important than the "hypoxic fraction" in determining tumor response to fractionated radiotherapy. Radiat Res 1997; 147(5):541–550.
79. Burgman P, Odonoghue JA, Humm JL, Ling CC. Hypoxia-induced increase in FDG uptake in MCF7 cells. J Nucl Med 2001; 42(1):170–175.
80. Clavo AC, Brown RS, Wahl RL. Fluorodeoxyglucose uptake in human cancer cell lines is increased by hypoxia. J Nucl Med 1995; 36(9):1625–1632.
81. Dearling JL, Flynn AA, Sutcliffe-Goulden J, Petrie IA, Boden R, Green AJ, et al. Analysis of the regional uptake of radiolabeled deoxyglucose analogs in human tumor xenografts. J Nucl Med 2004; 45(1):101–107.
82. Pugachev A, Ruan S, Carlin S, Larson SM, Campa J, Ling CC, et al. Dependence of FDG uptake on tumor microenvironment. Int J Radiat Oncol Biol Phys 2005; 62(2):545–553.
83. Cherk MH, Foo SS, Poon AM, Knight SR, Murone C, Papenfuss AT, et al. Lack of correlation of hypoxic cell fraction and angiogenesis with glucose metabolic rate in non-small cell lung cancer assessed by 18F-Fluoromisonidazole and 18F-FDG PET. J Nucl Med 2006; 47(12):1921–1926.
84. Zimny M, Gagel B, Dimartino E, Hamacher K, Coenen HH, Westhofen M, et al. FDG-a marker of tumour hypoxia? A comparison with [(18)F]fluoromisonidazole and pO (2)-polarography in metastatic head and neck cancer. Eur J Nucl Med Mol Imaging 2006; 33(12):1426–1431.
85. Rajendran JG, Mankoff DA, O'Sullivan F, Peterson LM, Schwartz DL, Conrad EU, et al. Hypoxia and glucose metabolism in malignant tumors: evaluation by [18F]fluoromisonidazole and [18F]fluorodeoxyglucose positron emission tomography imaging. Clin Cancer Res 2004; 10(7):2245–2252.
86. Thorwarth D, Eschmann SM, Holzner F, Paulsen F, Alber M. Combined uptake of [18F]FDG and [18F]FMISO correlates with radiation therapy outcome in head-and-neck cancer patients. Radiother Oncol 2006; 80(2):151–156.
87. Cher LM, Murone C, Lawrentschuk N, Ramdave S, Papenfuss A, Hannah A, et al. Correlation of hypoxic cell fraction and angiogenesis with glucose metabolic rate in gliomas using 18F-fluoromisonidazole, 18F-FDG PET, and immunohistochemical studies. J Nucl Med 2006; 47(3):410–418.
88. Dehdashti F, Mintun MA, Lewis JS, Bradley J, Govindan R, Laforest R, et al. In vivo assessment of tumor hypoxia in lung cancer with 60Cu-ATSM. Eur J Nucl Med Mol Imaging 2003; 30(6):844–850.
89. Lee N, Nehmeh S, Humm J, Cai S, Finn R, Schoder H. Reproducibility of fluorine-18-labeled fluoro-misonidazole positron emission tomography (FMISO PET) in detecting chronic hypoxia (CH) in Head/Neck cancer (HNC). Int J Radiat Oncol Biol Phys 2005; 63(2): S148–S149.
90. Koh WJ, Bergman KS, Rasey JS, Peterson LM, Evans ML, Graham MM, et al. Evaluation of oxygenation status during fractionated radiotherapy in human nonsmall cell lung cancers using [F-18]fluoromisonidazole positron emission tomography. Int J Radiat Oncol Biol Phys 1995; 33(2):391–398.
91. Wadsley JC, Bentzen SM. Investigation of relationship between change in locoregional control and change in overall survival in randomized controlled trials of modified radiotherapy in head-and-neck cancer. Int J Radiat Oncol Biol Phys 2004; 60(5):1405–1409.

4
Molecular and Functional Imaging in Radiation Oncology

Robert Jeraj and M. Elizabeth Meyerand

Introduction

Imaging has always played a very important role in radiation oncology. It started with the invention of X-rays over a century ago, through development of computed tomography (CT) imaging which significantly improved tumor localization and sensitivity [1–4] as well as enabled CT-based treatment planning of radiation therapy. Implementation of nuclear magnetic resonance techniques in medicine quickly led to an expanding field of magnetic resonance imaging (MRI) [5–7], which has further revolutionized clinical practice due to the improved soft-tissue contrast. Both, CT and MRI are primarily modalities for determining anatomical information. However, for complete assessment of disease status, monitoring tissue function is of a great importance because the disease processes typically start at the molecular and cellular level that only later lead to visible structural changes to the tissue. Similarly, anatomical changes in response to therapy come after the response on the molecular and cellular level, which becomes important in treatment outcome prediction as well as treatment efficacy assessment.

Functional imaging refers to either imaging of physiologic processes, such as blood flow to an organ or diseased tissue; visualizing ongoing biochemical and metabolic activities of normal and abnormal tissues; or using established pharmacologic methods to assess disease processes and develop new drugs [8]. Functional imaging is typically performed by the mainstream clinical radiology techniques like ultrasound, CT and MRI. On the other hand, the term *molecular imaging* typically refers to imaging specific molecular interactions and pathways, which reflect biochemical, physiological and pharmacological processes. The term molecular imaging was defined by the Commission on Molecular Imaging of the American College of Radiology as "the spatially localized and/or temporally resolved sensing of molecular and cellular processes in vivo." The main modalities for molecular imaging are positron emission tomography (PET), single photon emission tomography (SPECT), magnetic resonance spectroscopy (MRS) and optical imaging. Although they are based on quite different imaging processes, the terms functional and molecular imaging are often used interchangeably, due to a lack of consensus regarding their definitions.

M.P. Mehta et al. (eds.), *Radiation Oncology Advances.*

Applications of functional and molecular imaging in radiation oncology are numerous; however, at present the heaviest load relies on PET imaging. For a long time, PET imaging was primarily a research modality using radioactive isotopes of naturally occurring organic elements (carbon, nitrogen and oxygen). Because of their short lifetimes (20, 10 and 2 min, respectively) PET imaging was not clinically feasible. It was not until ^{18}F-2-deoxy-2-fluoro-D-glucose (FDG) was developed that PET imaging became practical in clinical oncology: in part because of the convenient half-life of ^{18}F of 110 min and in part because of the universality of increased glycolysis in malignant cells [9]. After 1998, when the Health Care Finance Administration and Medicare in the United States finally acknowledged that PET imaging is an invaluable tool in the differential diagnosis in several disease sites, FDG-PET imaging received wide clinical application [10]. Since then, the use of PET imaging in management of oncological disease has exploded. The most important applications of functional and molecular imaging are:

- *Diagnosis and staging*, typically performed in the initial phases of tumor assessment, with the main goal to establish if there is a tumor and if so, how advanced it is.
- *Treatment planning*, done prior to radiation therapy, where the extend of the tumor is determined.
- *Treatment assessment*, performed either during or after the treatment and where tumor response to treatment is established.

In the following sections, we will discuss various functional and molecular imaging modalities, the main imaging targets and corresponding imaging agents and modalities, review current applications and briefly discuss the future.

Molecular and Functional Imaging Modalities

While development of detectors for radioisotope decay detection goes back to the early 1950s [11, 12], the application of SPECT [13, 14] and PET [15–18] became clinically feasible in the 1970s in parallel with the development of computers that enabled tomographic reconstruction. Development of MRS started around the same time [19–21], which resulted in the first imaging of a tumor in early 1980s [22]. In the late 1980s a variety of functional magnetic resonance imaging (fMRI) techniques have been developed for imaging of physiologic phenomena, such as blood flow, perfusion or diffusion [23–27].

Positron Emission Tomography

In PET a short-lived positron-emitting radioactive tracer, which is chemically incorporated into a metabolically active molecule, is injected into the living subject. After decay, the positron annihilates with an electron, producing a pair of annihilation photons moving in opposite directions. These are detected when they reach a scintillator material in the scanning device, which is further converted into electrical signal. The technique depends on coincident detection of the pair of photons: photons, which do not arrive in pairs (i.e., within a few nanoseconds) are ignored. By measuring where the annihilation photons end up, their origin in the body can be plotted. This allows the uptake or activity of certain parts of the body to be determined. The resulting map shows the tissues in which the molecular probe has become concentrated. Radionuclides used in PET scanning are isotopes with a variety of half lives and chemical properties such as Carbon-11 (20 min), Nitrogen-13 (10 min), Oxygen-15 (2 min), Fluorine-18 (110 min), and Iodine-124 (4 days).

Single Photon Emission Tomography

SPECT is similar to PET, except that instead of a positron-emitting radioactive tracer, single photon emitting radioactive tracers are used, typically Technetium-99 (6 h), Iodine-123 (13.2 h), Iodine-131 (8 days) or Xenon-133 (5.3 days). SPECT images have less sensitivity and are less detailed than PET images, but the SPECT technique is less expensive than PET. In addition, SPECT centers are more accessible than PET centers because they do not have to be located near a particle accelerator.

Dynamic Contrast Enhanced Computer Tomography (DCE-CT)

DCE-CT is an extension of conventional CT, where a bolus injection of a contrast agent is used to follow dynamically redistribution of the agent in a patient body. In DCE-CT physiological parameters like tissue perfusion, relative blood volume, capillary permeability, and leakage can be measured. These parameters can provide physiological correlates for the microscopic changes that occur with tumor angiogenesis, for example.

Dynamic Contrast Enhanced Magnetic Resonance Imaging (DCE-MRI)

DCE-MRI has found several applications in radiation oncology like BOLD-MRI, which measures regional differences in oxygenated blood, perfusion MRI, which measures regional cerebral blood flow and diffusion-weighted MRI, which measures random movement of water molecules. It should be mentioned that, similar to other functional imaging techniques, functional MRI methods are prone to low sensitivity and specificity.

Magnetic Resonance Spectroscopy

MRS is an extension of conventional MRI, where high magnetic fields are used to manipulate spin states of certain nuclei that are tagged to a specific molecule and the resultant frequency response spectrum is measured. Because the electron cloud surrounding different chemical compounds shields the resonant atoms of spectroscopic interest to varying degrees depending on the specific compound and the specific position in the compound, the observed resonance frequency of the atoms in a magnetic field is slightly different and therefore identifiable with MRS. MRS can detect biochemically important compounds other than water and fat molecules and exploits the differences in the levels of cellular metabolites between normal and tumor tissues.

Optical Imaging

Optical imaging refers to any imaging technique employing visible or near-visible light as a detection source. While extremely promising because of the large amount of fluorescent probes for various biochemical markers currently used in cellular and molecular biology, optical techniques have the disadvantage of high light scattering, which typically confines them to surface probing or optical biopsy sampling. However, the importance of optical molecular imaging in preclinical research cannot be emphasized enough.

Comparison Between Different Imaging Modalities

Different modalities for functional and molecular imaging should be seen sometimes as competing, but more often, complementary modalities that can be used for various oncological applications. One should be aware though, that most of the modalities have been primarily developed for diagnostic imaging. This means that they were mainly developed to reliably identify and visualize a region of interest, which in radiation oncology applications most often refers to reliably identifying tumors and/or metastasis. In other words, most of the modalities were developed to optimize their binary response ("see" vs. "not see"). With the increased application of functional and molecular imaging for nondiagnostic applications, such as tumor microenvironment characterization and treatment response evaluation, image quantification is becoming more and more important. Table 1 is a summary of the physical characteristics of different modalities for functional and molecular imaging; for comparison, also anatomical imaging modalities like CT, MRI, and US are added.

The main advantage of functional and molecular imaging over the conventional anatomical imaging is that a much larger, almost infinite number of imaging targets are available. While anatomical imaging primarily relies on differences in either electron density (CT) or water (hydrogen) density (MRI) or tissue mechanical

Table 1 Comparison between different imaging modalities

Modality	Sensitivity	Specificity	Contrast	Spatial res.[a] (mm)	Temporal res.
PET	+++	+++	++	3–4	min
SPECT	++	++	+	10	min
DCE-CT	+	+	+	2	s
DCE-MRI	+	+	+	2	s
MRS	+	++	+	10	min
Optical	+++	++	+++	2[b]	ms
CT	+	+	++	0.5	s
MRI	+	+	+++	0.5	ms
US	+++	+	++	0.5	ms

Sensitivity and contrast are qualitatively scored as high (+++), medium (++) and low (+). Adapted from [57, 240]

[a]The quoted spatial resolution refers to clinical systems, while small animal systems, like micro-PET, micro-MRI, or micro-CT achieve much better resolution (~1 mm for micro-PET and micro-SPECT 10–50 μm for micro-CT, micro-MRI, and optical imaging)

[b]Spatial resolution of optical systems is dependent on the examined depth of the sample

properties (US), functional and molecular imaging explores either tumor or tissue specific properties, like changed metabolic rate, changed cell proliferation rate, changed hormone expression, changed gene expression, changed protein production, etc. Clearly, targeting tumor-specific functional and molecular expression increases the specificity of the method dramatically, as reflected in Table 1.

Naturally, the imaging targets have to be tailored to produce the highest possible imaging contrast, but furthermore they should measure the quantity of interest as closely as possible for a given application. For example, in order to monitor tissue response to treatment, one has to choose the tissue property that changes most in response to treatment, e.g., cell proliferation. Not all imaging modalities are optimal for all sites, e.g., application of a metabolitic marker for assessment of treatment response in brain, which has naturally high metabolic activity, will likely not give high image contrast. In other words, each application and each anatomical site require careful selection of the imaging target and imaging modality.

Molecular and Functional Imaging Targets

Some tumor imaging targets are generic in the sense that they explore some generic tumor property, like increased glycolysis in case of FDG-PET; others are targeting a specific property of the tumor microenvironment, like hypoxia in case of FMISO-PET. A brief review of the most important tumor imaging targets with the corresponding imaging agents is presented. While the effort is made to encompass a large variety of the most important imaging agents that have found its way into clinical radiation oncology, it should be noted that this area is under extremely intensive development and new, more or less promising imaging agents, are appearing frequently. While some of the agents are currently still under preclinical development, others, FDG-PET in particular, have gone through extensive clinical application and have become a part of the standard patient care.

A note of caution is appropriate here; almost all functional and molecular imaging agents are only *imaging surrogates* for the underlying biological processes [28–33]. Some are better and some are worse, but typically, one should be aware that "what you see is not what you get." No imaging agent is perfect and therefore, all functional and molecular images should be interpreted with appropriate skepticism. It is important to understand the limitations of each imaging agent and to be aware that even though certain imaging agents have been promoted as markers of certain tumor properties (e.g., FMISO-PET or BOLD-MRI as markers of hypoxia) this is in general a very simplified view. Most of these are not comparable with the much more specific biochemical markers used in cellular and molecular biology (e.g., TUNEL labeling for apoptosis).

Imaging agent *uptake kinetics and retention* can be relatively complicated and a complex compartmental kinetic analysis might be necessary to extract the information of interest [34–48]. While some molecular imaging agents have relatively simple uptake and retention kinetics (especially for cases with completely reversible or irreversible target binding), which can be dealt with by simple graphical methods like Logan [49] and Gjedde–Patlak analysis [50], some imaging agents require three- or four-compartment models to fit the kinetic parameters of clinical interest.

Another important consideration is that the *imaging techniques* are not perfect, nor are the imaging systems – it is known, for example, that different image reconstruction algorithms can lead to differences in the reconstructed PET images in excess of 20% [51–55]. For diagnostic applications, quantification is typically not important, since one is primarily interested in achieving the highest possible contrast; however, for quantitative assessment or for nonuniform treatment planning prescriptions one has to rely on absolute quantitative imaging information, which can become crucial.

There have been several very good reviews published recently that discuss various imaging targets and imaging agents [56, 57]; however, as the new imaging targets appear, these lists are expected to change significantly, with certain targets passing clinical validation tests and others not. The main molecular imaging targets are shown in Fig. 1.

Cellular Metabolism

By far the most important and widely used molecular imaging target is increased metabolism of tumor cells. Because of the relatively easy access to FDG, which is the main PET molecular imaging agent, the amount of clinical data and applications

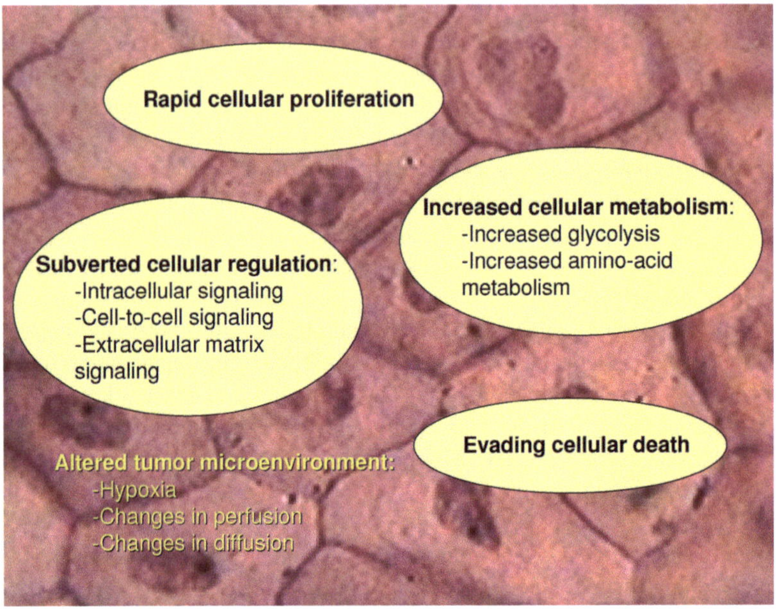

Fig. 1 Hallmarks of cancer targeted by molecular and functional imaging. Over 500 molecular imaging agents have been developed to target these processes. Interestingly, only a handful of the agents are commonly used in functional and molecular imaging

exceeds that of other molecular imaging applications. Even though FDG is not an ideal marker, as discussed below, it has been used for a variety of applications, including diagnosis and staging, treatment planning and treatment assessment. Two metabolic targets have been explored in molecular imaging – increased glucose metabolism and increased amino acid metabolism.

Glucose Metabolism

Discovery of the enhanced glycolytic rate in cancer cells [9] triggered a lot of inspiring research to determine whether a high glycolytic rate is essential for cancer cells or is a consequence of other metabolic processes. Subsequent research showed that increased glycolysis is neither an essential property of proliferating cells nor is it a distinguishing characteristic of malignancy [58]. Several factors are present as a result of the increased glycolysis and some of these are targeted in molecular imaging [9, 59, 60]. Because of the increased glycolysis, there is an increased number of glucose transporter molecules at the tumor cell surface, among which glut 1 and glut 3 were shown to be dominant in tumors [58, 61–63]. In addition, enhanced activity of some of the main enzymes controlling the glycolytic pathways, such as hexokinase can be found in malignant cells [64].

The main molecular imaging agent used for PET metabolic imaging is ^{18}F-2-deoxy-2-fluoro-D-glucose (FDG) [65–67]. FDG is transported into the cell through the glucose transporter protein at the cell membrane, depending on the concentration gradient of glucose from outside to inside the cell in a process that does not require energy. In the cell, FDG is phosphorylated to FDG-6-phosphate by hexokinase in a process that requires energy. FDG-6-phosphate is not a suitable substrate for the glycolytic enzymes that follow and therefore is not metabolized further in the glycolytic pathway. Because the cell membrane is not permeable to intermediate phosphorylated products, FDG-6-phosphate remains trapped inside the cell, proportionally to the overall glycolytic activity, which is the basis for FDG-PET imaging [58]. As FDG uptake depends on tumor growth-rate, it has been successfully used as a marker for tumor grade and malignancy. Interestingly, FDG uptake is also dependent on the cell cycle, with the highest uptake rate in the G_0/G_1 and G_2 phases, where the cells consume more glucose in preparation for the S and M phases, respectively [68].

By far the most extensive overview of the clinical application of FDG-PET imaging for tumor diagnostics and staging was compiled in the document submitted to the Health Care Financing Administration to request expanded Medicare reimbursement for FDG-PET [69]. Results from several new clinical studies have been published since then; however, the main conclusions remain the same and could be summarized by a simple statement: FDG-PET imaging significantly alters cancer management (on the average in over 30% of the cases) with sensitivity of PET around 85%, specificity around 90% and accuracy reaching almost 90%. Details are provided in Table 2.

Table 2 Sensitivity, specificity, accuracy, and effect on cancer management of FDG-PET imaging for cancer diagnostics and staging (in percent)

Cancer	Sensitivity	Specificity	Accuracy	Effect
Bladder	76/93	87/86	83/88	17/–
Brain	91/86	–/–	–/–	–/–
Breast	91/91	93/88	95/90	100/24
Colorectal	85/94	71/–	94/–	–/36
Gastroesoph	96/73	–/90	98/83	14/20
Head and neck	93/87	70/89	87/88	33/–
Hepatocellular	64/77	–/97	–/93	–/60
Lung	96/83	73/91	90/82	–/37
Lymphoma	100/90	–/93	–/88	–/21
Melanoma	–/83	–/91	–/91	–/26
Ovar/Uter/Cerv	66/54	77/96	77/–	–/–
Pancreas	94/90	90/93	92/91	50/36
Prostate	–/57	–/100	–/–	–/–
Renal	89/76	–/100	–/100	–/–
Testicular	–/82	–/94	–/92	–/22
Thyroid	68/69	67/89	100/84	9/22

The presented data refers to diagnostics/staging and is a summary of the data collected over the period of 1993–2000 [69]

Table 3 Prognostic relevance of FDG-PET imaging after therapy

Tumor	References	No pat	Survival resp (m)	Survival nonresp (m)	p
Head and neck	[241]	35	>60	18	0.002
Esophagus	[242]	36	>34	7	0.005
	[243]		>24	14	0.01
Lung	[244]	73	>36	<12	0.001
	[245]	47	56	19	<0.001
Cervix	[246]	152	>45	<20	<0.001

Table 4 Prognostic relevance of FDG-PET imaging during therapy

Tumor	References	No pat	Criter (ΔSUV) (%)	Survival resp (mo)	Survival nonresp (mo)	p
Head and neck	[247]	47	50	>120	40	0.004
Esophagus	[248]	37	35	>48	20	0.04
	[249]	20	30	>38	18	0.01
Lung	[250]	57	20	9	5	0.005
Stomach	[251]	35	35	>48	17	<0.001

Despite its limitations, change in glucose metabolism has often been used as a surrogate for determining viability of tumor cells and therefore for assessment of treatment efficacy and early posttreatment prognosis [44, 64, 70–81]. The quantitative treatment response assessment with FDG is limited, because FDG uptake does not relate to the proliferative activity of cancer cells, but only to the number of viable tumor cells. In addition, soon after radiation therapy, increased metabolism can still be seen because of apoptosis of tumor cells in response to therapy or decreased tumor density leaving normal cells with higher metabolism or inflammatory cells infiltrating where tumor cells are dying [82]. However, wide availability of FDG and relatively encouraging results have created a significant body of clinical data, which is summarized in Tables 3 and 4.

Amino Acid Metabolism

Even though glucose metabolism is the main molecular imaging target, increased metabolism of amino acids in tumors is also a very important and sometimes preferred target. Although all amino acids can diffuse into cells, the main transport is mediated by one of the two types of carriers (sodium mediated and sodium independent), which is typically increased in malignant transformation [83]. Imaging amino acid metabolism can have a higher sensitivity and specificity than glucose metabolism for anatomical sites with a high glucose metabolic background or is better able to differentiate tumor from inflammatory regions. Nearly all amino acids have been radiolabeled with ^{11}C and applied in a preclinical setting, of which mainly L-[methyl-^{11}C]-methionine (MET) and L-1-[^{11}C]-tyrosine (TYR) have been extensively studied clinically. In addition, several artificial amino acids such as L-3-[^{123}I]iodo-α-methyltyrosine (IMT), ^{18}F-fluoroethyl-L-tyrosine (FET) and ^{18}F-α-methyl-tyrosine (FMT) have been developed and applied clinically. Amino acid molecular imaging is particularly important in brain diagnostics and staging because of the high glucose metabolic activity, which limits the use of FDG-PET. The most frequently used amino acid for PET imaging in brain has been MET, even though some studies report success with other amino acids as well. The reported diagnostic accuracy is ranging from over 60% for low grade tumors to almost 100% for high grade tumors [84, 85]. For tumor grading, the reports are still controversial. This might be at least in part due to the fact that most of the studies rely on the standard assessment of the uptake (standardized uptake value (SUV) or tumor-to-brain ratio (T/N)), even though proper kinetic analysis can significantly increase the detection sensitivity and specificity [86, 87]. Amino acid imaging has been applied to other tumor sites like lung, head and neck, breast as well; however, the sensitivity and specificity are typically inferior to those of FDG-PET.

Cellular Proliferation

Another distinct feature of many tumors is rapid cellular proliferation, which is altered in response to antineoplastic therapies [88–94]. The current gold standards are various immunohistochemistry methods that detect proteins expressed primarily in proliferating cells. Examples include detection of the Ki-67 protein [95–97], which has become a gold standard in tissue proliferation assessment because of its presence in all proliferating cells that are in the active phases of the cell cycle (G_1, S, G_2, and mitosis), but absent in G_0 cells, or proliferating cell nuclear antigen (PCNA) [98].

In PET imaging the most commonly used proliferation markers are the *thymidine analogues*, such as 5-iodo-2′-deoxyuridine (IUdR) labeled with ^{124}I, 5-Bromo-2′-deoxyuridine (BrUdR), labeled with ^{76}Br, 5-Fluoro-2-deoxyuridine (FdUrd) labeled with ^{18}F [99–101] and adenosine or uracil analogues like ^{18}F-fluoro-deoxyadenosine (FAD) or ^{18}F-fluoro-ethyluracil (FEU) [102]. None of these markers has provided stable and completely satisfactory labeling of proliferation and therefore found only limited use. The most promising candidates for cell proliferation imaging are direct thymidine analogues, which can monitor thymidine transport into the cells. Higher thymidine activity is expected in malignant cells, because of the accelerated deoxyribonucleic acid synthesis. Initially, mostly ^{11}C-labeled thymidine was used for assessing cell proliferation [103–108]. The benefit of carbon thymidine labeling is diminished due to the short half-life of ^{11}C-thymidine and its rapid biodegradation. Recently the 3′-deoxy-3′-^{18}F-fluorothymidine (FLT) has been proposed as a new marker for imaging tumor proliferation by PET [74, 109–114]. Because the fluorine in FLT is placed in the 3′ position in deoxyribose, FLT works as a terminator of the growing DNA chain. Therefore, little FLT is actually accumulated in DNA, but it is retained intracellularly after phosphorylation by thymidine kinase 1 (TK1)

[115, 116]. This limitation may prove to be important in some situations, but so far, it has not been a problem. Interestingly, in cell lines, FLT retention correlated well with 3H-thymidine uptake, despite the fact that DNA incorporation was only 0.2% for FLT and over 90% for ^{3}H-thymidine [117]. Even though FLT uptake is correlated primarily to TK1 activity and not cell proliferation [113, 115], TK1 also shows an S-phase regulated expression [118] that can, for example, be altered by p53 gene regulation which can in turn be affected by ionizing radiation [119]. Direct correlation between FLT uptake and Ki-67 labeling index has also been observed [112, 120]; however, more extensive studies are needed to confirm direct correlation between FLT uptake and cell proliferation capacity for a variety of tumor types [121].

Another way of determining cell proliferation, particularly in the CNS is the use of ^{1}H MRS by detecting metabolic "fingerprint" of an entire tumor or regions within that tumor [122–129]. Metabolites that are detectable using ^{1}H MRS include choline at 3.2 ppm – generated in cell membrane production, creatine at 3.0 ppm – an indicator of cell energy metabolism, *N*-acetylaspartate at 2.0 ppm – produced by healthy neurons and lactate at 1.3 ppm – a byproduct of anaerobic metabolism. Several studies have postulated that the elevated choline may reflect an increase in the concentration of the spectroscopically detectable metabolites that are precursors of membrane phospholipids needed to support the increased cell turnover in neoplastic tissue [130–132]. A decreased NAA/creatine ratio is consistent with the replacement of healthy neurons by neoplastic cells [127]. Lactate, an end product of anaerobic glycolysis, is often elevated in rapidly growing tumors where hypoxic regions may exist [131, 132]. Studies have demonstrated a correlation between the ratio of these metabolites and the tumor grade. Several studies have shown that a common feature of many rapidly growing tumors is an increased choline to creatine ratio, decreased NAA to creatine ratio and an increased lactate to creatine ratio [122, 128, 131, 133]. It was showed that 104 of 105 different types of brain tumors could be correctly classified using multivoxel spectroscopy in which data were analyzed using peak heights [134].

Cellular Death

Several different cellular death events can occur after therapy, ranging from apoptosis, senescence to mitotic catastrophe. The senescence occurs when cells survive the exposure but lose the ability to proliferate; however, they are still metabolically active and may produce secreted proteins with potential tumor-promoting activities. Mitotic catastrophe is a result of abnormal mitosis and leads to the formation of interphase cells with multiple micronuclei. Apoptosis, or programmed cell death, is the major form of cell death, and very important for mechanism for elimination of damaged or immunologically recognized as harmful cells. The apoptosis process results in activation of a cascade of cysteine–aspartic acid proteases (caspases) that lead to irreversible changes that include cytoskeletal disruption, chromatin clumping, internucleosomal DNA cleavage, and, ultimately, disintegration of the cell into small membrane-bound remnants. These remnants are ultimately removed by macrophages.

The most important molecular imaging target for apoptosis is annexin V protein, which binds to the constitutive inner membrane-associated phosphatidylserine. Annexin V and its derivatives have been labeled with ^{99}Tc, several iodine isotopes, as well as ^{18}F [135–140] for use in SPECT or PET imaging. In addition to annexin V, there are several other potential molecular imaging apoptotic targets. The caspase enzymes, for example, also play a key role in the apoptotic pathway, which led to labeling of caspase activity inhibitors with ^{131}I or ^{99}Tc^{m} [141, 142]. The driving oncological application for apoptotic molecular imaging is assessment of treatment response. So far, most of the apoptosis imaging studies were done in preclinical models; however, the first human clinical studies have been reported [143]. Even though promising, there are still several technical limitations that prevent their use, like low tumor-to-background ratio and optimal imaging time. Recent labeling of annexin V with ^{18}F [135, 136] and continuous efforts to develop other alternative apoptotic targets warrants more attention in the near future.

Cellular Regulation

Inter- and intracellular communication is essential for each organ to function as a whole. In normally functioning cells, receptors and their cognate ligands collaborate and select one of a few mutually exclusive cellular events: temporary quiescence, cell division, terminal differentiation or activation of differential activities, senescence, or apoptosis (programmed cell death). In tumor cells, on the other hand, several receptor systems are subverted, ranging from upregulation, downregulation, and deregulation to deactivation, deletion, or constitutive activation [144] Even though it is possible to assess receptor status by ligand binding assays or immunohistological methods, in vivo molecular imaging has advantages, particularly if the receptor expression in the tumor is heterogeneous because of the variable local tumor microenvironment, or in case of metastatic or recurrent disease where the receptor status might be different from the primary tumor [145].

Molecular imaging of disturbed cellular regulation can be divided into targeting compounds and receptors for intracellular, cell-to-cell and extracellular matrix signaling. This is an area where most of the studies are still preclinical with only a limited number of clinical applications; therefore, we will limit the discussion to the most promising areas without providing much detail. For more details one should consult literature [144, 146].

Intracellular Signaling

Very important intracellular communication molecular imaging targets are estrogen and androgen receptors, which are often used as prognostic indicators in cancer management and predictive for targeted hormonal therapies.

A variety of halogenated derivatives of estradiol have been developed for *estrogen receptor* imaging, like 16α-^{18}F-fluoroestradiol (FES) [147–151], 16α-^{123}I-iodoestradiol (IES) [152–154] and methoxy-^{123}I-iodovinylestradiol (MIVE) [155, 156]. In general a rather good agreement between in vitro estrogen receptor assays and molecular imaging analysis has been observed, typically on the order of 90% [150, 151], resulting in the overall sensitivity of approximately 70% and specificity of 100% for the FES-PET imaging [149], which can have a significant impact on breast cancer management. However these results have to be confirmed in larger clinical trials. Estrogen receptor imaging has also proved to be very valuable for hormonal therapy assessment, where high accuracy was observed in limited clinical studies using tamoxifen treatment. Besides estrogen receptor imaging, tamoxifen has been directly labeled [157, 158], but more studies are needed to determine its clinical potential.

In contrast to estrogen receptors, *androgen receptors* have not proven to be a reliable predictor of hormonal therapy; however, they may still be of prognostic value [159, 160]. Most of the agents have been developed for PET imaging and are derivatives of testosterone, dihydrotestosterone and miboreline, typically labeled with ^{18}F. So far, only limited evaluation of these molecular agents has been done in humans, but because of their potential, particularly to improve staging and monitoring of prostate cancer, more studies are anticipated in the future [161–163].

Cell-to-Cell Signaling

Cell surface receptor-targeting molecular imaging agents target either G-protein-coupled receptors (generally affecting gene expression, but being responsible for also many immediate effects within the cell that do not involve gene expression), or cytokine receptors, most notably receptors tyrosine kinases.

The most commonly targeted *G-protein-coupled receptors* are somatostatin receptors, of which particularly subtypes 1 and 2 were shown to be prominent in overexpressing tumors [164]. While some tumors contain high numbers of somatostatin receptors, others have local accumulation of somatostatin receptor-positive activated mononuclear leucocytes, of which can be used as molecular imaging targets.^{111}In-diethylenetriamine pentaacetic acid octreotide (^{111}In-DTPA-octreotide) SPECT imaging [165] has been used for imaging of a variety of tumors. Results are variable, ranging from high specificity and sensitivity in the detection of primary tumors and distant spread (e.g., in gastrinoma, paraganglioma, Hodgin's lymphoma) [166–168], to mixed results (e.g., in small-cell lung cancer) [169] to rather low sensitivity and specificity (e.g., in non-Hodgkin's lymphoma) [170]. More research is needed before firm conclusions can be drawn. Development of PET imaging agents, like ^{68}Ga-DOTA-Tyr-octreotide (^{68}Ga-DOTA-TOC) is promising and these might replace SPECT imaging agents in the future because of higher sensitivity and better spatial resolution. Several other cell-surface receptors have been targeted because of their overexpression in different tumor types (e.g., cholecystokinin B receptors, sigma receptors), but again more clinical research is needed to establish their full clinical utility.

Another attractive and potentially very powerful target is *receptor tyrosine-kinases*. Epidermal growth factor receptors (EGFR), in particular, are attractive targets, because they are expressed in a large number of common cancers and are related to late stage of disease progression, high metastatic rate and increased cell proliferation [171]. Several EGFR molecular imaging agents have been developed, mostly for SPECT imaging, like ^{123}I-EGF, ^{131}I-EGF, ^{111}In-DTPA-EGF and ^{99m}Tc radiolabeled EGF monoclonal antibodies, but most of these are still in preclinical stage of development. Regardless, because of the strong interest, it is anticipated that more radiopharmaceutical development will be focused in this area, particularly on the development of novel PET imaging agents (e.g., ^{18}F-labeled monoclonal antibody Iressa).

Similarly strong interest surrounds imaging of vascular endothelial growth factor receptors (VEGFR) and fibroblast growth factor receptors (FGFR), because of the involvement of VEGF and FGF in angiogenesis. Upregulation of VEGF and FGF systems has been reported in virtually all human tumors examined, and correlates with standard histological indices of vascularity [172]. For molecular imaging VEGF subtypes 165 and 121 were labeled with ^{123}I for SPECT imaging [173], anti-VEGF monoclonal antibody VG76e with ^{124}I for PET imaging [174], FGF-1 with ^{99m}Tc [175] and FGF-2 with ^{111}In for SPECT imaging [176]. At the moment, all of the studies are preclinical, with mixed results, indicating that more basic research is needed before any of these molecular imaging agents will become clinically useful.

Extracellular-Matrix Signaling

Molecules that promote stable interactions between cells and their environment constitute another attractive target for molecular imaging. One of the most targeted groups is *integrins*, particularly those connected with angiogenesis. For example, $\alpha_v\beta_3$ integrin is expressed on vascular endothelial cells during angiogenesis and vascular remodeling enabling migration of activated endothelial cells through the basement membrane. Because it is not expressed in mature vessels or nonneoplastic epithelium, it is an attractive molecular imaging target with an expected high signal to background ratio. The $\alpha_v\beta_3$ integrin binds several ligands in the extracellular matrix, each containing the peptide sequence Arg-Gly-Asp (RGD). This forms the main basis for molecular imaging strategies that involve synthetic cyclic peptides containing these RGD sequences. These RGD peptides have initially been labeled primarily for SPECT imaging with ^{99m}Tc and ^{111}In, and labeling of the cyclic RGD peptide with ^{18}F and ^{64}Cu has been reported [177–183] indicating favorable biodistribution and high contrast. The compound is currently being translated into clinical applications.

Another important molecular imaging target, also involved in angiogenesis are *matrix metalloproteinases (MMP)*, which are the key enzymes involved in tumor invasiveness, metastasis, growth signaling and angiogenesis. Several MMP inhibitors have been labeled [184, 185]. While potentially promising targets, no clinical imaging has been reported. Because angiogenesis is such an important molecular imaging target due to the availability of a variety of antiangiogenic chemotherapies, significant developments in this area are anticipated in the near future.

Tumor Microenvironment

Hypoxia

Intratumoral oxygen levels may influence a multitude of biologic parameters that subsequently affect the malignant potential of a neoplasm [186]. Because of hypoxia, tumors might develop an increased potential for local invasive growth [187], as well as peripheral, regional and distant tumor cell spreading [188, 189]. Furthermore, intrinsic resistance to radiation and chemotherapy may be enhanced [190, 191]. It should be emphasized that tumor hypoxia is variable and that many tumors contain areas of low oxygenation that cannot be predicted by clinical size, stage, grade, histology, or site. There are several methods for assessing tumor hypoxia [192, 193], ranging from invasive methods like polarographic O_2 sensors [194] and luminescence-based optical sensors [195] to noninvasive methods such as near-infrared spectroscopy [196], phosphorescence imaging [197], fMRI [198] and PET imaging [33]. The most promising noninvasive in vivo methods for measuring hypoxia are fMRI and PET imaging. A problem with MRI imaging is that it does not necessarily measure tumor hypoxia directly but rather measures a combination of a reduction of deoxyhemoglobin in the blood as well as changes in blood flow [199, 200].

Several compounds have been synthesized for PET hypoxia imaging studies: [^{18}F]-fluoromisonidazole (F-MISO) [201–203], Cu-diacetyl-bis(N4-methylthiosemicarbazone) – ^{60}Cu-ATSM, ^{61}Cu-ATSM, ^{62}Cu-ATSM and ^{64}Cu-ATSM [204–214] or 2-nitroimidazoles based markers like 2-(2-nitroimidazol-1[H]-yl)-*N*-(3-^{18}F-fluoropropyl) acetamide (^{18}F-EF1) [215, 216], [2-(2-nitroimidazol-1-yl) -*N*-(3,3,3-trifluoropropyl)-acetamide] [217] and [2-(2-nitro-1[H]-imidazol-1-yl)-*N*-(2,2,3,3,3-penta-fluoropropyl)-acetamide] (^{18}F-EF5) [218, 219]. All these compounds diffuse into normally oxygenated and hypoxic cells but are retained in substantially higher concentrations in hypoxic issues. F-MISO, an analogue of 2-nitroimidazole, appears suboptimal for assessing hypoxia because of low uptake in hypoxic cells, and slow clearance from the normal tissues [220–223]. In contrast, Cu-ATSM appears to overcome these difficulties and may prove to be an effective agent for this purpose.

An indirect measure of potentially hypoxic regions is blood oxygen level dependent (BOLD) MRI imaging [26, 27], which is sensitive to the paramagnetic effects of deoxygenated hemoglobin [224, 225]. This imaging method has been used to indirectly assess oxygenation in tumors [226]. Because the amount of deoxyhemoglobin in blood is a function of the rates of delivery and utilization of oxygen, the BOLD effect is also an indirect indicator of tissue pO_2, metabolic rate and blood flow. Significant increases in T_2* in mammary tumors in response to hyperoxygenation [227] were demonstrated. BOLD MRI has the advantage of having a high spatial resolution and so is ideally suited to assessing the heterogeneity of responses within the tumor. Unfortunately, the complex patterns of signal intensity in MR images obtained on individual tumors has made it difficult to interpret the data. In particular, it has not been proven that dark regions have a relatively short T_2* predominantly because they are hypoxic and contain large amounts of deoxyhemoglobin. A short T_2* could also characterize an area of necrosis or dried blood which are also frequently found in rapidly growing tumors. This makes it important to add a physiological stimulus to the examination in order to monitor real-time responses of the tumor, thus using the tumor as its own control. When BOLD MRI is undertaken in conjunction with hyperoxygenation, regions that show an increase in T_2* are likely to have been oxygenated by the stimulus (lack of smooth muscles in tumor vessels → less vasoconstriction in tumor vessels → decreasing the relative vessel resistance → increased flow of oxygenated blood). Conversely, areas that appeared dark before the hyperoxygenation (short T_2*) and remain dark after the hyperoxygenation most likely correspond to regions of necrosis or dried blood and not viable tumor tissue [228]. So far, only a limited set of clinical data is applicable to correlate BOLD MRI imaging with hypoxia, and more studies are needed to determine usefulness of this potentially powerful and practical way of determining hypoxia.

Perfusion

Tumor perfusion is a very important functional imaging target, even though it is relatively nonspecific. The tumor typically needs an increased flow of nutrients from the blood. The diffusion into tissues is proportional to delivery, and can be used as a measure of perfusion. Several studies have demonstrated that tumor blood vessels are highly irregular, have arterial venous shunts, blind ends and lack smooth muscle. As a result, one would expect tumor blood flow to be highly irregular. Perfusion is sometimes used as a measure of tumor angiogenesis since changes in perfusion do occur at different stages in angiogenesis and further maturation of tumor vasculature [229]. Specifically, in the early stages of tumor growth new, leaky blood vessels are produced as a result of HIF-1α expression and the increase in VEGF resulting in low blood flow and relatively high vessel permeability. As the vessels mature and existing vessels are co-opted by the tumor we see an increased microvessel density resulting in an elevation in both blood flow and permeability. Finally, as these regions mature further, the vessels become less permeable so we see a relative increase in blood flow over permeability. However, in some tumors the blood perfusion observed in the tumor bed is lower than in normal tissue and get even further decreased as the tumor grows [230]. For this reason, neither perfusion nor permeability is completely adequate measures of angiogenesis, and therefore, more specific molecular markers are needed.

^{15}O-labeled water is one of the most extensively studied perfusion PET imaging agents [30, 231]. There is a relatively good correlation between perfusion and tracer accumulation. It should be emphasized that quantitative measurements of perfusion require determination of the blood time–activity curve, which can be obtained by arterial sampling or images of the left ventricle.

Perfusion MRI, or susceptibility contrast mapping, is another way for quantitative assessment of the blood volume and relative blood flow into regions within the brain [232, 233]. Perfusion MRI is typically performed with a bolus injection of the contrast agent, gadolinium diethylenetriaminepenta-acetic acid (Gd-DTPA), which changes magnetic properties proportionally to the density of blood vessels. Once the Gd-DTPA is injected, its uptake is monitored using echo-planar imaging (EPI) which produces high-resolution (1.5 mm) images in a time frame of less than 1 s per image. This technique is sensitive to changes in microvasculature at the capillary level, with hypervascular regions showing up as areas of high signal intensity. Malignancies are generally hypermetabolic and often exhibit pronounced neovascularization in regions of growth [234]. Perfusion MR has been successfully used to identify tumors of the breast [235] and CNS lymphomas [233] as well as malignant gliomas [236].

Similarly to perfusion MRI, DCE-CT can be used to assess perfusion. Even though CT can provide very high resolution, the microvessels are too small to be imaged directly (<0.1 mm), but their increased density translates in vivo to increased tumor perfusion and blood volume. DCE-CT has been used by various investigators to evaluate tumor microvessel density (MVD) [237].

Diffusion

In an isotropic environment (diffusion is the same in all directions), molecular mobility can be described by a scalar apparent diffusion coefficient (ADC) [238]. This ADC is essentially the constant of proportionality between the root-mean-square displacement of a water molecule and the square root of time during which the motion occurred. The ADC then characterizes the fluid being studied. Brain ADC changes are a function of the intraextracellular water homoeostasis. Therefore, changes in ADC reflect disturbances in ion and water homeostasis that can be present in pathological conditions such as brain ischemia and malignant lesions. Several studies have demonstrated the utility of diffusion imaging in the characterization of brain tumors. For example, it has been demonstrated that ADC's correlate with the degree of tumor cellularity [239]. In areas of rapid tumor cell growth, the extracellular space will decrease creating an environment where water motion is restricted outside the cells and in the more viscous intracellular space. Specifically, the ADC is affected by the translational movement of water that occurs in the extracellular space via swelling or increased cellularity. Therefore, the lowest ADC value indicates a high cellularity.

Diffusion weighted imaging (DWI) is a powerful MRI technique that provides a window into the microscopic structures and properties inside tissues as reflected by the motion of water molecules. Whereas conventional MRI demonstrates overall tissue contrast between cerebral gray matter (primarily neuronal cell bodies) and white matter (primarily neuronal axons), these methods cannot reveal the integrity of tissues. In brief, diffusion of water molecules in gray matter and cerebral spinal fluid (CSF) is largely isotropic (random due to unrestricted Brownian motion). By contrast, water molecules are directionally restricted when diffusing along the axons of neurons.

Future

Without any doubt, the use of functional and molecular imaging in radiation oncology is going to expand enormously over the next decades, mostly likely several-fold within the next 10 years. As an example – current growth of PET imaging studies performed in the United States is over 20% per year. Growth, even though less significant, is also observed in other functional and molecular imaging modalities. There are several reasons that will continue to drive this massive expansion in the future: (1) more widespread use of the already established molecular imaging procedures, (2) alternative uses of imaging modalities, (3) use of alternative molecular imaging agents, and (4) use of multiple and less commonly used molecular imaging modalities.

The expansion of current molecular imaging procedures will be driven by further clinical evidence for improved diagnostic in staging in a broad variety of tumors. The universal benefit has already resulted in full coverage of certain molecular imaging costs by medical insurance companies, for example FDG-PET. Interestingly, in the United States, in spite of the immense increase in PET imaging procedures only one-third of the centers providing PET scans own one or more PET scanners, while the other two-thirds rely on the mobile PET units. The mobile units are much less practical and not as readily assessable. It is not hard to image how the increased demand for PET scans will lead to further demand for in-house scanners, which will in turn provide more flexibility and stipulate even more scanning procedures.

The second reason for expansion is use of functional and molecular imaging for nontraditional uses, like repeat imaging for early treatment assessment and treatment outcome prediction. Currently, there are still several holdups preventing full expansion. The most important reason is insufficient clinical evidence to justify the cost–benefit of the increase scanning costs due to repeat imaging procedures. Therefore, most of the current studies are limited to research clinical trials, which are in turn building increased clinical evidence that will eventually lead to reimbursements for such procedure. However, before that happens, several questions await to be answered – for example, what is the optimal timing window of the repeat scans, which are the imaging modalities and agents that most effectively predict treatment outcome, what imaging-supported action levels should initiate change in cancer management and most importantly, what those actions should comprise. Before these questions are answered, the use of functional and molecular imaging for nontraditional uses will be limited solely to the well-defined clinical research protocols.

Currently there are only very few molecular imaging agents used in radiation oncology, with FDG-PET clearly leading the way. This is to some extend surprising, giving that there are over five hundred available molecular imaging agents available. The main bottleneck for the expansion is again lack of adequate clinical evidence, especially from large clinical trials, that would clearly define the boundaries and optimal use of these agents. Once enough firm clinical evidence is established, the reimbursement for clinical procedures will automatically follow. Unfortunately, clinical data accumulation is hampered with significant costs associated with typically on-site production of small quantities of molecular imaging agents. The cost difference between commercially produced agents and in-house production can be easily a factor of ten. In addition, the trials are consequently limited to only a few institutions that have, both the required infrastructure to produce molecular imaging agents (e.g., cyclotron), as well as the adequate expertise and interest to use them. However, it is only a matter of adequate resources and willingness, primarily from the funding agencies, which will initially have to carry the burden of increased clinical trial costs, when the rich spectrum of diverse molecular imaging agents will more aggressively enter the standard clinical practice. Molecular imaging agents assessing cell proliferation, apoptosis, angiogenesis and hypoxia are the likely the first newcomers.

Functional and molecular imaging is really only at the beginning of its wider application. As the interest for its more extensive use is building up, so is the response from academic community as well as medical imaging manufacturers. Both, improvements of the existing technology as well as development of novel imaging techniques will result from these efforts. Over the next few years, we can expect extensive investments in improvement of functional MRI and MRS spectroscopy, both in hardware and software. Parallel development of novel MRI contrast agents has a potential to change severely their molecular imaging capabilities with increased sensitivity and specificity. Development of combined multimodality molecular imaging, as PET/MRI is just at the doorstep of preclinical application. If proved successful, it will soon enter the clinical world as well, combining the best of functional MRI and molecular PET imaging. Improvements in optical imaging technology, particularly optical tomography, will enable exploration of the incredibly reach spectrum of optical molecular imaging agents, currently confined to preclinical research. Development of low dose CT systems will make functional CT methods, like perfusion CT, much more appealing and affordable in everyday clinical practice.

The main development in functional and molecular imaging in radiation oncology will be focused on the transition from generic to more application and/or tumor specific imaging. While we can expect that FDG-PET will continue to play one of the central roles in tumor diagnostics, the use of more specific molecular imaging agents, which will be able to more comprehensively assess biological signature of the tumors will become one of the main research focuses of the future. Identifying the level of overall tumor treatment resistance could provide basis for patient-specific therapy, where the required treatment dose would be defined according to patient-specific molecular imaging assessment. The main unknown is how to correlate the treatment response with molecular imaging information and which information is the most predictive of the response. As known from molecular tumor profiling, it is not possible to identify a single molecular target that would be completely predictive of the response. Perhaps, a combination of image and molecular marker assessment of pretreatment tumor condition, and in vivo assessment of its spatiotemporal response to therapy, will bring us a step further toward this ultimate goal.

Volumetric in vivo molecular imaging has also a potential to identify tumor subvolumes that are more or less radiotherapy resistant. Such assessment could provide basis for selective dose targeting of tumors, where parts of the tumors would receive either a higher or a lower dose, the approach most often termed "dose painting." While much talked about, such revolutionary approach has still a long way to go. There are too many unknowns at the moment. Neither we know how and when to access treatment resistance, nor which molecular imaging modality, nor which molecular imaging agent would be optimal. Is a single molecular imaging agent adequate, or multiple agents would be needed? We do not have enough data to know, whether a one-time pretreatment assessment is adequate, or a multiple imaging assessment is needed. If multiple imaging were needed, what would be the timing of the second or potentially even more imaging sessions? Is the early or late (residual tumor) treatment response most predictive? One should not overlook that both the molecular imaging modalities as well as molecular imaging agents have limitations, ranging from pure physical ones (e.g., partial volume effects) to biological ones (e.g., only approximate correlation to the imaged molecular processes). Nevertheless, the unprecedented capabilities of functional and molecular imaging to assess tumor biology in vivo, guarantee significant change in the radiation oncology treatment paradigm over the next decades.

References

1. New PF, Scott WR, Schnur JA, Davis KR, Taveras JM, Hochberg FH. Computed tomography with the EMI scanner in the diagnosis of primary and metastatic intracranial neoplasms. Radiology 1975; 114(1):75–87.
2. Baker HL Jr. The impact of computed tomography on neuroradiologic practice. Radiology 1975; 116(3):637–640.
3. Reich NE, Seidelmann FE. Computed tomography using the EMI scanner. Part II. Intracranial pathology. J Am Osteopath Assoc 1975; 74(12):1133–1138.
4. Seidelmann FE, Reich NE. Computed tomography using the EMI scanner. Part I. The apparatus, the normal scan, and its variants. J Am Osteopath Assoc 1975; 74(12):1125–1132.
5. Hawkes RC. Holland GN, Moore WS, Worthington BS. Nuclear magnetic resonance imaging – an overview. Radiography 1980; 46(551):253–255.
6. Crooks L, Herfkens R, Kaufman L, Hoenninger J, Arakawa M, McRee R, J. Watts. Nuclear magnetic resonance imaging. Prog Nucl Med 1981; 7:149–163.
7. Crooks LE, Ortendahl DA, Kaufman L, Hoenninger J, Arakawa M, Watts J, Cannon CR, Brant-Zawadzki M, Davis PL, Margulis AR. Clinical efficiency of nuclear magnetic resonance imaging. Radiology 1983; 146(1):123–128.

8. Alavi A, Kung JW, Zhuang H. Implications of PET based molecular imaging on the current and future practice of medicine. Semin Nucl Med 2004; 34(1):56–69.
9. Warburg O, Wind F, Negelein E. The metabolism of tumors in the body. J Gen Physiol 1927; 8(6):519–530.
10. Bar-Shalom R, Valdivia AY, Blaufox MD. PET imaging in oncology. Semin Nucl Med 2000; 30(3):150–185.
11. Anger HO. A multiple scintillation counter in vivo scanner. Am J Roentgenol Radium Ther Nucl Med 1953; 70(4):605–612.
12. Anger HO, Gottschalk A. Localization of brain tumors with the positron scintillation camera. J Nucl Med 1963; 4:326–330.
13. Kuhl DE, Edwards RQ. Cylindrical and section radioisotope scanning of the liver and brain. Radiology 1964; 83:926–936.
14. Kuhl DE, Edwards RQ, Ricci AR, Reivich M. Quantitative section scanning using orthogonal tangent correction. J Nucl Med 1973; 14(4):196–200.
15. Ter-Pogossian MM, Phelps ME, Hoffman EJ, Mullani NA. A positron-emission transaxial tomograph for nuclear imaging (PETT). Radiology 1975; 114(1):89–98.
16. Hoffmann EJ, Phelps ME, Mullani NA, Higgins CS, Ter-Pogossian MM. Design and performance characteristics of a whole-body positron transaxial tomograph. J Nucl Med 1976; 17(6):493–502.
17. Phelps ME, Hoffman EJ, Mullani NA, Ter-Pogossian MM. Application of annihilation coincidence detection to transaxial reconstruction tomography. J Nucl Med 1975; 16(3):210–224.
18. Phelps ME, Hoffman EJ, Huang SC, Ter-Pogossian MM. Effect of positron range on spatial resolution. J Nucl Med 1975; 16(7):649–652.
19. Hoult DI, Busby SJ, Gadian DG, Radda GK, Richards RE, Seeley PJ. Observation of tissue metabolites using 31P nuclear magnetic resonance. Nature 1974; 252(5481):285–287.
20. Moon RB, Richards JH. Conformation studies of various hemoglobins by natural-abundance 13 C NMR spectroscopy. Proc Natl Acad Sci USA 1972; 69(8):2193–2197.
21. Moon RB, Richards JH. Determination of intracellular pH by 31P magnetic resonance. J Biol Chem 1973; 248(20):7276–7278.
22. Griffiths JR, Stevens AN, Iles RA, Gordon RE, Shaw D. 31P-NMR investigation of solid tumours in the living rat. Biosci Rep 1981; 1(4):319–325.
23. Thomsen C, Henriksen O, Ring P. In vivo measurement of water self diffusion in the human brain by magnetic resonance imaging. Acta Radiol 1987; 28(3):353–361.
24. Singer JR, Crooks LE. Nuclear magnetic resonance blood flow measurements in the human brain. Science 1983; 221(4611):654–656.
25. Runge VM, Clanton JA, Price AC, Wehr CJ, Herzer WA, Partain CL, James AE Jr. The use of Gd DTPA as a perfusion agent and marker of blood–brain barrier disruption. Magn Reson Imaging 1985; 3(1):43–55.
26. Ogawa S, Lee TM, Kay AR, Tank DW. Brain magnetic resonance imaging with contrast dependent on blood oxygenation. Proc Natl Acad Sci USA 1990; 87(24):9868–9872.
27. Ogawa S, Lee TM, Nayak AS, Glynn P. Oxygenation-sensitive contrast in magnetic resonance image of rodent brain at high magnetic fields. Magn Reson Med 1990; 14(1):68–78.
28. Kelloff GJ, Hoffman JM, Johnson B, Scher HI, Siegel BA, Cheng EY, Cheson BD, Shaughnessy JO, Guyton KZ, Mankoff DA, Shankar L, Larson SM, Sigman CC, Schilsky RL, Sullivan DC. Progress and promise of FDG-PET imaging for cancer patient management and oncologic drug development. Clin Cancer Res 2005; 11(8):2785–2808.
29. Rehman S, Jayson GC. Molecular imaging of antiangiogenic agents. Oncologist 2005; 10(2):92–103.
30. Laking GR, Price PM. Positron emission tomographic imaging of angiogenesis and vascular function. Br J Radiol 2003; 76(Spec No. 1):S50–S59.
31. Becherer A, Karanikas G, Szabo M, Zettinig G, Asenbaum S, Marosi C, Henk C, Wunderbaldinger P, Czech T, Wadsak W, K. Kletter. Brain tumour imaging with PET: a comparison between [18F]fluorodopa and [11C]methionine. Eur J Nucl Med Mol Imaging 2003; 30(11):1561–1567.

32. Haberkorn U, Altmann A. Functional genomics and radioisotope-based imaging procedures. Ann Med 2003; 35(6):370–379.
33. Lewis JS, Welch MJ. PET imaging of hypoxia. Q J Nucl Med 2001; 45(2):183–188.
34. Thorwarth D, Eschmann SM, Paulsen F, Alber M. A kinetic model for dynamic [18F]-Fmiso PET data to analyse tumour hypoxia. Phys Med Biol 2005; 50(10):2209–2224.
35. Muzi M, Vesselle H, Grierson JR, Mankoff DA, Schmidt RA, Peterson L, Wells JM, Krohn KA. Kinetic analysis of 3′-deoxy-3′-fluorothymidine PET studies: validation studies in patients with lung cancer. J Nucl Med 2005; 46(2):274–282.
36. Tseng J, Dunnwald LK, Schubert EK, Link JM, Minoshima S, Muzi M, Mankoff DA. 18F-FDG kinetics in locally advanced breast cancer: correlation with tumor blood flow and changes in response to neoadjuvant chemotherapy. J Nucl Med 2004; 45(11):1829–1837.
37. Sutinen E, Nurmi M, Roivainen A, Varpula M, Tolvanen T, Lehikoinen P, Minn H. Kinetics of [(11)C]choline uptake in prostate cancer: a PET study. Eur J Nucl Med Mol Imaging 2004; 31(3):317–324.
38. Wells JM, Mankoff DA, Muzi M, O'Sullivan F, Eary JF, Spence AM, Krohn KA. Kinetic analysis of 2-[11C]thymidine PET imaging studies of malignant brain tumors: compartmental model investigation and mathematical analysis. Mol Imaging 2002; 1(3):151–159.
39. Lehtio K, Oikonen V, Gronroos T, Eskola O, Kalliokoski K, Bergman J, Solin O, Grenman R, Nuutila P, Minn H. Imaging of blood flow and hypoxia in head and neck cancer: initial evaluation with [(15)O]H(2)O and [(18)F]fluoroerythronitroimidazole PET. J Nucl Med 2001; 42(11):1643–1652.
40. Weber WA, Schwaiger M, Avril N. Quantitative assessment of tumor metabolism using FDG-PET imaging. Nucl Med Biol 2000; 27(7):683–687.
41. Mineura K, Shioya H, Kowada M, Ogawa T, Hatazawa J, Uemura K. Blood flow and metabolism of oligodendrogliomas: a positron emission tomography study with kinetic analysis of 18F-fluorodeoxyglucose. J Neurooncol 1999; 43(1):49–57.
42. Mankoff DA, Shields AF, Link JM, Graham MM, Muzi M, Peterson LM, Eary JF, Krohn KA. Kinetic analysis of 2-[11C]thymidine PET imaging studies: validation studies. J Nucl Med 1999; 40(4):614–624.
43. Mankoff DA, Shields AF, Graham MM, Link JM, Eary JF, Krohn KA. Kinetic analysis of 2-[carbon-11]thymidine PET imaging studies: compartmental model and mathematical analysis. J Nucl Med 1998; 39(6):1043–1055.
44. Tsuyuguchi N. Kinetic analysis of glucose metabolism by FDG-PET versus proliferation index of Ki-67 in meningiomas–comparison with gliomas. Osaka City Med J 1997; 43(2):209–223.
45. Minn H, Zasadny KR, Quint LE, Wahl RL. Lung cancer: reproducibility of quantitative measurements for evaluating 2-[F-18]-fluoro-2-deoxy-D-glucose uptake at PET. Radiology 1995; 196(1):167–173.
46. Minn H, Leskinen-Kallio S, Lindholm P, Bergman J, Ruotsalainen U, Teras M, Haaparanta M. [18F]fluorodeoxyglucose uptake in tumors: kinetic vs. steady-state methods with reference to plasma insulin. J Comput Assist Tomogr 1993; 17(1):115–123.
47. Hawkins RA, Choi Y, Huang SC, Hoh CK, Dahlbom M, Schiepers C, Satyamurthy N, Barrio JR, Phelps ME. Evaluation of the skeletal kinetics of fluorine-18-fluoride ion with PET. J Nucl Med 1992; 33(5):633–642.
48. Yamaguchi T, Sasaki H, Ogawa T, Mineura K, Uemura K, Kanno I, Shishido F, Murakami M, Inugami A, Higano S. Relation between tissue nature and (18F) fluorodeoxyglucose kinetics evaluated by dynamic positron emission tomography in human brain tumors. Acta Radiol Suppl 1986; 369:415–418.
49. Logan J. Graphical analysis of PET data applied to reversible and irreversible tracers. Nucl Med Biol 2000; 27(7):661–670.
50. Patlak CS, Blasberg RG. Graphical evaluation of blood-to-brain transfer constants from multiple-time uptake data. Generalizations. J Cereb Blood Flow Metab 1985; 5(4):584–590.
51. Boellaard R, van Lingen A, Lammertsma AA. Experimental and clinical evaluation of iterative reconstruction (OSEM) in dynamic PET: quantitative characteristics and effects on kinetic modeling. J Nucl Med 2001; 42(5):808–817.

52. Oda K, Toyama H, Uemura K, Ikoma Y, Kimura Y, Senda M. Comparison of parametric FBP and OS-EM reconstruction algorithm images for PET dynamic study. Ann Nucl Med 2001; 15(5):417–423.
53. Jaskowiak CJ, Bianco JA, Perlman SB, Fine JP. Influence of reconstruction iterations on 18F-FDG PET/CT standardized uptake values. J Nucl Med 2005; 46(3):424–428.
54. Lartizien C, Kinahan PE, Swensson R, Comtat C, Lin M, Villemagne V, Trebossen R. Evaluating image reconstruction methods for tumor detection in 3-dimensional whole-body PET oncology imaging. J Nucl Med 2003; 44(2):276–290.
55. Etchebehere EC, Macapinlac HA, Gonen M, Humm K, Yeung HW, Akhurst T, Scher HI, Larson SM. Qualitative and quantitative comparison between images obtained with filtered back projection and iterative reconstruction in prostate cancer lesions of (18)F-FDG PET. Q J Nucl Med 2002; 46(2):122–130.
56. Cook GJ. Oncological molecular imaging: nuclear medicine techniques. Br J Radiol 2003; 76(Spec No. 2): S152–S158.
57. Apisarnthanarax S, Chao KS. Current imaging paradigms in radiation oncology. Radiat Res 2005; 163(1):1–25.
58. Pauwels EK, Ribeiro MJ, Stoot JH, McCready VR, Bourguignon M, Maziere B. FDG accumulation and tumor biology. Nucl Med Biol 1998; 25(4):317–322.
59. Weber G. Enzymology of cancer cells (first of two parts). N Engl J Med 1977; 296(9):486–492.
60. Weber G. Enzymology of cancer cells (second of two parts). N Engl J Med 1977; 296(10):541–551.
61. Brown RS, Wahl RL. Overexpression of Glut-1 glucose transporter in human breast cancer. An immunohistochemical study. Cancer 1993; 72(10):2979–2985.
62. Higashi T, Tamaki N, Honda T, Torizuka T, Kimura T, Inokuma T, Ohshio G, Hosotani R, Imamura M, Konishi J. Expression of glucose transporters in human pancreatic tumors compared with increased FDG accumulation in PET study. J Nucl Med 1997; 38(9):1337–1344.
63. Yamamoto T, Seino Y, Fukumoto H, Koh G, Yano H, Inagaki N, Yamada Y, Inoue K, Manabe T, Imura H. Over-expression of facilitative glucose transporter genes in human cancer. Biochem Biophys Res Commun 1990; 170(1):223–230.
64. Kubota K. From tumor biology to clinical Pet: a review of positron emission tomography (PET) in oncology. Ann Nucl Med 2001; 15(6):471–486.
65. Brownell GL, Ackerman RH, Strauss HW, Elmaleh DR, Cochavi S, Alpert N, Correia JA, Kearfott KJ, Taveras J. Preliminary imaging results with 18F-2-fluoro-2-deoxy-D-glucose. J Comput Assist Tomogr 1980; 4(4):473–477.
66. Som P, Atkins HL, Bandoypadhyay D, Fowler JS, MacGregor RR, Matsui K, Oster ZH, Sacker DF, Shiue CY, Turner H, Wan CN, Wolf AP, Zabinski SV. A fluorinated glucose analog, 2-fluoro-2-deoxy-D-glucose (F-18): nontoxic tracer for rapid tumor detection. J Nucl Med 1980; 21(7):670–675.
67. Tewson TJ, Welch MJ, Raichle ME. [18F]-labeled 3-deoxy-3-fluoro-D-glucose: synthesis and preliminary biodistribution data. J Nucl Med 1978; 19(12):1339–1345.
68. Kubota R, Kubota K, Yamada S, Tada M, Ido T, Tamahashi N. Active and passive mechanisms of [fluorine-18] fluorodeoxyglucose uptake by proliferating and prenecrotic cancer cells in vivo: a microautoradiographic study. J Nucl Med 1994; 35(6):1067–1075.
69. Gambhir SS, Czernin J, Schwimmer J, Silverman DH, Coleman RE, Phelps ME. A tabulated summary of the FDG PET literature. J Nucl Med 2001; 42(5 Suppl):1S–93S.
70. Higashi K, Ueda Y, Yagishita M, Arisaka Y, Sakurai A, Oguchi M, Seki H, Nambu Y, Tonami H, Yamamoto I. FDG PET measurement of the proliferative potential of non-small cell lung cancer. J Nucl Med 2000; 41(1):85–92.
71. Smith TA. FDG uptake, tumour characteristics and response to therapy: a review. Nucl Med Commun 1998; 19(2):97–105.
72. Kole AC, Plaat BE, Hoekstra HJ, Vaalburg W, Molenaar WM. FDG and L-[1–11C]-tyrosine imaging of soft-tissue tumors before and after therapy. J Nucl Med 1999; 40(3):381–386.

73. Vansteenkiste JF, Stroobants SG, Dupont PJ, De Leyn PR, Verbeken EK, Deneffe GJ, Mortelmans LA, Demedts MG. Prognostic importance of the standardized uptake value on (18)F-fluoro-2-deoxy-glucose-positron emission tomography scan in non-small-cell lung cancer: an analysis of 125 cases. Leuven Lung Cancer Group. J Clin Oncol 1999; 17(10):3201–3206.
74. Wagner M, Seitz U, Buck A, Neumaier B, Schultheiss S, Bangerter M, Bommer M, Leithauser F, Wawra E, Munzert G, Reske SN. 3′-[18F]fluoro-3′-deoxythymidine ([18F]-FLT) as positron emission tomography tracer for imaging proliferation in a murine B-Cell lymphoma model and in the human disease. Cancer Res 2003; 63(10):2681–2687.
75. Weber WA, Avril N, Schwaiger M. Relevance of positron emission tomography (PET) in oncology. Strahlenther Onkol 1999; 175(8):356–373.
76. Higashi K, Clavo AC, Wahl RL. Does FDG uptake measure proliferative activity of human cancer cells? In vitro comparison with DNA flow cytometry and tritiated thymidine uptake. J Nucl Med 1993; 34(3):414–419.
77. Mankoff DA, Dehdashti F, Shields AF. Characterizing tumors using metabolic imaging: PET imaging of cellular proliferation and steroid receptors. Neoplasia 2000; 2(1–2):71–88.
78. Mandelkern M, Raines J. Positron emission tomography in cancer research and treatment. Technol Cancer Res Treat 2002; 1(6):423–439.
79. Francis DL, Freeman A, Visvikis D, Costa DC, Luthra SK, Novelli M, Taylor I, Ell PJ. In vivo imaging of cellular proliferation in colorectal cancer using positron emission tomography. Gut 2003; 52(11):1602–1606.
80. Hoffmann M, Kletter K, Becherer A, Jager U, Chott A, Raderer M. 18F-fluorodeoxyglucose positron emission tomography (18F-FDG-PET) for staging and follow-up of marginal zone B-cell lymphoma. Oncology 2003; 64(4):336–340.
81. Lind P, Kresnik E, Kumnig G, Gallowitsch HJ, Igerc I, Matschnig S, Gomez I. 18F-FDG-PET in the follow-up of thyroid cancer. Acta Med Austriaca 2003; 30(1):17–21.
82. Spence AM, Muzi M, Graham MM, O'Sullivan F, Link JM, Lewellen TK, Lewellen B, Freeman SD, Mankoff DA, Eary JF, Krohn KA. 2-[(18)F]Fluoro-2-deoxyglucose and glucose uptake in malignant gliomas before and after radiotherapy: correlation with outcome. Clin Cancer Res 2002; 8(4):971–979.
83. Jager PL, Vaalburg W, Pruim J, de Vries EG, Langen KJ, Piers DA. Radiolabeled amino acids: basic aspects and clinical applications in oncology. J Nucl Med 2001; 42(3):432–445.
84. Ogawa T, Shishido F, Kanno I, Inugami A, Fujita H, Murakami M, Shimosegawa E, Ito H, Hatazawa J, Okudera T, et al. Cerebral glioma: evaluation with methionine PET. Radiology 1993; 186(1):45–53.
85. Mosskin M, Bergstrom M, Collins VP, Ehrin E, Eriksson L, von Holst H, G. Noren. Positron emission tomography with 11C-methionine of intracranial tumours compared with histology of multiple biopsies. Acta Radiol Suppl 1986; 369:157–160.
86. Popperl G, Goldbrunner R, Gildehaus FJ, Kreth FW, Tanner P, Holtmannspotter M, Tonn JC, Tatsch K. O-(2-[18F]fluoroethyl)-L-tyrosine PET for monitoring the effects of convection-enhanced delivery of paclitaxel in patients with recurrent glioblastoma. Eur J Nucl Med Mol Imaging 2005; 32(9):1018–1025.
87. Weckesser M, Langen KJ, Rickert CH, Kloska S, Straeter R, Hamacher K, Kurlemann G, Wassmann H, Coenen HH, Schober O. O-(2-[18F]fluorethyl)-L-tyrosine PET in the clinical evaluation of primary brain tumours. Eur J Nucl Med Mol Imaging 2005; 32(4):22–429.
88. Sherley JL, Kelly TJ. Regulation of human thymidine kinase during the cell cycle. J Biol Chem 1988; 263(17):8350–8358.
89. Begg AC. Prediction of repopulation rates and radiosensitivity in human tumours. Int J Radiat Biol 1994; 65(1):103–108.
90. Hall EJ. Radiobiology for the radiologist. 5th ed. 2000, Philadelphia, USA: Lippincot Williams & Wilkins. p. 588.
91. Haustermans K, Fowler JF. Is there a future for cell kinetic measurements using IdUrd or BdUrd? Int J Radiat Oncol Biol Phys 2001; 49(2):505–511.

92. Krohn KA, Mankoff DA, Eary JF. Imaging cellular proliferation as a measure of response to therapy. J Clin Pharmacol 2001; Suppl:96S–103S.
93. Steel GG. Basic clinical radiobiology. 3rd ed. 2002, London, UK: Arnold, Hodder Headline Group. p. 262.
94. Kyle AH, Huxham LA, Baker JH, Burston HE, Minchinton AI. Tumor distribution of bromodeoxyuridine-labeled cells is strongly dose dependent. Cancer Res 2003; 63(18):5707–5711.
95. Gerdes J, Lemke H, Baisch H, Wacker HH, Schwab U, Stein H. Cell cycle analysis of a cell proliferation-associated human nuclear antigen defined by the monoclonal antibody Ki-67. J Immunol 1984; 133(4):1710–1715.
96. Gerdes J. Ki-67 and other proliferation markers useful for immunohistological diagnostic and prognostic evaluations in human malignancies. Semin Cancer Biol 1990; 1(3):199–206.
97. Scholzen T, Gerdes J. The Ki-67 protein: from the known and the unknown. J Cell Physiol 2000; 182(3):311–322.
98. Landberg G, Roos G. Expression of proliferating cell nuclear antigen (PCNA) and Ki-67 antigen in human malignant hematopoietic cells. Acta Oncol 1991; 30(8):917–921.
99. Ryser JE, Blauenstein P, Remy N, Weinreich R, Hasler PH, Novak-Hofer I, Schubiger PA. [76Br]Bromodeoxyuridine, a potential tracer for the measurement of cell proliferation by positron emission tomography, in vitro and in vivo studies in mice. Nucl Med Biol 1999; 26(6):673–679.
100. Blasberg RG, Roelcke U, Weinreich R, Beattie B, von Ammon K, Yonekawa Y, Landolt H, Guenther I, Crompton NE, Vontobel P, Missimer J, Maguire RP, Koziorowski J, Knust EJ, Finn RD, Leenders KL. Imaging brain tumor proliferative activity with [124I]iododeoxyuridine. Cancer Res 2000; 60(3):624–635.
101. Buchmann I, Vogg AT, Glatting G, Schultheiss S, Moller P, Leithauser F, Schulte M, Gfrorer W, Kotzerke J, Reske SN. [18F]5-fluoro-2-deoxyuridine-PET for imaging of malignant tumors and for measuring tissue proliferation. Cancer Biother Radiopharm 2003; 18(3):327–337.
102. Kim CG, Yang DJ, Kim EE, Cherif A, Kuang LR, Li C, Tansey W, Liu CW, Li SC, Wallace S, Podoloff DA. Assessment of tumor cell proliferation using [18F]fluorodeoxyadenosine and [18F]fluoroethyluracil. J Pharm Sci 1996; 85(3):339–344.
103. Shields AF, Larson SM, Grunbaum Z, Graham MM. Short-term thymidine uptake in normal and neoplastic tissues: studies for PET. J Nucl Med 1984; 25(7):759–764.
104. Martiat P, Ferrant A, Labar D, Cogneau M, Bol A, Michel C, Michaux JL, Sokal G. In vivo measurement of carbon-11 thymidine uptake in non-Hodgkin's lymphoma using positron emission tomography. J Nucl Med 1988; 29(10):1633–1637.
105. Goethals P, Lameire N, van Eijkeren M, Kesteloot D, Thierens H, Dams R. [Methyl-carbon-11] thymidine for in vivo measurement of cell proliferation. J Nucl Med 1996; 37(6):1048–1052.
106. Shields AF, Mankoff DA, Link JM, Graham MM, Eary JF, Kozawa SM, Zheng M, Lewellen B, Lewellen TK, Grierson JR, Krohn KA. Carbon-11-thymidine and FDG to measure therapy response. J Nucl Med 1998; 39(10):1757–1762.
107. Eary JF, Mankoff DA, Spence AM, Berger MS, Olshen A, Link JM, O'Sullivan F, Krohn KA. 2-[C-11]thymidine imaging of malignant brain tumors. Cancer Res 1999; 59(3):615–621.
108. Wells P, Gunn RN, Alison M, Steel C, Golding M, Ranicar AS, Brady F, Osman S, Jones T, Price P. Assessment of proliferation in vivo using 2-[(11)C]thymidine positron emission tomography in advanced intra-abdominal malignancies. Cancer Res 2002; 62(20):5698–5702.
109. Shields AF, Grierson JR, Dohmen BM, Machulla HJ, Stayanoff JC, Lawhorn-Crews JM, Obradovich JE, Muzik O, Mangner TJ. Imaging proliferation in vivo with [F-18]FLT and positron emission tomography. Nat Med 1998; 4(11):1334–1336.
110. Grierson JR, Shields AF. Radiosynthesis of 3′-deoxy-3′-[(18)F]fluorothymidine: [(18)F]FLT for imaging of cellular proliferation in vivo. Nucl Med Biol 2000; 27(2):143–156.

111. Mier W, Haberkorn U, Eisenhut M. [18F]FLT; portrait of a proliferation marker. Eur J Nucl Med Mol Imaging 2002; 29(2):165–169.
112. Buck AK, Halter G, Schirrmeister H, Kotzerke J, Wurziger I, Glatting G, Mattfeldt T, Neumaier B, Reske SN, Hetzel M. Imaging proliferation in lung tumors with PET: 18F-FLT versus 18F-FDG. J Nucl Med 2003; 44(9):1426–1431.
113. Schwartz JL, Tamura Y, Jordan R, Grierson JR, Krohn KA. Monitoring tumor cell proliferation by targeting DNA synthetic processes with thymidine and thymidine analogs. J Nucl Med 2003; 44(12):2027–2032.
114. Vesselle H, Grierson J, Peterson LM, Muzi M, Mankoff DA, Krohn KA. 18F-Fluorothymidine radiation dosimetry in human PET imaging studies. J Nucl Med 2003; 44(9):1482–1488.
115. Rasey JS, Grierson JR, Wiens LW, Kolb PD, Schwartz JL. Validation of FLT uptake as a measure of thymidine kinase-1 activity in A549 carcinoma cells. J Nucl Med 2002; 43(9):1210–1217.
116. Barthel H, Cleij MC, Collingridge DR, Hutchinson OC, Osman S, He Q, Luthra SK, Brady F, Price PM, Aboagye EO. 3′-deoxy-3′-[18F]fluorothymidine as a new marker for monitoring tumor response to antiproliferative therapy in vivo with positron emission tomography. Cancer Res 2003; 63(13):3791–3798.
117. Toyohara J, Waki A, Takamatsu S, Yonekura Y, Magata Y, Fujibayashi Y. Basis of FLT as a cell proliferation marker: comparative uptake studies with [3H]thymidine and [3H]arabinothymidine, and cell-analysis in 22 asynchronously growing tumor cell lines. Nucl Med Biol 2002; 29(3):281–287.
118. Munch-Petersen B, Cloos L, Jensen HK, Tyrsted G. Human thymidine kinase 1. Regulation in normal and malignant cells. Adv Enzyme Regul 1995; 35:69–89.
119. Schwartz JL, Tamura Y, Jordan R, Grierson JR, Krohn KA. Effect of p53 activation on cell growth, thymidine kinase-1 activity, and 3′-deoxy-3′fluorothymidine uptake. Nucl Med Biol 2004; 31(4):419–423.
120. Vesselle H, Grierson J, Muzi M, Pugsley JM, Schmidt RA, Rabinowitz P, Peterson LM, Vallieres E, Wood DE. In vivo validation of 3′deoxy-3′-[(18)F]fluorothymidine ([(18)F]FLT) as a proliferation imaging tracer in humans: correlation of [(18)F]FLT uptake by positron emission tomography with Ki-67 immunohistochemistry and flow cytometry in human lung tumors. Clin Cancer Res 2002; 8(11):3315–3323.
121. Shields AF. PET imaging with 18F-FLT and thymidine analogs: promise and pitfalls. J Nucl Med 2003; 44(9):1432–1434.
122. Rand SD, Prost R, Haughton V, Mark L, Strainer J, Johansen J, Kim TA, Chetty VK, Mueller W, Meyer G, Krouwer H. Accuracy of single-voxel proton MR spectroscopy in distinguishing neoplastic from nonneoplastic brain lesions. AJNR Am J Neuroradiol 1997; 18(9):1695–1704.
123. Butzen J, Prost R, Chetty V, Donahue K, Neppl R, Bowen W, Li SJ, Haughton V, Mark L, Kim T, Mueller W, Meyer G, Krouwer H, Rand S. Discrimination between neoplastic and nonneoplastic brain lesions by use of proton MR spectroscopy: the limits of accuracy with a logistic regression model. AJNR Am J Neuroradiol 2000; 21(7):1213–1219.
124. Allen JR, Prost RW, Griffith OW, Erickson SJ, Erickson BA. In vivo proton (H1) magnetic resonance spectroscopy for cervical carcinoma. Am J Clin Oncol 2001; 24(5):522–529.
125. Majos C, Julia-Sape M, Alonso J, Serrallonga M, Aguilera C, Acebes JJ, Arus C, Gili J. Brain tumor classification by proton MR spectroscopy: comparison of diagnostic accuracy at short and long TE. AJNR Am J Neuroradiol 2004; 25(10):1696–1704.
126. Kim JH, Chang KH, Na DG, Song IC, Kwon BJ, Han MH, Kim K. 3T 1H-MR spectroscopy in grading of cerebral gliomas: comparison of short and intermediate echo time sequences. AJNR Am J Neuroradiol 2006; 27(7):1412–1418.
127. Luan W, Zhang J. In vivo hydrogen-1 magnetic resonance spectroscopy study of human intracranial tumors. Chin Med J (Engl) 1998; 111(1):56–58.
128. Tedeschi G, Lundbom N, Raman R, Bonavita S, Duyn JH, Alger JR, Di Chiro G. Increased choline signal coinciding with malignant degeneration of cerebral gliomas: a serial proton magnetic resonance spectroscopy imaging study. J Neurosurg 1997; 87(4): 516–524.

129. Virta A, Patronas N, Raman R, Dwyer A, Barnett A, Bonavita S, Tedeschi G, Lundbom N. Spectroscopic imaging of radiation-induced effects in the white matter of glioma patients. Magn Reson Imaging 2000; 18(7):851–857.
130. Ott D, Hennig J, Ernst T. Human brain tumors: assessment with in vivo proton MR spectroscopy. Radiology 1993; 186(3):745–752.
131. Yamagata NT, Miller BL, McBride D, Chang L, Chiang F, Nikas D, Osborne D, Buchthal SD. In vivo proton spectroscopy of intracranial infections and neoplasms. J Neuroimaging 1994; 4(1):23–28.
132. Meyerand ME, Pipas JM, Mamourian A, Tosteson TD, Dunn JF. Classification of biopsy-confirmed brain tumors using single-voxel MR spectroscopy. AJNR Am J Neuroradiol 1999; 20(1):117–123.
133. Bruhn H, Frahm J, Gyngell ML, Merboldt KD, Hanicke W, Sauter R, Hamburger C. Noninvasive differentiation of tumors with use of localized H-1 MR spectroscopy in vivo: initial experience in patients with cerebral tumors. Radiology 1989; 172(2):541–548.
134. Preul MC, Caramanos Z, Collins DL, Villemure JG, Leblanc R, Olivier A, Pokrupa R, Arnold DL. Accurate, noninvasive diagnosis of human brain tumors by using proton magnetic resonance spectroscopy. Nat Med 1996; 2(3):323–325.
135. Murakami Y, Takamatsu H, Taki J, Tatsumi M, Noda A, Ichise R, Tait JF, Nishimura S. 18F-labelled annexin V: a PET tracer for apoptosis imaging. Eur J Nucl Med Mol Imaging 2004; 31(4):469–474.
136. Grierson JR, Yagle KJ, Eary JF, Tait JF, Gibson DF, Lewellen B, Link JM, Krohn KA. Production of [F-18]fluoroannexin for imaging apoptosis with PET. Bioconjug Chem 2004; 15(2):373–379.
137. Toretsky J, Levenson A, Weinberg IN, Tait JF, Uren A, Mease RC. Preparation of F-18 labeled annexin V: a potential PET radiopharmaceutical for imaging cell death. Nucl Med Biol 2004; 31(6):747–752.
138. Keen HG, Dekker BA, Disley L, Hastings D, Lyons S, Reader AJ, Ottewell P, Watson A, Zweit J. Imaging apoptosis in vivo using 124I-annexin V and PET. Nucl Med Biol 2005; 32(4):395–402.
139. van de Wiele C, Lahorte C, Vermeersch H, Loose D, Mervillie K, Steinmetz ND, Vanderheyden JL, Cuvelier CA, Slegers G, Dierck RA. Quantitative tumor apoptosis imaging using technetium-99m-HYNIC annexin V single photon emission computed tomography. J Clin Oncol 2003; 21(18):3483–3487.
140. Belhocine TZ, Blankenberg FG. 99mTc-Annexin A5 uptake and imaging to monitor chemosensitivity. Methods Mol Med 2005; 111:363–380.
141. Haberkorn U, Kinscherf R, Krammer PH, Mier W, Eisenhut M. Investigation of a potential scintigraphic marker of apoptosis: radioiodinated Z-Val-Ala-DL-Asp(O-methyl)-fluoromethyl ketone. Nucl Med Biol 2001; 28(7):793–798.
142. Haberkorn U, Mier W, Eisenhut M. Scintigraphic imaging of gene expression and gene transfer. Curr Med Chem 2005; 12(7):779–794.
143. Belhocine T, Steinmetz N, Hustinx R, Bartsch P, Jerusalem G, Seidel L, Rigo P, Green A. Increased uptake of the apoptosis-imaging agent (99m)Tc recombinant human Annexin V in human tumors after one course of chemotherapy as a predictor of tumor response and patient prognosis. Clin Cancer Res 2002; 8(9):2766–2774.
144. Van Den Bossche B, Van de Wiele C. Receptor imaging in oncology by means of nuclear medicine: current status. J Clin Oncol 2004; 22(17):3593–3607.
145. Holdaway IM, Bowditch JV. Variation in receptor status between primary and metastatic breast cancer. Cancer 1983; 52(3):479–485.
146. Katzenellenbogen JA, Coleman RE, Hawkins RA, Krohn KA, Larson SM, Mendelsohn J, Osborne CK, Piwnica-Worms D, Reba RC, Siegel BA, et al. Tumor receptor imaging: proceedings of the National Cancer Institute workshop, review of current work, and prospective for further investigations. Clin Cancer Res 1995; 1(8):921–932.
147. McGuire AH, Dehdashti F, Siegel BA, Lyss AP, Brodack JW, Mathias CJ, Mintun MA, Katzenellenbogen JA, Welch MJ. Positron tomographic assessment of 16 alpha-[18F]

fluoro-17 beta-estradiol uptake in metastatic breast carcinoma. J Nucl Med 1991; 32(8):1526–1531.
148. Mortimer JE, Dehdashti F, Siegel BA, Trinkaus K, Katzenellenbogen JA, Welch MJ. Metabolic flare: indicator of hormone responsiveness in advanced breast cancer. J Clin Oncol 2001; 19(11):2797–2803.
149. Mortimer JE, Dehdashti F, Siegel BA, Katzenellenbogen JA, Fracasso P, Welch MJ. Positron emission tomography with 2-[18F]Fluoro-2-deoxy-D-glucose and 16alpha-[18F]fluoro-17beta-estradiol in breast cancer: correlation with estrogen receptor status and response to systemic therapy. Clin Cancer Res 1996; 2(6):933–939.
150. Dehdashti F, Mortimer JE, Siegel BA, Griffeth LK, Bonasera TJ, Fusselman MJ, Detert DD, Cutler PD, Katzenellenbogen JA, Welch M.J. Positron tomographic assessment of estrogen receptors in breast cancer: comparison with FDG-PET and in vitro receptor assays. J Nucl Med 1995; 36(10):1766–1774.
151. Mintun MA, Welch MJ, Siegel BA, Mathias CJ, Brodack JW, McGuire AH, Katzenellenbogen JA. Breast cancer: PET imaging of estrogen receptors. Radiology 1988; 169(1):45–48.
152. Scheidhauer K, Muller S, Smolarz K, Brautigam P, Briele B. [Tumor scintigraphy using 123I-labeled estradiol in breast cancer–receptor scintigraphy]. Nuklearmedizin 1991; 30(3):84–99.
153. Scheidhauer K, Scharl A, Schicha H. Estrogen receptor scintigraphy. Q J Nucl Med 1998; 42(1):26–32.
154. Schober O, Scheidhauer K, Jackisch C, Schicha H, Smolarz K, Bolte A, Reiners C, Hoffken K, Biersack HJ, Briele B, et al. Breast cancer imaging with radioiodinated oestradiol. Lancet 1990; 335(8704):1522.
155. Bennink RJ, Rijks LJ, van Tienhoven G, Noorduyn LA, Janssen AG, Sloof GW. Estrogen receptor status in primary breast cancer: iodine 123-labeled cis-11beta-methoxy-17alpha-iodovinyl estradiol scintigraphy. Radiology 2001; 220(3):774–779.
156. Bennink RJ, van Tienhoven G, Rijks LJ, Noorduyn AL, Janssen AG, Sloof GW. In vivo prediction of response to antiestrogen treatment in estrogen receptor-positive breast cancer. J Nucl Med 2004; 45(1):1–7.
157. Inoue T, Kim EE, Wallace S, Yang DJ, Wong FC, Bassa P, Cherif A, Delpassand E, Buzdar A, Podoloff DA. Positron emission tomography using [18F]fluorotamoxifen to evaluate therapeutic responses in patients with breast cancer: preliminary study. Cancer Biother Radiopharm 1996; 11(4):235–245.
158. Yang D, Kuang LR, Cherif A, Tansey W, Li C, Lin WJ, Liu CW, Kim EE, Wallace S. Synthesis of [18F]fluoroalanine and [18F]fluorotamoxifen for imaging breast tumors. J Drug Target 1993; 1(3):259–267.
159. Trachtenberg J, Walsh PC. Correlation of prostatic nuclear androgen receptor content with duration of response and survival following hormonal therapy in advanced prostatic cancer. J Urol 1982; 127(3):466–471.
160. Trachtenberg J, Bujnovszky P, Walsh P.C. Androgen receptor content of normal and hyperplastic human prostate. J Clin Endocrinol Metab 1982; 54(1):17–21.
161. Liu A, Carlson KE, Katzenellenbogen JA. Synthesis of high affinity fluorine-substituted ligands for the androgen receptor. Potential agents for imaging prostatic cancer by positron emission tomography. J Med Chem 1992; 35(11):2113–2129.
162. Katzenellenbogen JA. Designing steroid receptor-based radiotracers to image breast and prostate tumors. J Nucl Med 1995; 36(6 Suppl):8S–13S.
163. Choe YS, Lidstrom PJ, Chi DY, Bonasera TA, Welch MJ, Katzenellenbogen JA. Synthesis of 11 beta-[18F]fluoro-5 alpha-dihydrotestosterone and 11 beta-[18F]fluoro-19-nor-5 alpha-dihydrotestosterone: preparation via halofluorination-reduction, receptor binding, and tissue distribution. J Med Chem 1995; 38(5):816–825.
164. Reubi JC, Waser B, Schaer JC, Laissue JA. Somatostatin receptor sst1-sst5 expression in normal and neoplastic human tissues using receptor autoradiography with subtype-selective ligands. Eur J Nucl Med 2001; 28(7):836–846.

165. Krenning EP, Kwekkeboom DJ, Reubi JC, van Hagen PM, van Eijck CH, Oei HY, Lamberts S.W. 111In-octreotide scintigraphy in oncology. Digestion 1993; 54 Suppl 1:84–87.
166. van den Anker-Lugtenburg PJ, Lowenberg B, Lamberts SW, Krenning EP. The relevance of somatostatin receptor expression in malignant lymphomas. Metabolism 1996; 45(8 Suppl 1):96–97.
167. Kwekkeboom DJ, van Urk H, Pauw BK, Lamberts SW, Kooij PP, Hoogma RP, Krenning EP. Octreotide scintigraphy for the detection of paragangliomas. J Nucl Med 1993; 34(6):873–878.
168. Gibril F, Reynolds JC, Doppman JL, Chen CC, Venzon DJ, Termanini B, Weber HC, Stewart CA, Jensen RT. Somatostatin receptor scintigraphy: its sensitivity compared with that of other imaging methods in detecting primary and metastatic gastrinomas. A prospective study. Ann Intern Med 1996; 125(1):26–34.
169. Berenger N, Moretti JL, Boaziz C, Vigneron N, Morere JF, Breau JL. Somatostatin receptor imaging in small cell lung cancer. Eur J Cancer 1996; 32A(8):1429–1431.
170. Lugtenburg PJ, Lowenberg B, Valkema R, Oei HY, Lamberts SW, Eijkemans MJ, van Putten WL, Krenning EP. Somatostatin receptor scintigraphy in the initial staging of low-grade non-Hodgkin's lymphomas. J Nucl Med 2001; 42(2):222–229.
171. Herbst RS. Review of epidermal growth factor receptor biology. Int J Radiat Oncol Biol Phys 2004; 59(2 Suppl):21–26.
172. Ferrara N, Davis-Smyth T. The biology of vascular endothelial growth factor. Endocr Rev 1997; 18(1):4–25.
173. Li S, Peck-Radosavljevic M, Koller E, Koller F, Kaserer K, Kreil A, Kapiotis S, Hamwi A, Weich HA, Valent P, Angelberger P, Dudczak R, Virgolini I. Characterization of (123)I-vascular endothelial growth factor-binding sites expressed on human tumour cells: possible implication for tumour scintigraphy. Int J Cancer 2001; 91(6):789–796.
174. Collingridge DR, Carroll VA, Glaser M, Aboagye EO, Osman S, Hutchinson OC, Barthel H, Luthra SK, Brady F, Bicknell R, Price P, Harris AL. The development of [(124)I]iodinated-VG76e: a novel tracer for imaging vascular endothelial growth factor in vivo using positron emission tomography. Cancer Res 2002; 62(20):5912–5919.
175. Zinn KR, Kelpke S, Chaudhuri TR, Sugg T, Mountz JM, Thompson JA. Imaging Tc-99m-labeled FGF-1 targeting in rats. Nucl Med Biol 2000; 27(4):407–414.
176. Kobayashi H, Sakahara H, Hosono M, Shirato M, Konishi J, Takahashi JA, Oda Y, Kikuchi H, Endo K, Kozai Y, Scintigraphic detection of xenografted tumors producing human basic fibroblast growth factor. Cancer Immunol Immunother 1993; 37(5):281–285.
177. Beer AJ, Haubner R, Goebel M, Luderschmidt S, Spilker ME, Wester HJ, Weber WA, Schwaiger M. Biodistribution and pharmacokinetics of the alphavbeta3-selective tracer 18F-galacto-RGD in cancer patients. J Nucl Med 2005; 46(8):1333–1341.
178. Chen X, Tohme M, Park R, Hou Y, Bading JR, Conti PS. Micro-PET imaging of alphavbeta3-integrin expression with 18F-labeled dimeric RGD peptide. Mol Imaging 2004; 3(2):96–104.
179. Chen X, Park R, Hou Y, Khankaldyyan V, Gonzales-Gomez I, Tohme M, Bading JR, Laug WE, Conti PS. MicroPET imaging of brain tumor angiogenesis with 18F-labeled PEGylated RGD peptide. Eur J Nucl Med Mol Imaging 2004; 31(8):1081–1089.
180. Zhang X, Xiong Z, Wu Y, Cai W, Tseng JR, Gambhir SS, Chen X. Quantitative PET Imaging of Tumor Integrin {alpha}v{beta}3 Expression with 18F-FRGD2. J Nucl Med 2006; 47(1):113–121.
181. Chen X. Multimodality imaging of tumor integrin alphavbeta3 expression. Mini Rev Med Chem 2006; 6(2):227–234.
182. Chen X, Sievers E, Hou Y, Park R, Tohme M, Bart R, Bremner R, Bading JR, Conti PS. Integrin alpha v beta 3-targeted imaging of lung cancer. Neoplasia 2005; **7**(3):271–279.
183. Chen X, Park R, Khankaldyyan V, Gonzales-Gomez I, Tohme M, Moats RA, Bading JR, Laug WE, Conti P.S. Longitudinal microPET imaging of brain tumor growth with F-18-labeled RGD peptide. Mol Imaging Biol 2006; 8(1):9–15.

184. Zheng QH, Fei X, Liu X, Wang JQ, Bin Sun H, Mock BH, Lee Stone K, Martinez TD, Miller KD, Sledge GW, Hutchins GD. Synthesis and preliminary biological evaluation of MMP inhibitor radiotracers [11C]methyl-halo-CGS 27023A analogs, new potential PET breast cancer imaging agents. Nucl Med Biol 2002; 29(7):761–770.
185. Furumoto S, Takashima K, Kubota K, Ido T, Iwata R, Fukuda H. Tumor detection using 18F-labeled matrix metalloproteinase-2 inhibitor. Nucl Med Biol 2003; 30(2):119–125.
186. Brown JM, Giaccia AJ. The unique physiology of solid tumors: opportunities (and problems) for cancer therapy. Cancer Res 1998; 58(7):1408–1416.
187. Graham CH, Forsdike J, Fitzgerald CJ, Macdonald-Goodfellow S. Hypoxia-mediated stimulation of carcinoma cell invasiveness via upregulation of urokinase receptor expression. Int J Cancer 1999; 80(4):617–623.
188. Hockel M, Schlenger K, Hockel S, Vaupel P. Hypoxic cervical cancers with low apoptotic index are highly aggressive. Cancer Res 1999; 59(18):4525–4528.
189. Graeber TG, Osmanian C, Jacks T, Housman DE, Koch CJ, Lowe SW, Giaccia AJ. Hypoxia-mediated selection of cells with diminished apoptotic potential in solid tumours. Nature 1996; 379(6560):88–91.
190. Brown JM. The hypoxic cell: a target for selective cancer therapy–eighteenth Bruce F. Cain Memorial Award lecture. Cancer Res 1999; 59(23):5863–5870.
191. Zhivotovsky B, Joseph B, Orrenius S. Tumor radiosensitivity and apoptosis. Exp Cell Res 1999; 248(1):10–17.
192. Chapman JD. Measurement of tumor hypoxia by invasive and non-invasive procedures: a review of recent clinical studies. Radiother Oncol 1991; 20(Suppl 1):13–19.
193. Chapman JD, Engelhardt EL, Stobbe CC, Schneider RF, Hanks GE. Measuring hypoxia and predicting tumor radioresistance with nuclear medicine assays. Radiother Oncol 1998; 46(3):229–237.
194. Kallinowski F, Zander R, Hoeckel M, Vaupel P. Tumor tissue oxygenation as evaluated by computerized-pO2-histography. Int J Radiat Oncol Biol Phys 1990; 19(4):953–961.
195. Griffiths JR, Robinson SP. The OxyLite: a fibre-optic oxygen sensor. Br J Radiol 1999; 72(859):627–630.
196. Hull EL, Conover DL, Foster TH. Carbogen-induced changes in rat mammary tumour oxygenation reported by near infrared spectroscopy. Br J Cancer 1999; 79(11–12):1709–1716.
197. Wilson DF, Cerniglia GJ. Localization of tumors and evaluation of their state of oxygenation by phosphorescence imaging. Cancer Res 1992; 52(14):3988–3993.
198. Dunn JF, Swartz HM. Blood oxygenation. Heterogeneity of hypoxic tissues monitored using bold MR imaging. Adv Exp Med Biol 1997; 428:645–650.
199. Robinson SP, Howe FA, Rodrigues LM, Stubbs M, Griffiths JR. Magnetic resonance imaging techniques for monitoring changes in tumor oxygenation and blood flow. Semin Radiat Oncol 1998; 8(3):197–207.
200. Kannurpatti SS, Biswal BB, Hudetz AG. Regional dynamics of the fMRI-BOLD signal response to hypoxia-hypercapnia in the rat brain. J Magn Reson Imaging 2003; 17(6):641–647.
201. Koh WJ, Rasey JS, Evans ML, Grierson JR, Lewellen TK, Graham MM, Krohn KA, Griffin TW. Imaging of hypoxia in human tumors with [F-18]fluoromisonidazole. Int J Radiat Oncol Biol Phys 1992; 22(1):199–212.
202. Koh WJ, Bergman KS, Rasey JS, Peterson LM, Evans ML, Graham MM, Grierson JR, Lindsley KL, Lewellen TK, Krohn KA, et al. Evaluation of oxygenation status during fractionated radiotherapy in human nonsmall cell lung cancers using [F-18]fluoromisonidazole positron emission tomography. Int J Radiat Oncol Biol Phys 1995; 33(2):391–398.
203. Rasey JS, Koh WJ, Evans ML, Peterson LM, Lewellen TK, Graham MM, Krohn KA. Quantifying regional hypoxia in human tumors with positron emission tomography of [18F]fluoromisonidazole: a pretherapy study of 37 patients. Int J Radiat Oncol Biol Phys 1996; 36(2):417–428.

204. Fujibayashi Y, Taniuchi H, Yonekura Y, Ohtani H, Konishi J, Yokoyama A. Copper-62-ATSM: a new hypoxia imaging agent with high membrane permeability and low redox potential. J Nucl Med 1997; 38(7):1155–1160.
205. Lewis JS, McCarthy DW, McCarthy TJ, Fujibayashi Y, Welch MJ. Evaluation of 64Cu-ATSM in vitro and in vivo in a hypoxic tumor model. J Nucl Med 1999; 40(1):177–183.
206. Takahashi N, Fujibayashi Y, Yonekura Y, Welch MJ, Waki A, Tsuchida T, Sadato N, Sugimoto K, Itoh H. Evaluation of 62Cu labeled diacetyl-bis(N4-methylthiosemicarbazone) as a hypoxic tissue tracer in patients with lung cancer. Ann Nucl Med 2000; 14(5):323–328.
207. Lewis J, Laforest R, Buettner T, Song S, Fujibayashi Y, Connett J, Welch M. Copper-64-diacetyl-bis(N4-methylthiosemicarbazone): an agent for radiotherapy. Proc Natl Acad Sci USA 2001; 98(3):1206–1211.
208. Obata A, Yoshimi E, Waki A, Lewis JS, Oyama N, Welch MJ, Saji H, Yonekura Y, Fujibayashi Y. Retention mechanism of hypoxia selective nuclear imaging/radiotherapeutic agent cu-diacetyl-bis(N4-methylthiosemicarbazone) (Cu-ATSM) in tumor cells. Ann Nucl Med 2001; 15(6):499–504.
209. Takahashi N, Fujibayashi Y, Yonekura Y, Welch MJ, Waki A, Tsuchida T, Sadato N, Sugimoto K, Nakano A, Lee JD, Itoh H. Copper-62 ATSM as a hypoxic tissue tracer in myocardial ischemia. Ann Nucl Med 2001; 15(3):293–296.
210. Maurer RI, Blower PJ, Dilworth JR, Reynolds CA, Zheng Y, Mullen GE. Studies on the mechanism of hypoxic selectivity in copper bis(thiosemicarbazone) radiopharmaceuticals. J Med Chem 2002; 45(7):1420–1431.
211. Dehdashti F, Grigsby PW, Mintun MA, Lewis JS, Siegel BA, Welch MJ. Assessing tumor hypoxia in cervical cancer by positron emission tomography with 60Cu-ATSM: relationship to therapeutic response – a preliminary report. Int J Radiat Oncol Biol Phys 2003; 55(5):1233–1238.
212. Dehdashti F, Mintun MA, Lewis JS, Bradley J, Govindan R, Laforest R, Welch MJ, Siegel BA. In vivo assessment of tumor hypoxia in lung cancer with 60Cu-ATSM. Eur J Nucl Med Mol Imaging 2003; 30(6):844–850.
213. Obata A, Kasamatsu S, Lewis JS, Furukawa T, Takamatsu S, Toyohara J, Asai T, Welch MJ, Adams SG, Saji H, Yonekura Y, Fujibayashi Y. Basic characterization of (64)Cu-ATSM as a radiotherapy agent. Nucl Med Biol 2005; 32(1):21–28.
214. Obata A, Yoshimoto M, Kasamatsu S, Naiki H, Takamatsu S, Kashikura K, Furukawa T, Lewis JS, Welch MJ, Saji H, Yonekura Y. Fujibayashi Y. Intra-tumoral distribution of (64)Cu-ATSM: a comparison study with FDG. Nucl Med Biol 2003; 30(5):529–534.
215. Kachur AV, Dolbier WR Jr, Evans SM, Shiue CY, Shiue GG, Skov KA, Baird IR, James BR, Li AR, Roche A, Koch CJ. Synthesis of new hypoxia markers EF1 and [18F]-EF1. Appl Radiat Isot 1999; 51(6):643–650.
216. Evans SM, Kachur AV, Shiue CY, Hustinx R, Jenkins WT, Shive GG, Karp JS, Alavi A, Lord EM, Dolbier WR Jr, Koch CJ. Noninvasive detection of tumor hypoxia using the 2-nitroimidazole [18F]EF1. J Nucl Med 2000; 41(2):327–336.
217. Josse O, Labar D, Georges B, Gregoire V, Marchand-Brynaert J. Synthesis of [18F]-labeled EF3 [2-(2-nitroimidazol-1-yl)-N-(3,3,3-trifluoropropyl)-acetamide], a marker for PET detection of hypoxia. Bioorg Med Chem 2001; 9(3):665–675.
218. Dolbier WR Jr, Li AR, Koch CJ, Shiue CY, Kachur AV. [18F]-EF5, a marker for PET detection of hypoxia: synthesis of precursor and a new fluorination procedure. Appl Radiat Isot 2001; 54(1):73–80.
219. Ziemer LS, Evans SM, Kachur AV, Shuman AL, Cardi CA, Jenkins WT, Karp JS, Alavi A, Dolbier WR Jr, Koch CJ. Noninvasive imaging of tumor hypoxia in rats using the 2-nitroimidazole 18F-EF5. Eur J Nucl Med Mol Imaging 2003; 30(2):259–266.
220. Bentzen L, Keiding S, Horsman MR, Gronroos T, Hansen SB, Overgaard J. Assessment of hypoxia in experimental mice tumours by [18F]fluoromisonidazole PET and pO2 electrode measurements. Influence of tumour volume and carbogen breathing. Acta Oncol 2002; 41(3):304–312.

221. Bentzen L, Keiding S, Nordsmark M, Falborg L, Hansen SB, Keller J, Nielsen OS, Overgaard J. Tumour oxygenation assessed by 18F-fluoromisonidazole PET and polarographic needle electrodes in human soft tissue tumours. Radiother Oncol 2003; 67(3):339–344.
222. Rajendran JG, Wilson DC, Conrad EU, Peterson LM, Bruckner JD, Rasey JS, Chin LK, Hofstrand PD, Grierson JR, Eary JF, Krohn KA. [(18)F]FMISO and [(18)F]FDG PET imaging in soft tissue sarcomas: correlation of hypoxia, metabolism and VEGF expression. Eur J Nucl Med Mol Imaging 2003; 30(5):695–704.
223. Rajendran JG, Mankoff DA, O'Sullivan F, Peterson LM, Schwartz DL, Conrad EU, Spence AM, Muzi M, Farwell DG, Krohn KA. Hypoxia and glucose metabolism in malignant tumors: evaluation by [18F]fluoromisonidazole and [18F]fluorodeoxyglucose positron emission tomography imaging. Clin Cancer Res 2004; 10(7):2245–2252.
224. Pauling L, Coryell CD. The magnetic properties and structure of hemoglobin, oxyhemoglobin and carbonmonoxyhemoglobin. Proc Natl Acad Sci USA 1936; 22(4):210–216.
225. Thulborn KR, Waterton JC, Matthews PM, Radda GK. Oxygenation dependence of the transverse relaxation time of water protons in whole blood at high field. Biochim Biophys Acta 1982; 714(2):265–270.
226. Robinson SP, Howe FA, Griffiths JR. Noninvasive monitoring of carbogen-induced changes in tumor blood flow and oxygenation by functional magnetic resonance imaging. Int J Radiat Oncol Biol Phys 1995; 33(4):855–859.
227. Karczmar GS, River JN, Li J, Vijayakumar S, Goldman Z, Lewis MZ. Effects of hyperoxia on T2* and resonance frequency weighted magnetic resonance images of rodent tumours. NMR Biomed 1994; 7(1–2):3–11.
228. Dewhirst MW, Tso CY, Oliver R, Gustafson CS, Secomb TW, Gross JF. Morphologic and hemodynamic comparison of tumor and healing normal tissue microvasculature. Int J Radiat Oncol Biol Phys 1989; 17(1):91–99.
229. Law M, Yang S, Babb JS, Knopp EA, Golfinos JG, Zagzag D. Johnson G. Comparison of cerebral blood volume and vascular permeability from dynamic susceptibility contrast-enhanced perfusion MR imaging with glioma grade. AJNR Am J Neuroradiol 2004; 25(5):746–755.
230. Costouros NG, Diehn FE, Libutti SK. Molecular imaging of tumor angiogenesis. J Cell Biochem Suppl 2002; 39:72–78.
231. Bacharach SL, Libutti SK, Carrasquillo JA. Measuring tumor blood flow with H(2)(15)O: practical considerations. Nucl Med Biol 2000; 27(7):671–676.
232. Thomas DL, Lythgoe MF, Pell GS, Calamante F, Ordidge RJ. The measurement of diffusion and perfusion in biological systems using magnetic resonance imaging. Phys Med Biol 2000; 45(8):R97–R138.
233. Luypaert R, Boujraf S, Sourbron S, Osteaux M. Diffusion and perfusion MRI: basic physics. Eur J Radiol 2001; 38(1):19–27.
234. Aronen HJ, Gazit IE, Louis DN, Buchbinder BR, Pardo FS, Weisskoff RM, Harsh GR, Cosgrove GR, Halpern EF, Hochberg FH, et al. Cerebral blood volume maps of gliomas: comparison with tumor grade and histologic findings. Radiology 1994; 191(1):41–51.
235. Kuhl CK, Mielcareck P, Klaschik S, Leutner C, Wardelmann E, Gieseke J, Schild HH. Dynamic breast MR imaging: are signal intensity time course data useful for differential diagnosis of enhancing lesions? Radiology 1999; 211(1):101–110.
236. Pardo FS, Aronen HJ, Kennedy D, Moulton G, Paiva K, Okunieff P, Schmidt EV, Hochberg FH, Harsh GR, Fischman AJ, et al. Functional cerebral imaging in the evaluation and radiotherapeutic treatment planning of patients with malignant glioma. Int J Radiat Oncol Biol Phys 1994; 30(3):663–669.
237. Miles KA. Tumour angiogenesis and its relation to contrast enhancement on computed tomography: a review. Eur J Radiol 1999; 30(3):198–205.
238. Le Bihan D. Molecular diffusion nuclear magnetic resonance imaging. Magn Reson Q 1991; 7(1):1–30.
239. Sugahara T, Korogi Y, Kochi M, Ikushima I, Shigematu Y, Hirai T, Okuda T, Liang L, Ge Y, Komohara Y, Ushio Y, Takahashi M. Usefulness of diffusion-weighted MRI with echo-planar

technique in the evaluation of cellularity in gliomas. J Magn Reson Imaging 1999; 9(1):53–60.

240. Pomper MG. Molecular imaging: an overview. Acad Radiol 2001; 8(11):1141–1153.
241. Kunkel M, Reichert TE, Benz P, Lehr HA, Jeong JH, Wieand S, Bartenstein P, Wagner W, Whiteside TL. Overexpression of Glut-1 and increased glucose metabolism in tumors are associated with a poor prognosis in patients with oral squamous cell carcinoma. Cancer 2003; 97(4):1015– 1024.
242. Flamen P, Van Cutsem E, Lerut A, Cambier JP, Haustermans K, Bormans G, De Leyn P, Van Raemdonck D, De Wever W, Ectors N, Maes A, Mortelmans L. Positron emission tomography for assessment of the response to induction radiochemotherapy in locally advanced oesophageal cancer. Ann Oncol 2002; 13(3):361–368.
243. Swisher SG, Erasmus J, Maish M, Correa AM, Macapinlac H, Ajani JA, Cox JD, Komaki RR, Hong D, Lee HK, Putnam JB Jr, Rice DC, Smythe WR, Thai L, Vaporciyan AA, Walsh GL, Wu TT, Roth JA. 2-Fluoro-2-deoxy-D-glucose positron emission tomography imaging is predictive of pathologic response and survival after preoperative chemoradiation in patients with esophageal carcinoma. Cancer 2004; 101(8):1776–1785.
244. MacManus MR, Hicks R, Fisher R, Rischin D, Michael M, Wirth A, Ball DL. FDG-PET-detected extracranial metastasis in patients with non-small cell lung cancer undergoing staging for surgery or radical radiotherapy–survival correlates with metastatic disease burden. Acta Oncol 2003; 42(1):48–54.
245. Hellwig D, Graeter TP, Ukena D, Georg T, Kirsch CM, Schafers HJ. Value of F-18-fluorodeoxyglucose positron emission tomography after induction therapy of locally advanced bronchogenic carcinoma. J Thorac Cardiovasc Surg 2004; 128(6):892–899.
246. Grigsby PW, Siegel BA, Dehdashti F, Rader J, Zoberi I. Posttherapy [18F] fluorodeoxyglucose positron emission tomography in carcinoma of the cervix: response and outcome. J Clin Oncol 2004; 22(11):2167–2171.
247. Brun E, Kjellen E, Tennvall J, Ohlsson T, Sandell A, Perfekt R, Wennerberg J, Strand SE. FDG PET studies during treatment: prediction of therapy outcome in head and neck squamous cell carcinoma. Head Neck 2002; 24(2):127–135.
248. Weber WA, Ott K, Becker K, Dittler HJ, Helmberger H, Avril NE, Meisetschlager G, Busch R, Siewert JR, Schwaiger M. Fink U. Prediction of response to preoperative chemotherapy in adenocarcinomas of the esophagogastric junction by metabolic imaging. J Clin Oncol 2001; 19(12):3058–3065.
249. Weber WA, Ott K. Imaging of esophageal and gastric cancer. Semin Oncol 2004; 31(4):530–541.
250. Weber WA, Petersen V, Schmidt B, Tyndale-Hines L, Link T, Peschel C. Schwaiger M. Positron emission tomography in non-small-cell lung cancer: prediction of response to chemotherapy by quantitative assessment of glucose use. J Clin Oncol 2003; 21(14):2651–2667.
251. Ott K, Fink U, Becker K, Stahl A, Dittler HJ, Busch R, Stein H, Lordick F, Link T, Schwaiger M, Siewert JR,Weber WA. Prediction of response to preoperative chemotherapy in gastric carcinoma by metabolic imaging: results of a prospective trial. J Clin Oncol 2003; 21(24):4604–4610.

5 Prognostic and Predictive Markers in Radiation Therapy: Focus on Prostate Cancer

Mark A. Ritter

Introduction

Biomarkers are molecular characteristics that provide clinically useful information in addition to that currently available via standard clinical and pathological testing. Continued development of molecular techniques has aided the discovery of new potential biomarkers for cancer and it is hoped that these will develop into tests useful in diagnosing as well as in defining prognosis and prognostic markers and predicting response to specific therapies, so-called predictive markers. Perhaps, even more importantly, the identification of predictive biomarkers may serve to identify molecular pathways of treatment resistance that might be selectively targeted or, when that is not possible, might be circumvented by choosing an alternative form of treatment with nonoverlapping modes of action.

While biomarker development continues across the entire spectrum of cancer types, this review will focus upon developments in the field of prostate cancer. Furthermore, the emphasis will be on biomarkers relating to prognosis and prediction of response to radiation therapy in local, regionally confined prostate cancer. Biomarker-enhanced early detection will not be considered here.

The Need for Biomarkers of Radiation Response in Prostate Cancer

Prostate cancer remains the second leading cause of cancer deaths in males in the US. Optimal treatment for clinically localized prostate cancer has not been determined, but radiation therapy plays a major role in the management of localized disease. In spite of a favorable toxicity profile and outcomes that appear to be comparable to those obtained with radical prostatectomy, clinical outcomes after radiation therapy still suggest that local and regional tumor recurrence remains a numerically and clinically important mode of treatment failure, one that can lead to subsequent disease dissemination [1].

M.P. Mehta et al. (eds.), *Radiation Oncology Advances.*

Recognition of the need to improve tumor control has led to investigations of combined radiation and androgen deprivation therapy [2, 3] and of conformal dose escalation [4–8]. These approaches have improved clinical outcome for patients with locally advanced and/or high grade tumors, but further progress may require a better understanding of how alterations in radiation and androgen deprivation response pathways can influence outcome.

In spite of PSA screening-powered earlier detection of prostate cancer, it is evident that a significant proportion of diagnosed patients still go on to failure of treatment, with some eventually succumbing to their disease. Furthermore, it has become increasingly evident that local failure continues to be a frequent cause of failure. While the classical clinical triad of stage, grade, and pretreatment PSA provides a useful initial prognostic snapshot, it is also clear that its prognostic accuracy has significant limitations. While most patients with favorable characteristics (low T stage, grade, and PSA) do have favorable outcomes independent of treatment modality, some continue to fail therapy. Similarly, at the other end of the spectrum, those with combinations of these factors conferring high risk frequently but not invariably fail. The widest prognostic uncertainties, however, fall within the group of so-called intermediate risk patients – generally although variably defined as having PSAs of greater than 10 ng/ml or Gleason scores of 7 or more or T stages of T2b or greater. These are patients with a wide range of outcomes and in whom a better ability to prognosticate outcome and a better understanding of the pathways of treatment response could present an ability to optimally select and individualize therapy. In addition, the value of proven biomarkers, whether predictive or prognostic, simply as stratification factors should not be overlooked. The identification and stratification of previously unappreciated treatment group heterogeneity can significantly enhance a study's power to detect real outcome differences between randomized treatment arms [9].

This review will focus on radiation therapy and prostate cancer and will discuss choice of markers and patient cohorts for study, strengths and limitations of existing correlative studies, measurement methodologies, and future directions and opportunities.

Optimal Biomarkers and Patient Cohort Characteristics

As with other primary tumors, there is evidence that prostate cancers can have molecular alterations that render them poorly responsive to radiation therapy, thus contributing to many of the treatment failures observed. If such radioresponse-altering molecular changes could be conclusively identified and reproducibly measured, their routine measurement could supplement the medical decision-making process and allow a better tailoring of treatment to the biological characteristics of each patient's tumor.

The key to identifying useful markers of radiation response lies in the proper selection of both of the markers to be tested and the patient cohort to test them in.

The ideal candidate marker should (1) have a biological rationale, including supportive preclinical data; (2) have sufficient prevalence to be practical as a predictor, and (3) be associated with or be amenable to a therapeutic solution, potentially some form of targeted therapy. At the clinical correlative level, the crucial test of a biomarker is whether it offers clinically useful information that is independent of that provided by well-recognized clinical prognosticators of recurrence and death, prognosticators such as clinical stage, Gleason score and pretreatment PSA in the case of prostate cancer.

Markers need to be judiciously and selectively chosen for testing, limiting the number studied in any given investigation, so as not to statistically compromise the ability of the study to separately identify each marker. Furthermore, the amount of pretreatment diagnostic tissue available may limit the analysis options available. In the case of prostate cancer, the small amount of tissue generally available from needle biopsies available in a radiotherapy setting significantly limits the type of testing that is feasible.

Gene expression panels that correlate with clinical outcome are an alternative to this individual candidate biomarker-specific approach. Such panels, discussed later, are potentially useful in providing prognostic and possibly predictive information but are less readily applicable to devising a molecular targeting approach that improves outcomes. Expression analyses can, however, be extremely useful in identifying individual biomarkers that warrant further investigation [10].

The clinical profile of patients included in correlative studies is equally important and must be matched with the goals of the study. The studied patient cohort must have been uniformly treated. Furthermore, patients need to have had a low likelihood of occult, distant disease at the time of diagnosis if response to localized radiation therapy is the clinical endpoint. In radiotherapy-treated prostate cancer, for example, follow-up policies usually do not include needle rebiopsy of the prostate in biochemically failing patients. This fact, together with the limited accuracy of needle rebiopsies even when carried out, make it imperative that attempts to correlate biomarker status with radiation-induced tumor control be performed in patient populations initially at low risk for occult metastatic disease. Favorable-to-intermediate risk patients comprise the optimal patient cohort for such studies.

Evaluation of Candidate Markers

Biological Rationale

In an effort to identify biomarkers that specifically predict treatment outcomes after radiotherapy, it is most logical to focus upon radiation response pathways and that will be the emphasis here. Numerous studies have indicated that the status of biologic markers associated with cell cycle control, DNA repair and apoptosis, such as p53, bcl-2, mdm2 or epidermal growth factor receptor (EGFr), can influence in vitro response to radiation in tumor cells from cancers of the breast [11–14], head and neck [15–19], and lung [20, 21]. Specifically for prostate cancer cells, the status of p53 has been found to alter the in vitro chemotherapy or radiation response [22–24] and to be directly or indirectly involved in DNA repair, cell cycle control, repopulation, and apoptosis [25]. mdm2 status has been found to alter the in vitro response of prostate cancer cells to radiation, antiandrogen treatment, or the two combined [26–28]. Bcl-2 status, as well, alters the radiation response of prostate cancer cells in vitro [29–31]. In addition, evidence supporting the role of prostaglandin signaling during cancer development and growth has led to studies combining Cox-2 inhibitors with radiation. An in vivo animal study found that the combination of radiotherapy with COX-2 inhibitors produced an improved response when compared to radiotherapy alone. The TCD 50 values in a xenograft tumor were found to be reduced by 50% with combined treatment [32].

Thus, there are good preclinical, biological rationales supporting a potential role of biomarkers involved in cell cycle control, DNA repair, or apoptosis as predictors of clinical radiation response. The focus of this review will be on biomarkers identified in clinical correlative studies as being associated with outcomes of radiation treatment. A brief description of the biological role of some of the most promising markers follows:

p53. The tumor suppressor gene, p53 has been extensively described as a central mediator of a cell's response to DNA damaging agents, with involvement in induction of the apoptotic response, DNA repair, and cell cycle delay [25]. DNA damage induces an increase in p53 protein levels, resulting in the potential activation of numerous molecular pathways. These include transcriptional activation of the cyclin-dependent kinase inhibitor p21WAF1/CIP1, which potentiates cell cycle arrest [33] as well as activation of GADD45 and its DNA repair-related actions [34]. p53 also induces transcriptional activation of mdm2, one of the main negative cellular regulators of p53 [35].

Numerous in vitro studies that have manipulated cellular p53 status have found increased resistance to the cytotoxic effects of radiation or chemotherapy when p53 function is disabled [36, 37] or increased sensitivity when p53 function is augmented [22–24]. Additionally, compromise of p53 function have been shown to shorten cell doubling times [38, 39], a change that might promote tumor clonogen repopulation during multiple fraction radiation therapy. These findings strongly imply that p53 dysfunction will reduce the effectiveness of radiation in controlling prostate cancer. However, since response to ionizing radiation could well involve a number of p53-mediated events, which require the integration of both intracellular and extracellular signals, the precise impact of p53 status upon radiosensitivity could vary with and should be determined in each type of tumor.

There also appear to be interactions between p53 status and response to antiandrogen therapy. It is well known that hormone refractory prostate cancers have a higher incidence of p53 mutations. Additionally, Berchardt et al. [40] found that antisense p53 cDNA transfected into LNCaP cells rendered these cells tumorogenic in castrated nude mice, implying a role for p53 in maintaining androgen dependence.

In prostate cancer, the majority of p53 mutations result in an over-accumulation of the functionally inactive p53 protein because of a prolonged protein half-life [41], an accumulation that can be conveniently detected using an immunohistochemical (IHC) approach [42]. Thus, a high p53 IHC staining intensity and labeling index correlates strongly with p53 mutations and could present an adequate, clinically practical alternative to a more time consuming, detailed mutational analysis.

Bcl-2 and bax. Apoptosis is a key molecular pathway of radiation-induced cell killing in many tumor types. Apoptosis is thought to play an important role in cell death in prostate cancer [43], both during antiandrogen and cytotoxic treatment [44]. The baseline apoptotic index has been found to predict for radiation response in bladder cancer [45], although no such direct evidence is currently available for prostate cancer. Bcl-2 is a key regulator of the apoptotic pathway and, thus, likely plays both p53-dependent and independent roles in modifying response to radiation. Specifically, bcl-2 antagonizes apoptosis primarily by blocking the release of cytochrome C from the mitochondria [46]. Given the contribution of apoptosis to radiation-induced cell killing, bcl-2, as a regulator of apoptosis, could well play an important role in tumor radiation response. Numerous prostate cancer studies have associated androgen-independent growth with bcl-2 overexpression and studies comparing tumorogenic growth in bcl-2 expressing and non-expressing LNCaP cell have found that bcl-2 expression confers androgen independence [47]. These studies suggest that bcl-2-overexpressing prostate tumors will be less responsive to androgen deprivation therapy. As will be discussed, there are some correlative data suggesting a role for bcl-2 as a predictor of radiation response in prostate cancer. Should such findings be verified, the current availability of anti-bcl-2 agents offers a roadmap for targeted therapeutic intervention.

mdm2. This is a particularly intriguing potential marker. mdm2 is under transcriptional control of p53 and in turn binds to p53 thereby promoting its degradation and inhibiting its transcriptional activation of genes related to cell cycle arrest and apoptosis [48]. Overexpression of mdm2 is found in many different tumors including bladder [49], bronchogenic [50], and prostate [51, 52] and appears to be a common mechanism of p53 inactivation contributing to transformation. In addition, mdm2 has been shown to bind to pRB, E2F, and RNA, suggesting that mdm2 has p53-independent activities that may also be associated with its transforming properties and may contribute to progression.

Several studies [26, 28] have found that specific antihuman-mdm2, mixed-backbone oligonucleotides had significant antitumor activity in both in vitro and in vivo prostate cancer models, regardless of p53 status, and increased response to certain chemotherapeutic agents. These data support the concept that mdm2 has a role in cancer progression and resistance to therapy through both p53-dependent and independent mechanisms. Furthermore, Pollack et al. [27] have found that antisense oligonucleotide-based suppression of mdm2 leads to increased in vitro sensitivity of LNCaP cells to radiation, androgen deprivation therapy, and both treatments combined. Similarly, Grunbaum et al. have found that antisense mdm2 produces radiosensitization and increased apoptosis, although this was in a sarcoma cell line [53].

Should mdm2 prove to be predictive of response to radiation and androgen ablation, systemically delivered antisense oligonucleotides [54] could become a feasible therapeutic intervention. The ability of mdm2 to create resistance to both radiation and androgen deprivation together with its frequent overexpression in prostate cancer suggests a promising potential as a predictive biomarker and therapeutic target.

Biomarker Frequency

An infrequently abnormal marker, even if highly correlated with radiosensitivity, will have poor efficiency as a predictor or prognosticator. Similarly, a very high frequency of abnormality will have limited usefulness, although involvement in an important response pathway could still provide selective targeting opportunities. Thus, from a predictive usefulness standpoint, the most effective potential predictive markers will be those with neither low nor high but moderate prevalence in the identified patient cohort. Table 1 summarizes report frequencies for some of the markers discussed above and it is noted that the prevalence of many of these markers appear satisfactory for use in predictive testing.

Table 1 Frequency of the presence of abnormal biomarker levels in early stage prostate cancer

Marker	% abnormal	Reference
p53	20–40	[55–58]
Bcl-2	16–25	[55, 59, 60]
Bax	21	[59]
mdm2	32–44	[51, 52, 62]
Ki-67	27–33	[52, 59]
Cox-2	83	[62]
p16	27<25% labeling	[63]
pRB	73>20% labeling	

Biomarker Assessment Methods

A number of approaches, including immunohistochemistry, mass spectroscopy, mutational analysis, and expression analysis are now actively being applied in developing diagnostic and prognostic biomarkers in a variety of cancers including prostate [64]. Recent expression analysis studies have found intriguing correlations between expression of sets of genes and clinical outcome in prostate cancer [10, 65, 66]. Some of the identified genes serve dual functions, providing growth advantages in the primary tumor as well as facilitating metastasis. However, all such studies to date include only patients drawn from radical prostatectomy cohorts and, thus, do not speak directly to radiation therapy-specific prognosis. Preliminary investigations utilizing comparative genomic hybridization have also suggested the ability to identify markers that specifically identify metastatic lymph node risk [67] with early results suggesting predictive accuracy rates of about 75%, similar to the accuracy of standard prognostic nomograms. Another differential gene expression profiling study of clinically localized prostate tumors from relapsing and nonrelapsing patients identified a set of four genes with a pattern of expression that could predict recurrence [68].

Most biomarker-clinical correlation information available for radiation-treated prostate cancer patients has been obtained using an immunohistochemical approach, a direct consequence of the limited tissue available from diagnostic needle biopsies. Methods employing laser capture microdissection of needle biopsy specimens followed by expression analysis are currently under development, but again are hindered by the small amount of tissue readily available as well as by reduced RNA recovery from formalin-fixed tissues. Similarly, retrospective mass spectroscopy-based proteomic studies are hindered both by limited tissue and formalin fixation [69]. Also of potential concern is the risk that core needle biopsies may not always fully represent the majority of the cancer in the prostate, but needle biopsies are the only specimens generally available for predictive assays in patients treated with radiation therapy. However, as will be described, there are correlative studies using such samples that do suggest considerable predictive or prognostic promise. It should be noted that Gleason scores are also subject to core biopsy-related sampling errors, yet are highly correlated with outcome after primary radiation therapy.

The challenges presented by limited tissue and formalin fixation have forced a heavy reliance on immunohistochemistry in such correlative studies of outcome in radiation-treated prostate cancer; it is therefore useful to briefly discuss the strengths and limitations of the technology.

Immunohistochemistry

While being the most commonly used method for detecting antigen levels in tissue, IHC is subject to potential artifacts throughout all stages of the process, including fixation, storage, staining, and scoring. Variable fixation procedures can influence antigen availability, as can differing antigen retrieval methods. The use of different antibodies and staining procedures for the same biomarker can make interstudy comparisons difficult. Finally, the scoring methodology itself, whether employed with suitable controls and whether manual or image analysis assisted, can also significantly influence outcomes.

Automated digital microscopy-based analysis of immunohistochemical stains (with appropriate staining controls and optimized staining) may provide a more quantitative and reproducible means of analysis of protein expression in formalin-fixed tissues than does manual counting alone. Studies comparing digital microscopy-assisted counting to manual counting indicate excellent correlation between the two and suggest better accuracy at the very low and very high ends of the labeling index spectrum [70]. Perhaps the strongest rationale for using such systems is their potential to assist in standardizing marker analysis methodologies so that clinically useful markers can be more fully exploited throughout the oncology community. Biomarkers must be reproducible (both within and between institutes) in order to have any significant impact on clinical management. Tissue microarrays would ideally be used in such studies, given their cost and time effectiveness [71], but unfortunately their use is challenging when tissue specimens are limited to that available from core needle biopsies.

Clinical Correlative Data in Prostate Cancer

There exists a growing body of clinical correlative data for prostate cancer linking clinical outcomes after radiation therapy with several molecular markers involved in cell cycle control, DNA repair, apoptosis, and proliferation. A summary of biomarker correlative studies in radiation-treated prostate cancer patients is contained in Table 2 and is described below.

Table 2 Abnormal marker expression vs. clinical outcomes after radiation therapy for early stage prostate cancer

Marker	# patients	Predicts failure?	When assessed?	Reference
p53	129	+(high labeling)	Pretreatment	[57]
p53	13	+(high labeling)	At recurrence	[72]
p53	53	+(high labeling)	Pretreatment	[58]
p53	55	+(high labeling)	At recurrence	[56]
GST-pi		+(high labeling)		
p53	54	+(high labeling)	Pretreatment	[55]
Bcl-2		+(high labeling)		
Bcl-2	43 Pre-RT;	+(high labeling) ±(high labeling)	Pretreatment and at recurrence	[73]
p53	53 Post-RT			
Bcl-2	42	+(low labeling)	Pretreatment	[74]
Bcl-2	77	+(high labeling)	Pretreatment	[59]
Bcl-2; bax	119	No	Pretreatment	[75]
Bcl-2	20	+(high labeling)	At recurrence	[76]
Bcl-2/bax ratio	41	+(high ratio)	Pretreatment	[77]
Bax	77	+(low labeling)	Pretreatment	[59]
Ki-67	108	+(high labeling)	Pretreatment	[78, 79]
mdm-2	108	+(high labeling)	Pretreatment	[61]
p16	67	+(low labeling)	Pretreatment	[63]
pRb		±(high labeling)		
Cox-2	586	+(>intensity)	Pretreatment	[80]

Markers of Cell Cycle Control, DNA Repair and Apoptosis

We have reported a strong, independent correlation between p53 overaccumulation and poor radiation therapy outcome in early-to-intermediate risk prostate cancer patients [58], consistent with the reports of others [55, 56, 72]. Correlation between poor radiation therapy outcome and elevated bcl-2 or reduced bax status have been reported by Pollack [59] and others [55, 73, 76, 77], but the relationships have not been confirmed in all studies [74, 75], leaving the status of bcl-2 and bax as radiation biomarkers in doubt.

In addition, mdm2 overexpression has been found to independently correlate with poor outcome in a group of patients with locally advanced prostate cancer treated with radiation with or without hormonal therapy [61]. Low expression of the marker, p16, has also been found to correlate independently with increased recurrence rates [63], while increased intensity of staining of Cox-2 has been found to correlate independently with outcome in radiation therapy-treated patients as well [80].

Marker status in all of these studies was determined using immunohistochemical analyses and primarily performed on pretreatment biopsies, with abnormal levels of these selected markers correlating with increased risk of recurrence.

Proliferation

Since disregulation of proliferation is an essential element of malignant progression, biomarkers of proliferation might therefore be expected to provide prognostic information. The Ki-67 index, for example, in spite of some correlation with tumor grade, has been found to be independently prognostic for outcome in patients with clinically localized disease treated with radiotherapy [59, 78]. In addition, another clinical correlative study has linked high Ki-67 labeling index to poor clinical outcomes in patients treated with combined androgen deprivation and radiation [79]. The clinical trial studied, RTOG 92-02, included 537 intermediate-to-high risk prostate cancer patients. The Ki-67 index was investigated as a continuous variable vs. the clinical endpoints of local control, biochemical control, disease-specific survival, and overall survival. In multivariate analyses that included PSA, Gleason score, and T-stage, Ki-67 staining index was associated with local failure ($p = 0.08$), biochemical failure ($p = 0.0445$), distant metastases ($p = 0.0001$), cause specific mortality ($p = 0.0001$), and overall mortality ($p = 0.0094$). In fact, Ki67 was the most significant determinant of metastasis and cause specific mortality.

A high Ki-67 labeling index has also, however, been found to be correlated with poorer outcome in patient cohorts treated with radical prostatectomy [81] as well as in patients who were primarily expectantly managed [82, 83], implying that Ki-67 may be more of a global prognosticator than a radiation-specific predictor of outcome.

Hypoxia

Molecular assessments of hypoxia can serve as biomarkers. Hypoxia has long been understood as a physiologic state that occurs frequently in solid tumors and that can significantly protect tumor cells from the cytotoxic effects of radiation, with a more recent recognition that hypoxia can also serve as a promoter of malignant progression. Hypoxia has been found in a microelectrode study to predict for poor outcome in patients with localized prostate cancer treated with radiotherapy [84]. There is both direct microelectrode and indirect immunihistochemical and hypoxic imaging evidence that prostate cancers as well as prostatic hyperplasia can contain significant areas of hypoxia [85]. Furthermore, several studies demonstrate correlations between hypoxia and other markers of tumor aggressiveness, such as high Gleason score and vessel density, suggesting that a hypoxic microenvironment promotes malignant progression to more aggressive cell phenotypes, potentially conferring greater radioresistance as well as greater propensity to metastasize [85]. Such a relationship in prostate cancer would not be unexpected, given the mounting evidence for tumors in other anatomic sites, particularly head and neck, that tumor hypoxia can have a profound negative influence both on local tumor control and overall survival [86, 87].

Tumor hypoxia can be assessed prospectively using systemically administered hypoxia markers such as the 2-nitroimidazole, pimonidazole, followed by immunohistochemical detection [85], or with PET-based hypoxia imaging agents such [18F]-fluoromisonidazole [88] or Cu-ATSM [89]. Retrospective analyses in tissue sections using intrinsic hypoxia-induced markers such as Hif-1a, Hif-2a, and CA-IX have also shown promise, with the majority of studies taking place in head and neck cancer patients [90]. In addition, there has been some success in correlating serum osteopontin, a secreted phosphoglycoprotein, both with tumor microelectrode O2 levels as well as with clinical outcomes in radiation-treated head and neck patients [91–93].

To date, with the exception of the microelectrode study [84], the role of hypoxia in radio resistance and recurrence of prostate cancer has not been explored in clinical studies. The ready availability of intrinsic hypoxia markers applicable to biopsy specimens makes such studies attractive.

Limitations of Existing Studies

While studies such as those described above have provided useful hypothesis-building insights, many of these cited in Table 2 are from single institutions and involved relatively small numbers of patients. Furthermore, some permitted the inclusion of patients with a broad range of pretreatment prognoses (including very high PSAs, high tumor grades, and even hormonally resistant disease in some cases) or focused on more locally advanced prostate cancer. Our study [58] did limit eligibility to early-to-intermediate risk patients who were uniformly treated with radiation alone.

The studies cited in Table 2 that have employed biopsy specimens from Radiation Therapy Oncology Group (RTOG) prostate trials in studying p53 [57], mdm2 [61], p16 [63], Ki-67 [79], and Cox-2 [80] are exceptions that offer the advantage of larger patient numbers along with narrowly defined clinical and treatment characteristics. These trials, however, have focused on patients with more locally advanced, high-risk disease than is typically seen contemporarily in the era of PSA screening. Thus, although these studies provide provocative evidence for the predictive value of many of these markers, further validation of these correlative relationships in contemporarily relevant, early-to-intermediate risk patients is needed. Furthermore, information remains limited concerning the predictive power of these markers in the context of combined radiation/androgen deprivation therapy.

Additionally, all of these studies have been carried out in patient cohorts that have received radiation doses of 66–70 Gy, doses now generally considered suboptimal, with the question being whether higher radiation doses would overcome at least in part the poor prognostic impact associated with these markers at lower radiation doses. Finally, virtually all of these studies have included only patients treated with radiotherapy, leaving unresolved whether the correlations observed between outcome and biomarkers are specifically linked to radiation response or rather, simply reflect a prognostic power independent of treatment modality. In that regard, we have reported a strong, independent correlation between p53 status and radiation therapy outcome in early-to-intermediate risk prostate cancer patients [58]. This correlation was found to be highly significant for 80 radiation-treated patients, but not for 84 clinically matched, surgery-treated patients [60], suggesting that, for radiation, p53 is truly a predictive rather than a prognostic marker.

Future Studies and Directions

Large Prospective Clinical Trials

Additional studies are needed that focus on large groups of patients with long follow-up and with narrowly defined pretreatment characteristics that decrease the likelihood of distant disease at the time of treatment (PSA ≤20 ng/ml and Gleason score ≤7), characteristics that better match those of patients most commonly diagnosed today. A focus on earlier stage disease also reduces the risk of occult metastatic disease at presentation, thereby enhancing the ability to test marker predictive value for a local modality such as radiation therapy. It is only through such large, well-controlled studies that biomarkers preliminarily identified as promising can be validated.

The Radiation Therapy Oncology Group (RTOG) began in the 1980s to acquire and centrally store diagnostic biopsy specimens from a variety of primary tumors from patients enrolled on a number of RTOG studies, including many for prostate cancer. While earlier RTOG prostate trials, as previously discussed, focused on patients with locally advanced, higher risk disease, more recent studies have increasingly addressed management of intermediate and low risk patients. Using this valuable tissue repository resource containing paraffin-embedded core biopsy specimens, a number of new biomarker studies are currently underway in addition to the RTOG-derived studies cited above. These include ongoing studies of p53, bcl-2, bax, Ki-67, mdm-2, Survivin, AKT, and Stat3. It will ultimately be necessary to rank and prioritize these markers based upon how strongly they demonstrate independent correlations with clinical outcome.

Biomarker-Based Adaptive Therapy

The most straightforward approach in prostate cancer patients identified through prognostic markers as having radioresistant tumors would be to simply escalate dose or, when medically feasible, to redirect patients to surgery. However, the identification of clinically relevant radiation response biomarkers would also provide tremendous insight into a specific tumor's mechanisms of resistance to radiation (or androgen deprivation therapy), an insight that could potentially allow novel biologic/molecular therapeutic approaches to be administered in an individualized fashion.

There are numerous examples of potential molecular or chemotherapy targeting strategies currently in either preclinical or early clinical development that could form the rationale for future biomarker-guided, protocol-based investigations. These include antisense, gene replacement, and small molecule inhibitor approaches. For p53, examples include targeting with gene replacement [94], p53 mutant targeting oncolytic viruses [95] or taxanes, which, unlike many other chemotherapeutics, maintain activity against p53 mutant tumors [96]. There also are emerging small molecule-based strategies that either induce conformational changes in mutant p53 protein that restore its functional activity or interfere with the mdm2–p53 interaction that promotes p53 destruction [97]. Another alternative is a small molecule, pifithrin, that inhibits p53 function in p53 wild type cells, offering the potential of protecting normal tissues from radiation during dose escalation while leaving mutant p53 tumor radiosensitivity unchanged [98]. Examples of targeting other biomarkers include bcl-2 [30, 31, 99] or mdm-2 [28] antisense approaches. Since androgen deprivation therapy is often given adjunctively with radiotherapy in prostate cancer, biomarker studies might also dictate when a selective application of androgen deprivation is warranted. For example, androgen deprivation therapy might be found to eliminate a suboptimal radiation-only outcome associated with a particular biomarker abnormality.

Conclusion

The immense potential of predictive biomarkers for improving prostate cancer treatment has stimulated the investigation of numerous molecular marker candidates. Several that have undergone individual testing have shown considerable promise, among them p53, Ki-67, mdm-2, p16 and Cox-2, most of which have shown correlations with clinical outcome independent of standard clinical prognostic parameters. However, the field still remains in its early phase, with no biomarker to date having undergone rigorous validation. A number of other markers have shown promise in radical prostatectomy patients, including p16INK4A, p27Kip1, c-Myc, AR, E-cadherin, and VEGF, diminishing their likelihood of being useful as radiation-specific biomarkers. By the same reasoning, markers that have been shown to influence outcome after radiation therapy should be tested in paired studies of radiation and surgery patients to explore their degree of radiation specificity.

In addition, further progress in identifying and validating biomarkers of occult metastatic disease could permit modeling of the competitive risks of tumor local recurrence vs. occult lymph node metastases, allowing more informed decisions regarding treatment modifications such as androgen ablation therapy and pelvic lymph node irradiation.

For further progress to be maximized, immunostaining analysis methods must become more quantitative and reproducible and archived pathology specimens from large, controlled clinical trials should be employed. Clinical tissue repositories should routinely store frozen tissue and plasma to increase analysis options. Testing must adapt to the tissue quantity limitations inherent in core needle biopsy specimens and move beyond its focus on individual candidate markers and imunohistochemistry to employ high volume gene expression and proteomic techniques. These methods, together with bioinformatics methodology, could not only identify new, individual biomarkers, but also help better define radioresponse pathways and their elements, so that markers that occupy functionally parallel or serial pathways can be identified. Such information will be necessary before predictive biomarker strategies can be optimized.

References

1. Fuks Z, Leibel SA, Wallner KE, et al. The effect of local control on metastatic dissemination in carcinoma of the prostate: long-term results in patients treated with 125I implantation. Int J Radiat Oncol Biol Phys 1991; 21(3):537–547.
2. Pilepich MV, Krall JM, al-Sarraf M, et al. Androgen deprivation with radiation therapy compared with radiation therapy alone for locally advanced prostatic carcinoma: a randomized comparative trial of the Radiation Therapy Oncology Group. Urology 1995; 45(4):616–623.
3. Bolla M, Gonzalez D, Warde P, et al. Improved survival in patients with locally advanced prostate cancer treated with radiotherapy and goserelin. N Engl J Med 1997; 337(5):295–300.

4. Hanks GE, Lee WR, Hanlon AL, et al. Conformal technique dose escalation for prostate cancer: biochemical evidence of improved cancer control with higher doses in patients with pretreatment prostate-specific antigen > or = 10 NG/ML [see comments]. Int J Radiat Oncol Biol Phys 1996; 35(5):861–868.
5. Zelefsky MJ, Leibel SA, Gaudin PB, et al. Dose escalation with three-dimensional conformal radiation therapy affects the outcome in prostate cancer [see comments]. Int J Radiat Oncol Biol Phys 1998; 41(3):491–500.
6. Roach M 3rd, Meehan S, Kroll S, et al. Radiotherapy for high grade clinically localized adenocarcinoma of the prostate [see comments]. J Urol 1996; 156(5):1719–1723.
7. Vicini FA, Kestin LL, Martinez AA. The importance of adequate follow-up in defining treatment success after external beam irradiation for prostate cancer. Int J Radiat Oncol Biol Phys 1999; 45(3):553–561.
8. Pollack A, Zagars GK, Starkschall G, et al. Prostate cancer radiation dose response: results of the M. D. Anderson phase III randomized trial. Int J Radiat Oncol Biol Phys 2002; 53(5):1097–1105.
9. Betensky RA, Louis DN, Cairncross JG. Influence of unrecognized molecular heterogeneity on randomized clinical trials. J Clin Oncol 2002; 20(10):2495–2499.
10. Henshall SM, Afar DE, Hiller J, et al. Survival analysis of genome-wide gene expression profiles of prostate cancers identifies new prognostic targets of disease relapse. Cancer Res 2003; 63(14):4196–4203.
11. Chiarugi V, Magnelli L, Cinelli M. Role of p53 mutations in the radiosensitivity status of tumor cells. Tumori 1998; 84(5):517–520.
12. Meyn MS. Ataxia-telangiectasia and cellular responses to DNA damage. Cancer Res 1995; 55(24):5991–6001.
13. Meyn RE, Stephens LC, Mason KA, Medina D. Radiation-induced apoptosis in normal and pre-neoplastic mammary glands in vivo: significance of gland differentiation and p53 status. Int J Cancer 1996; 65(4):466–472.
14. Sakakura C, Sweeney EA, Shirahama T, et al. Overexpression of bax sensitizes human breast cancer MCF-7 cells to radiation-induced apoptosis. Int J Cancer 1996; 67(1):101–105.
15. Huang SM, Bock JM, Harari PM. Epidermal growth factor receptor blockade with C225 modulates proliferation, apoptosis, and radiosensitivity in squamous cell carcinomas of the head and neck [In Process Citation]. Cancer Res 1999; 59(8):1935–1940.
16. Nogueira CP, Dolan RW, Gooey J, et al. Inactivation of p53 and amplification of cyclin D1 correlate with clinical outcome in head and neck cancer. Laryngoscope 1998; 108(3):345–350.
17. Raybaud-Diogene H, Fortin A, Morency R, Roy J, Monteil RA, Tetu B. Markers of radioresistance in squamous cell carcinomas of the head and neck: a clinicopathologic and immunohistochemical study. J Clin Oncol 1997; 15(3):1030–1038.
18. Servomaa K, Kiuru A, Grenman R, Pekkola-Heino K, Pulkkinen JO, Rytomaa T. p53 mutations associated with increased sensitivity to ionizing radiation in human head and neck cancer cell lines. Cell Prolif 1996; 29(5):219–230.
19. Sheridan MT, O'Dwyer T, Seymour CB, Mothersill CE. Potential indicators of radiosensitivity in squamous cell carcinoma of the head and neck. Radiat Oncol Investig 1997; 5(4):180–186.
20. Biard DS, Martin M, Rhun YL, et al. Concomitant p53 gene mutation and increased radiosensitivity in rat lung embryo epithelial cells during neoplastic development. Cancer Res 1994; 54(13):3361–3364.
21. Sirzen F, Zhivotovsky B, Nilsson A, Bergh J, Lewensohn R. Spontaneous and radiation-induced apoptosis in lung carcinoma cells with different intrinsic radiosensitivities. Anticancer Res 1998; 18(2A):695–699.
22. Ahmed MM, Sells SF, Venkatasubbarao K, et al. Ionizing radiation-inducible apoptosis in the absence of p53 linked to transcription factor EGR-1. J Biol Chem 1997; 272(52):33056–33061.

23. Colletier PJ, Ashoori F, Cowen D, et al. Adenoviral-mediated p53 transgene expression sensitizes both wild-type and null p53 prostate cancer cells in vitro to radiation. Int J Radiat Oncol Biol Phys 2000; 48(5):1507–1512.
24. Sasaki R, Shirakawa T, Zhang ZJ, et al. Additional gene therapy with Ad5CMV-p53 enhanced the efficacy of radiotherapy in human prostate cancer cells. Int J Radiat Oncol Biol Phys 2001; 51(5):1336–1345.
25. Cuddihy AR, Bristow RG. The p53 protein family and radiation sensitivity: Yes or no? Cancer Metastasis Rev 2004; 23(3–4):237–257.
26. Wang H, Yu D, Agrawal S, Zhang R. Experimental therapy of human prostate cancer by inhibiting MDM2 expression with novel mixed-backbone antisense oligonucleotides: in vitro and in vivo activities and mechanisms. Prostate 2003; 54(3):194–205.
27. Mu Z, Hachem P, Agrawal S, Pollack A. Antisense MDM2 sensitizes prostate cancer cells to androgen deprivation, radiation, and the combination. Int J Radiat Oncol Biol Phys 2004; 58(2):336–343.
28. Zhang Z, Li M, Wang H, Agrawal S, Zhang R. Antisense therapy targeting MDM2 oncogene in prostate cancer: Effects on proliferation, apoptosis, multiple gene expression, and chemotherapy. Proc Natl Acad Sci USA 2003.
29. An J, Chervin AS, Nie A, Ducoff HS, Huang Z. Overcoming the radioresistance of prostate cancer cells with a novel Bcl-2 inhibitor. Oncogene 2006.
30. Mu Z, Hachem P, Pollack A. Antisense Bcl-2 sensitizes prostate cancer cells to radiation. Prostate 2005; 65(4):331–340.
31. Scott SL, Higdon R, Beckett L, et al. BCL2 antisense reduces prostate cancer cell survival following irradiation. Cancer Biother Radiopharm 2002; 17(6):647–656.
32. Kishi K, Petersen S, Petersen C, et al. Preferential enhancement of tumor radioresponse by a cyclooxygenase-2 inhibitor. Cancer Res 2000; 60(5):1326–1331.
33. Dulic V, Kaufmann WK, Wilson SJ, et al. p53-dependent inhibition of cyclin-dependent kinase activities in human fibroblasts during radiation-induced G1 arrest. Cell 1994; 76(6):1013–1023.
34. Smith ML, Chen IT, Zhan Q, et al. Interaction of the p53-regulated protein Gadd45 with proliferating cell nuclear antigen. Science 1994; 266(5189):1376–1380.
35. Momand J, Wu HH, Dasgupta G. MDM2–master regulator of the p53 tumor suppressor protein. Gene 2000; 242(1–2):15–29.
36. Siles E, Villalobos M, Valenzuela MT, et al. Relationship between p53 status and radiosensitivity in human tumour cell lines. Br J Cancer 1996; 73(5):581–588.
37. Li CY, Nagasawa H, Dahlberg WK, Little JB. Diminished capacity for p53 in mediating a radiation-induced G1 arrest in established human tumor cell lines. Oncogene 1995; 11(9):1885–1892.
38. Langendijk JA, Thunnissen FB, Lamers RJ, de Jong JM, ten Velde GP, Wouters EF. The prognostic significance of accumulation of p53 protein in stage III non-small cell lung cancer treated by radiotherapy. Radiother Oncol 1995; 36(3):218–224.
39. Bourhis J, Bosq J, Wilson GD, et al. Correlation between p53 gene expression and tumor-cell proliferation in oropharyngeal cancer. Int J Cancer 1994; 57(4):458–462.
40. Burchardt M, Burchardt T, Shabsigh A, et al. Reduction of wild type p53 function confers a hormone resistant phenotype on LNCaP prostate cancer cells. Prostate 2001; 48(4):225–230.
41. Rovinski B, Benchimol S. Immortalization of rat embryo fibroblasts by the cellular p53 oncogene. Oncogene 1988; 2(5):445–452.
42. Wertz IE, Deitch AD, Gumerlock PH, Gandour-Edwards R, Chi SG, de Vere White RW. Correlation of genetic and immunodetection of TP53 mutations in malignant and benign prostate tissues. Hum Pathol 1996; 27(6):573–580.
43. Sklar GN, Eddy HA, Jacobs SC, Kyprianou N. Combined antitumor effect of suramin plus irradiation in human prostate cancer cells: the role of apoptosis. J Urol 1993; 150(5 Pt 1): 1526–1532.

44. Bruckheimer EM, Gjertsen BT, McDonnell TJ. Implications of cell death regulation in the pathogenesis and treatment of prostate cancer. Semin Oncol 1999; 26(4):382–398.
45. Chyle V, Pollack A, Czerniak B, et al. Apoptosis and downstaging after preoperative radiotherapy for muscle- invasive bladder cancer [see comments]. Int J Radiat Oncol Biol Phys 1996; 35(2):281–287.
46. Shimizu S, Narita M, Tsujimoto Y. Bcl-2 family proteins regulate the release of apoptogenic cytochrome c by the mitochondrial channel VDAC. Nature 1999; 399(6735):483–487.
47. Beham AW, Sarkiss M, Brisbay S, Tu SM, von Eschenbach AC, McDonnell TJ. Molecular correlates of bcl-2-enhanced growth following androgen-ablation in prostate carcinoma cells in vivo. Int J Mol Med 1998; 1(6):953–959.
48. Momand J, Zambetti GP, Olson DC, George D, Levine AJ. The mdm-2 oncogene product forms a complex with the p53 protein and inhibits p53-mediated transactivation. Cell 1992; 69(7):1237–1245.
49. Lianes P, Orlow I, Zhang ZF, et al. Altered patterns of MDM2 and TP53 expression in human bladder cancer. J Natl Cancer Inst 1994; 86(17):1325–1330.
50. Gorgoulis VG, Rassidakis GZ, Karameris AM, et al. Immunohistochemical and molecular evaluation of the mdm-2 gene product in bronchogenic carcinoma. Mod Pathol 1996;9(5):544–554.
51. Leite KR, Franco MF, Srougi M, et al. Abnormal expression of MDM2 in prostate carcinoma. Mod Pathol 2001; 14(5):428–436.
52. Osman I, Drobnjak M, Fazzari M, Ferrara J, Scher HI, Cordon-Cardo C. Inactivation of the p53 pathway in prostate cancer: impact on tumor progression. Clin Cancer Res 1999; 5(8):2082–2088.
53. Grunbaum U, Meye A, Bache M, et al. Transfection with mdm2-antisense or wtp53 results in radiosensitization and an increased apoptosis of a soft tissue sarcoma cell line. Anticancer Res 2001; 21(3B):2065–2071.
54. Agrawal S, Kandimalla ER, Yu D, et al. Potentiation of antitumor activity of irinotecan by chemically modified oligonucleotides. Int J Oncol 2001; 18(5):1061–1069.
55. Ritter MA, Gilchrist KW, Voytovich M, Chappell RJ, Verhoven BM. The role of p53 in radiation therapy outcomes for favorable-to-intermediate-risk prostate cancer. Int J Radiat Oncol Biol Phys 2002; 53(3):574–580.
56. Scherr DS, Vaughan ED Jr, Wei J, et al. BCL-2 and p53 expression in clinically localized prostate cancer predicts response to external beam radiotherapy. J Urol 1999; 162(1):12–16; discussion 6–7.
57. Cheng L, Sebo TJ, Cheville JC, et al. p53 protein overexpression is associated with increased cell proliferation in patients with locally recurrent prostate carcinoma after radiation therapy. Cancer 1999; 85(6):1293–1299.
58. Grignon DJ, Caplan R, Sarkar FH, et al. p53 status and prognosis of locally advanced prostatic adenocarcinoma: a study based on RTOG 8610. J Natl Cancer Inst 1997; 89(2):158–165.
59. Pollack A, Cowen D, Troncoso P, et al. Molecular markers of outcome after radiotherapy in patients with prostate carcinoma: Ki-67, bcl-2, bax, and bcl-x. Cancer 2003; 97(7):1630–1638.
60. Ritter MA. Unpublished. 2006.
61. Khor LY, Desilvio M, Al-Saleem T, et al. MDM2 as a predictor of prostate carcinoma outcome: an analysis of Radiation Therapy Oncology Group Protocol 8610. Cancer 2005; 104(5):962–967.
62. Lee LM, Pan CC, Cheng CJ, Chi CW, Liu TY. Expression of cyclooxygenase-2 in prostate adenocarcinoma and benign prostatic hyperplasia. Anticancer Res 2001; 21(2B):1291–1294.
63. Chakravarti A, Heydon K, Wu CL, et al. Loss of p16 expression is of prognostic significance in locally advanced prostate cancer: an analysis from the Radiation Therapy Oncology Group protocol 86–10. J Clin Oncol 2003; 21(17):3328–3334.
64. Calvo A, Gonzalez-Moreno O, Yoon CY, et al. Prostate cancer and the genomic revolution: Advances using microarray analyses. Mutat Res 2005; 576(1–2):66–79.

65. Lapointe J, Li C, Higgins JP, et al. Gene expression profiling identifies clinically relevant subtypes of prostate cancer. Proc Natl Acad Sci USA 2004; 101(3):811–816.
66. Singh D, Febbo PG, Ross K, et al. Gene expression correlates of clinical prostate cancer behavior. Cancer Cell 2002; 1(2):203–209.
67. Paris PL, Weinberg V, Simko J, et al. Preliminary evaluation of prostate cancer metastatic risk biomarkers. Int J Biol Markers 2005; 20(3):141–145.
68. Latil A, Bieche I, Chene L, et al. Gene expression profiling in clinically localized prostate cancer: a four-gene expression model predicts clinical behavior. Clin Cancer Res 2003; 9(15):5477–5485.
69. Ornstein DK, Tyson DR. Proteomics for the identification of new prostate cancer biomarkers. Urol Oncol 2006; 24(3):231–236.
70. Hilbe W, Gachter A, Duba HC, et al. Comparison of automated cellular imaging system and manual microscopy for immunohistochemically stained cryostat sections of lung cancer specimens applying p53, ki-67 and p120. Oncol Rep 2003; 10(1):15–20.
71. Milanes-Yearsley M, Hammond ME, Pajak TF, et al. Tissue micro-array: a cost and time-effective method for correlative studies by regional and national cancer study groups. Mod Pathol 2002; 15(12):1366–1373.
72. Grossfeld GD, Olumi AF, Connolly JA, et al. Locally recurrent prostate tumors following either radiation therapy or radical prostatectomy have changes in Ki-67 labeling index, p53 and bcl- 2 immunoreactivity. J Urol 1998; 159(5):1437–1443.
73. Huang A, Gandour-Edwards R, Rosenthal SA, Siders DB, Deitch AD, White RW. p53 and bcl-2 immunohistochemical alterations in prostate cancer treated with radiation therapy. Urology 1998; 51(2):346–351.
74. Bylund A, Stattin P, Widmark A, Bergh A. Predictive value of bcl-2 immunoreactivity in prostate cancer patients treated with radiotherapy. Radiother Oncol 1998; 49(2):143–148.
75. Khor LY, Desilvio M, Li R, et al. Bcl-2 and bax expression and prostate cancer outcome in men treated with radiotherapy in Radiation Therapy Oncology Group protocol 86–10. Int J Radiat Oncol Biol Phys 2006; 66(1):25–30.
76. Rosser CJ, Reyes AO, Vakar-Lopez F, et al. Bcl-2 is significantly overexpressed in localized radio-recurrent prostate carcinoma, compared with localized radio-naive prostate carcinoma. Int J Radiat Oncol Biol Phys 2003; 56(1):1–6.
77. Mackey TJ, Borkowski A, Amin P, Jacobs SC, Kyprianou N. bcl-2/bax ratio as a predictive marker for therapeutic response to radiotherapy in patients with prostate cancer. Urology 1998; 52(6):1085–1090.
78. Cowen D, Troncoso P, Khoo VS, et al. Ki-67 staining is an independent correlate of biochemical failure in prostate cancer treated with radiotherapy. Clin Cancer Res 2002; 8(5):1148–1154.
79. Pollack A, DeSilvio M, Khor LY, et al. Ki-67 staining is a strong predictor of distant metastasis and mortality for men with prostate cancer treated with radiotherapy plus androgen deprivation: Radiation Therapy Oncology Group Trial 92–02. J Clin Oncol 2004; 22(11):2133–2140.
80. Khor L-Y, Bae K, Pollack A, et al. Cox-2 Expression Predicts Prostate Cancer Outcome: An Analysis of RTOG 92–02. Int J Radiat Oncol Biol Phys 2006; 66(3):S202.
81. Bubendorf L, Sauter G, Moch H, et al. Ki67 labelling index: an independent predictor of progression in prostate cancer treated by radical prostatectomy. J Pathol 1996; 178(4):437–441.
82. Borre M, Bentzen SM, Nerstrom B, Overgaard J. Tumor cell proliferation and survival in patients with prostate cancer followed expectantly. J Urol 1998; 159(5):1609–1614.
83. Bubendorf L, Tapia C, Gasser TC, et al. Ki67 labeling index in core needle biopsies independently predicts tumor-specific survival in prostate cancer. Hum Pathol 1998; 29(9):949–954.
84. Movsas B, Chapman JD, Hanlon AL, et al. Hypoxic prostate/muscle pO2 ratio predicts for biochemical failure in patients with prostate cancer: preliminary findings. Urology 2002; 60(4):634–639.

85. Carnell DM, Smith RE, Daley FM, Saunders MI, Bentzen SM, Hoskin PJ. An immunohistochemical assessment of hypoxia in prostate carcinoma using pimonidazole: implications for radioresistance. Int J Radiat Oncol Biol Phys 2006; 65(1):91–99.
86. Nordsmark M, Bentzen SM, Rudat V, et al. Prognostic value of tumor oxygenation in 397 head and neck tumors after primary radiation therapy. An international multi-center study. Radiother Oncol 2005; 77(1):18–24.
87. Meng AX, Jalali F, Cuddihy A, et al. Hypoxia down-regulates DNA double strand break repair gene expression in prostate cancer cells. Radiother Oncol 2005; 76(2):168–176.
88. Rischin D, Hicks RJ, Fisher R, et al. Prognostic significance of [18F]-misonidazole positron emission tomography-detected tumor hypoxia in patients with advanced head and neck cancer randomly assigned to chemoradiation with or without tirapazamine: a substudy of Trans-Tasman Radiation Oncology Group Study 98.02. J Clin Oncol 2006; 24(13):2098–2104.
89. Chao KS, Bosch WR, Mutic S, et al. A novel approach to overcome hypoxic tumor resistance: Cu-ATSM-guided intensity-modulated radiation therapy. Int J Radiat Oncol Biol Phys 2001; 49(4):1171–1182.
90. Koukourakis MI, Bentzen SM, Giatromanolaki A, et al. Endogenous markers of two separate hypoxia response pathways (hypoxia inducible factor 2 alpha and carbonic anhydrase 9) are associated with radiotherapy failure in head and neck cancer patients recruited in the CHART randomized trial. J Clin Oncol 2006; 24(5):727–735.
91. Bache M, Reddemann R, Said HM, et al. Immunohistochemical detection of osteopontin in advanced head-and-neck cancer: prognostic role and correlation with oxygen electrode measurements, hypoxia-inducible-factor-1alpha-related markers, and hemoglobin levels. Int J Radiat Oncol Biol Phys 2006; 66(5):1481–1487.
92. Overgaard J, Eriksen JG, Nordsmark M, Alsner J, Horsman MR. Plasma osteopontin, hypoxia, and response to the hypoxia sensitiser nimorazole in radiotherapy of head and neck cancer: results from the DAHANCA 5 randomised double-blind placebo-controlled trial. Lancet Oncol 2005; 6(10):757–764.
93. Petrik D, Lavori PW, Cao H, et al. Plasma osteopontin is an independent prognostic marker for head and neck cancers. J Clin Oncol 2006; 24(33):5291–5297.
94. Nishizaki M, Meyn RE, Levy LB, et al. Synergistic inhibition of human lung cancer cell growth by adenovirus-mediated wild-type p53 gene transfer in combination with docetaxel and radiation therapeutics in vitro and in vivo. Clin Cancer Res 2001; 7(9):2887–2897.
95. Hamid O, Varterasian ML, Wadler S, et al. Phase II trial of intravenous CI-1042 in patients with metastatic colorectal cancer. J Clin Oncol 2003; 21(8):1498–1504.
96. Weinstein JN, Myers TG, O'Connor PM, et al. An information-intensive approach to the molecular pharmacology of cancer. Science 1997; 275(5298):343–349.
97. Wiman KG. Strategies for therapeutic targeting of the p53 pathway in cancer. Cell Death Differ 2006; 13(6):921–926.
98. Komarov PG, Komarova EA, Kondratov RV, et al. A chemical inhibitor of p53 that protects mice from the side effects of cancer therapy. Science 1999; 285(5434):1733–1737.
99. Morris MJ, Tong WP, Cordon-Cardo C, et al. Phase I trial of BCL-2 antisense oligonucleotide (G3139) administered by continuous intravenous infusion in patients with advanced cancer. Clin Cancer Res 2002; 8(3):679–683.

Section II
Advances in Molecular Biology and Targeted Therapies

6
Overview of Cancer Molecular Radiobiology

Jann N. Sarkaria and Robert G. Bristow

Introduction

The first recorded use of X-rays for the treatment of cancer occurred within about 1 year of their discovery in the late 1800s by Roentgen. The study of X-rays and other ionizing radiations, and their clinical application to cancer treatment, has become increasingly sophisticated. This chapter will provide an overview of the molecular responses induced in cells by ionizing radiation and will discuss how molecularly targeted inhibitors can be used to enhance the efficacy of therapeutic radiation.

Interaction of Radiation with Living Cells

X-rays, in the form of high-energy photons, deposit energy into tissue by indirect ionization. This is a process where photons interact with and accelerate electrons out of their atomic orbitals. These accelerated electrons then directly interact with matter to generate free radicals (molecules with unpaired electrons). Most of the electron energy deposited in cells is initially in water (because the cell is about 80% water), leading to the rapid production (i.e., within 10^{-14} to 10^{-4} s) of reactive radical intermediates which interact with DNA, RNA or protein molecules in the cell. The [$OH^{\bullet}$] radical, an oxidizing agent, is probably the most damaging. The cell contains naturally occurring thiol compounds (e.g., glutathione, cysteine, and cysteamine) containing sulfhydryl (SH) groups that react chemically with the free radicals to decrease their damaging effects. The intracellular levels of thiols and antioxidative molecules may differ between normal and tumor tissues. One clinical strategy to protect normal tissues from radiotherapy-induced damage is the use of the drug, amifostine (a thiol-containing compound), to protect against radiotherapy-induced xerostomia (i.e., dry mouth after irradiation of salivary glands).

Biochemical processes in cells, such as DNA, RNA, or protein synthesis, respiration, or other metabolism can be inhibited by irradiation but this usually requires quite large doses of radiation of the order of 10–100 Gy. DNA is a major target of

M.P. Mehta et al. (eds.), *Radiation Oncology Advances.*

ionizing radiation and even-relatively small amounts of DNA damage can lead to cell death. Ward [1] has described clusters of ionizations within a few nanometers of the DNA called "local multiply damaged sites" (LMDS). These include combinations of single- or double-strand breaks in the sugar-phosphate backbone of the molecule, alteration or loss of DNA bases, and formation of cross-links (between the DNA strands or between DNA and chromosomal proteins). It has been estimated that approximately 10^5 ionizations can occur within the cell per gray of absorbed radiation dose, leading to approximately: 1,000–3,000 DNA–DNA or DNA–protein cross-links, 1,000 damaged DNA bases, 500–1,000 single-strand and 25–50 double-strand DNA break. These DNA lesions are repaired by a variety of DNA repair pathways, which probably act together to repair clustered LMDS-associated lesions.

Cellular Response to Ionizing Radiation

Cells respond to radiation damage by arresting progression through the cell cycle, and then either repairing the DNA damage or invoking cell death pathways. This highly coordinated cellular response to damage is orchestrated by a complex signaling network that is comprised of proteins that can be broadly categorized as (1) sensors, (2) integrators, and (3) effectors. Sensors, such as the MRE11-RAD50-NBS1 (MRN) complex are recruited to sites of DNA damage, and, in turn, recruit integrator proteins such as the ATM protein. Integrating proteins then direct the cellular response to damage by activating specific effector responses such as cell cycle arrest, DNA repair, and apoptosis.

Cell Cycle Arrest

Mammalian cells respond to ionizing radiation by delaying their progression through the cell cycle which allows for repair of DNA damage in cells prior to DNA replication or mitosis. This also prevents genetic instability in future cell generations [2] (Fig. 1). Central to the activation of the IR-checkpoints is the initial sensing of DNA breaks by the telomeric protein TRF2 and the MRE11-RAD50-NBS1 (MRN) complex with subsequent activation of the ATM kinase [3, 4]. ATM is a member of the phosphatidlylinositol 3-kinase-like family of serine/threonine protein kinases (PIKKs), and serves to integrate the cellular response to DNA damage by coordinating cell cycle arrest, DNA damage and cell death. Other members of this family include the ATM-and Rad3-related (ATR) kinase that responds to single-stranded DNA, and stalled or collapsed DNA replication forks, the DNA-dependent protein kinase catalytic subunit (DNA-PKcs), which is a DNA-dsb repair protein, and the mammalian target of rapamycin (mTOR), which is involved in nutrient stress response [3]. ATM, together with DNA-PKcs, phosphorylates the histone H2AX (called γ-H2AX when phosphorylated on serine residue 139) along

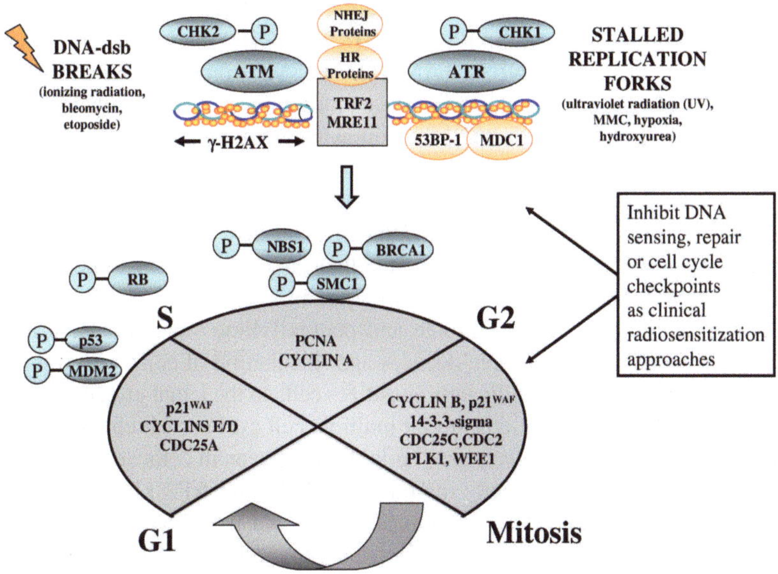

Fig. 1 Radiosensitization by inhibiting cell cycle checkpoints. Initial DNA-dsbs caused by radiotherapy are sensed by the telomeric protein TRF2 within 2 s following DNA damage and followed by binding of the MRN (MRE11-RAD50-NBS1) repair complex. This acts like a beacon for the recruitment of the PI3K-like kinases ATM. The ATR kinase responds to stalled DNA replication forks following some chemotherapy agents (e.g., MMC or gemcitabine). ATM activation triggers the G1, S and G2 checkpoints within the cell cycle. These include spatiotemporal phosphorylation of the histone H2AX and the p53, CHK2, NBS1, BRCA1 and SMC1 proteins close to the DNA-dsb. For the G1 checkpoint, p53 becomes fully stabilized with acquired resistance to MDM2-mediated proteasomal degradation. This leads to upregulation of the $p21^{WAF}$ protein which inhibits the action of both CyclinD-CDK4 and CyclinE-CDK2 complexes. This causes a cell cycle block in late G1 and early S phases, respectively, and maintains the RB protein in a hypo-phosphorylated state bound to E2F to prevent DNA replication. A second more rapid G1-S checkpoint can also be facilitated directly by CHK2 through the CDC25A kinase. 14–3–3 family members are small acidic proteins that are able to bind and sequester CDC25C, whose phosphatase activity is required for the G2 to M transition. Practically every cell cycle checkpoint has been inhibited by the use of RNA antisense (AS) or silencing RNA (siRNA) strategies and this approach has successfully targeted ATM, ATR and MRN in vitro with resultant radiosensitivity. Reconstitution of normal wild type p53 function in tumors in which p53 function is abrogated can be achieved through gene therapy (adenoviralp53 or ONXY-015) or agents that reactivate normal p53 function by altering mutant p53 conformation (e.g., CP-31398, PRIMA1). Finally, there are a number of ATM (KU55953), CDK (e.g., CYC-202 (roscovitine), BMS-387032), CHK1 (e.g., UCN-01) inhibitors which radiosensitize abrogating DNA repair and checkpoint control

megabase-length tracks surrounding a DNA break. MRN acts as initial damage "sensor" for DNA-dsb repair proteins or proteins involved in signal transduction of the damage including BRCA1, MDC1, p53, MDM2, 53BP1, CHK2 and CHK1, which engage G1, S and G2 cell cycle arrests (see Fig. 1) [3, 5].

The ATM-dependent G1 checkpoint is mediated by the p53 tumor suppressor protein and the CHK2 kinase. Their concerted actions through $p21^{WAF}$ and CDC25A alter the activity of CyclinE-CDK and RB (retinoblastoma) protein complexes at the

G1-S interface and initiation of DNA replication. The ATM-dependent intra-S-phase checkpoint is controlled by both ATM-CHK2-CDC25A signaling and alternate phosphorylation of BRCA1, NBS1, FANCD2, and SMC1 proteins. The p53, 53BP-1, CHK1, and CHK2 proteins act as downstream mediators of ATM and ATR in the G2 checkpoint mediated by CyclinB-CDC2. Following DNA damage, CHK2 and CHK1 phosphorylate CDC25C to inhibit its activity towards CyclinB-CDC2 and the cell arrests in G2/M. p53 also up-regulates 14–3–3-σ, which subsequently sequesters CDC25C into the cytoplasm also culminating in an inactive CyclinB-CDC2 complex. Together the ATM and ATR pathways, and their associated checkpoints, represent exciting targets for therapy if tumor-specificity can be achieved.

Methyl xanthines, such as caffeine and pentoxifylline were first described as radiosensitizing agents over three decades ago. Incubation of cells with 0.5–2 mM caffeine or pentoxifylline significantly sensitizes cells to the lethal effects of ionizing radiation. Similar concentrations inhibit multiple cell cycle arrest checkpoints, and some of these checkpoint defects are similar to those seen in cells deficient in ATM function. In fact, caffeine directly inhibits both ATM and ATR kinase activities at concentrations associated with radiosensitization, and these data suggest that the radiosensitizing effects of caffeine are secondary to inhibition of ATM and possibly ATR. Intriguingly, caffeine is a much more effective sensitizing agent in cells that lack normal p53 function. This has been demonstrated convincingly in a series of five studies examining the radiosensitization of paired cell lines that differed only by their p53 status [6]. Caffeine reproducibly increased the radiosensitivity of cells lacking normal p53 function by 1.4 to 2.8-fold but had minimal to no effect on the sensitivity of the wild type p53 cell lines. Although radiosensitizing concentrations of caffeine cannot be achieved in humans, more selective and potent ATM inhibitors are in development, and the caffeine data suggest that these ATM inhibitors might selectively radiosensitize tumors lacking wild type p53 function, while sparing normal tissues (reviewed in Choudhury et al. 2005) [6]. Because the majority of epithelial human tumors have lost normal p53 function, such a p53-selective sensitizing strategy would be widely applicable in clinical radiation therapy.

DNA Repair

Two major pathways repair potentially lethal DNA double-strand breaks (dsb) in mammalian cells. The imprecise nonhomologous end-joining (NHEJ) pathway is the predominant repair process for cells in G_0, G_1 or early S-phase, and mutant cell lines lacking key components of this pathway all exhibit impaired kinetics of DNA dsb repair and exquisite radiosensitivity [6]. Homologous recombination (HR) is a more precise repair mechanism and is more important for the repair of dsb in late-S and G_2 when a sister chromatid is available for the recombination reaction [6]. Cell lines with defects in HR exhibit moderate radiosensitivity and decreased fidelity of repair but do not demonstrate the profound defects in DNA repair kinetics characteristic of the NHEJ mutant cells following ionizing radiation.

There is no simple relationship between expression of DNA repair genes or proteins and the relative radiosensitivity among unselected normal or tumor cells that do not have a recognized genetic defect in DNA repair [7]. However, in defined cell models, DNA repair capacity can influence cellular radiosensitivity as indicated by the extreme radiosensitivity of cells from some patients with DNA repair deficiency syndromes such as Ataxia Telangiectasia and the Nijmegen Breakage Syndrome [5]. Similarly, isogenic cells defective in the expression of the BRCA1 and BRCA2 can have decreased HR-related repair of DNA-dsbs and decreased radiation cell survival [8]. A reduced capacity for repair of DNA double-strand breaks is also observed among X-ray-sensitive mutant Chinese hamster ovary (CHO) cells and among radiosensitive fibroblasts derived from severe combined immunodeficiency (SCID) in which the deficient NHEJ was correlated to a lack of DNA-PKcs, Ku70 or XRCC4 proteins. These cells also have defective V(D)J recombination which also requires appropriate repair of DNA-dsbs for clonal expansion of mature T and B cell subsets during immune responses [9]. Indeed, mouse cells made deficient for NHEJ (i.e., mouse knockouts for DNA-PKcs or Ku70 genes) have exquisite radiosensitivity and defective DNA dsb rejoining. A number of clinical radiosensitization strategies are now being explored which take advantage of the differences in DNA-dsb repair in malignant and normal cells [6].

Apoptosis

For the majority of normal and tumor cells, death secondary to mitotic catastrophe accounts for most of the cell kill following irradiation. However, in some radiosensitive cells and the cancers that arise from them – notably lymphocytes, spermatocytes, thymocytes, and salivary gland epithelium – irradiation causes the cells to undergo apoptosis within hours of exposure. The biochemical and morphologic characteristics of apoptosis include cell membrane blebbing, the formation of nuclear apoptotic bodies, and specific DNA fragmentation. Depending on the type of cell, the intracellular target(s) for the induction of the apoptotic response may be either the cell membrane or the DNA or both. The timing of radiation-induced apoptosis may relate to the relative expression and function of proteins which trigger an apoptotic response. For example, radiation can lead to upregulation of genes (e.g., *fas*, *bax*, and *caspase-3*), which can facilitate apoptosis and/or downregulation of genes (e.g., *bcl-2*), which act to prevent apoptosis [10].

The involvement of the cell membrane in triggering radiation-induced apoptosis is illustrated by the sphingomyelin-dependent signaling pathway within the cell membrane which can induce apoptosis in the absence of DNA damage [11, 12]. In certain cells, such as endothelial, lymphoid and haematopoietic cells, ceramide mediates apoptosis. Ceramide is generated from sphingomyelin (SM) by the action of acid sphingomyelinase (ASM), or by de novo synthesis coordinated through the enzyme ceramide synthase. In the radiation response, ceramide serves as a second messenger in initiating apoptosis, while some of its metabolites block apoptosis.

Radiation-induced crypt damage, organ failure, and death from a gastrointestinal syndrome were reduced when endothelial apoptosis in the supporting, vasculature was inhibited pharmacologically by intravenous basic fibroblast growth factor (bFGF) or genetically by deletion of the ASM gene [13]. Altering the apoptotic response of tumor cells may be one strategy to sensitize tumors to radiotherapy. As selected tumors may evade RT-induced apoptosis by overexpressing bcl-2 or by lacking p53 expression or function or decreasing bcl-2 function. Therefore, restoration of wild type p53 function using gene therapy might potentiate radiation cell killing.

Cell Survival Signaling

There is evidence that the aberrant expression of oncogenes or tumor suppressor genes may increase the intrinsic cellular radioresistance of human and rodent cells. For example, increased radiation survival has been observed in selected cell lines following the transfection of a single oncogene, such as activated *ras*, *src*, or *raf* [14, 15]. This has led to studies designed to radiosensitize tumor cells by the inhibition of oncogene function using inhibitors of intracellular signaling pathways or antisense (or siRNA) to decrease oncogene overexpression [16]. Other approaches have utilized the reintroduction of a normal tumor suppressor gene into resistant cells containing a mutated tumor suppressor gene, such as p53.

Ras Signaling

When the *ras* oncogene undergoes mutation, it is permanently activated in the GTP-bound signaling state, providing proliferative signals in the absence of growth factor ligands. This leads to increasing cell proliferation, transformation and relative radioresistance. Increased radioresistance is also observed in cells transfected with an activated *ras* gene in combination with a nuclear co-operating oncogene, such as c-*myc* or mutant *p53* [17, 18]. Inhibitors of *ras* protein prenylation or function (farnesyl transferase inhibitors) have been reported to enhance radiation-induced cytotoxicity amongst preclinical models of human breast, lung, colon, and bladder cancer cells expressing mutated *H*- or *K-ras* genes. Although improvements in *ras*-pathway specificity are required for future development of farnesyl transferase inhibitors in the radiotherapy clinic, at least one early Phase I trial has shown clinical success with minimal toxicity using these drugs, in the treatment of advanced lung and head and neck cancers [19].

Downstream to *ras*, the *raf-MEK-ERK* and phosphatidylinositol-3 kinase (*PI3K*)-*Akt/PKB* pathways are two separate signaling pathways that have been linked to tumor radioresistance. Using antisense oligonucleotides against human *raf*, increased radiosensitivity has been observed in a human squamous cancer cell line (SQ-20B). *Ras*-mediated radioresistance in rat cells appears to be dependent on *PI3K* and *raf* signaling pathways, and less on the *MEK* signaling pathway [15]. Inhibitors of *PI3K* signaling such as LY294002 and wortmannin significantly enhances the response to radiation in lung, bladder, colon, breast, HNSCC and cervical cancer cells. These compounds are relatively non-specific and not suitable for clinical use, but many major pharmaceutical companies have more selective and potent PI3K and/or Akt inhibitors in development that will be exciting to test in combination with radiation and chemotherapeutic agents.

Receptor Tyrosine Kinases

Constitutive signaling from receptor tyrosine kinases are implicated in modulating radiation resistance in epithelial tumors. The most prominent example of this effect is with the epidermal growth factor receptor (EGFR) family of RTKs and is the subject of a subsequent chapter. In addition to the EGFR family, the *insulin-like growth factor-1 receptor (IGF-1R)* is a cell surface receptor with tyrosine kinase activity which has been linked to increased radioresistance. Mouse embryo fibroblasts in which the IGF-1R gene has been knocked out exhibit increased sensitivity to radiation compared to wildtype cells [20]. Mouse monoclonal antibodies have also been used to block IGF-1R signaling in cell culture and xenograft tumor models. An in vitro colon cancer model of chemoradiation demonstrated enhanced cyotoxicity when exposed to the anti-IGF-1R mouse monoclonal antibody αIR3 [21]. Similar results were observed in mouse melanoma cells where IGF-1R was downregulated by an antisense construct [22]. More recently, antitumor efficacy and potentiation of radiation-induced apoptosis was demonstrated for the fully human anti-IGF-1R antibody A12 in a model of non-small cell lung cancer [23] (Fig. 3). IGF-1R tyrosine kinase inhibition strategies yield similar radiosensitizing effects; breast cancer cells treated with kinase inhibitor tyrophostin AG 1024 were more sensitive to radiation than untreated controls [24]. Although the mechanism of receptor tyrosine kinase inhibitor-mediated radiosensitization is not completely understood, the promising preclinical studies have stimulated strong interest in investigating this approach in the clinic.

mTOR Signaling

The mTOR signaling network is important for driving cell growth and proliferation in multiple tumor types. mTOR signaling is activated by mitogenic stimuli through the PI3K/Akt signaling pathway and by the Rheb1 GTPase. Rheb1-mediated activation of mTOR signaling is suppressed during nutrient–stress by the tuberous sclerosis complex-2 (TSC2) protein, which in turn is regulated by the LKB1 protein (mutation of *LKB1* is the cause of Puetz–Jeghers syndrome) [25–30]. mTOR signals downstream to multiple components of the protein translation machinery involved in translating protein transcripts with complex 5′ untranslated regions. Many of these transcripts are involved in promoting tumor cell proliferation and angiogenesis, and pharmacologic inhibition of mTOR signaling by the selective inhibitor rapamycin results in growth arrest and inhibition of tumor angiogenesis.

Angiogenesis and tumor cell proliferation have been implicated as important mediators that can influence the efficacy of traditional cytotoxic cancer therapies; therefore, significant research effort has focused on the evaluation of combinations of mTOR inhibitors with standard cancer therapies. Rapamycin potentiates cisplatin-induced apoptosis in multiple cell lines including HL-60 leukemia cells and SKOV3 ovarian cancer cells [31]. Likewise, insulin-like growth factor-induced resistance to cisplatin in Rh30 rhabdomyosarcoma cells can be reversed by rapamycin treatment [32]. Geoerger et al. demonstrated that combinations of rapamycin with either cisplatin or camptothecin provide additive growth inhibition in the rapamycin-sensitive DAOY medulloblastoma cell line but not in the rapamycin-resistant D283 cell line [33]. Consistent with this in vitro data, CCI-779 therapy provides for additive tumor growth inhibition in animals when combined with doxorubicin or cisplatin in PC3 or DAOY xenografts, respectively [33]. A recent study suggests that mTOR inhibition results in enhanced cytotoxicity through prevention of p21 translation, which then leads to increased p53-dependent apoptosis [34]. Taken together, these data suggest that mTOR-dependent signaling may be important for resistance to chemotherapy-induced apoptosis and may provide a rationale for selecting certain tumor genotypes for combination therapy with rapamycin and cisplatin.

Rapamycin also can enhance the efficacy of radiation therapy. Based on preclinical and clinical data demonstrating that tumor proliferation during fractionated radiotherapy contributes to clinical radiation resistance [35, 36], rapamycin-mediated inhibition of tumor proliferation during radiotherapy might enhance the efficacy of radiation [37]. Consistent with the idea that mTOR is not involved in DNA damage responses, unlike the related ATM, ATR and DNA-PKcs kinases, rapamycin had no effect on the in vitro radiation sensitivity of several glioma cell lines including U87 cells. In contrast, intermittent dosing with rapamycin throughout a fractionated course of radiation significantly enhanced the efficacy of treatment in radioresistant U87 xenografts. Phase I clinical trials are now evaluating the combination of definitive radiation therapy, cisplatin, and rapamycin in patients with unresectable lung cancer.

Targeting Housekeeping Proteins

The oncogenic signaling pathways mediating radiation resistance are complex and interconnected, and there is a growing appreciation that targeting more than one component within these pathways may be of benefit. While this can be achieved through combinations of selective pathway inhibitors, disrupting the activities of key house-keeping proteins also can be used to simultaneously downregulate multiple proteins involved in radiation response. In this section, the radiosensitizing effects of HSP90 inhibitors, proteosome inhibitors, and histone deacetylase inhibitors will be discussed.

HSP90 Inhibitors

HSP90 is a highly abundant protein playing a role in the cellular stress response. HSP90 plays a regulatory role under normal physiologic conditions by maintaining the conformational stability and maturation of a number of specific proteins involved in a variety of oncogenic processes including cellular proliferation, cell cycle regulation and apoptosis. Inhibition of HSP90 function is known to cause selective degradation of these proteins, placing it at an interface with multiple oncogenic processes and thereby making it a promising target for cancer therapy [38]. Several proteins including EGFR, ErbB2, Raf-1, extracellular signal-regulated kinase-1 (ERK1), vascular epithelial growth factor (VEGF), and protein kinase B (PKB)/AKT, are known to promote radiation resistance, providing rationale for the combination of these agents with radiation [39–41].

HSP90 inhibitors have demonstrated the capacity to enhance radiation response both in vitro and in vivo in a diverse panel cancer cell lines including glioma, prostate, cervical, pancreatic, colon, and lung cancer [39–43]. The heterogeneity of cell lines studied supports the multitargeted approach offered by HSP90 inhibitors in enhancing radiation sensitivity. Enmon et al. have shown that the combination of the HSP90 inhibitor 17AAG and radiation produce synergistic growth suppression in human prostate carcinoma spheroids [43]. Similarly, Bisht et al. demonstrated the capacity of 17AAG to potentate radiation response through what was described as a chemically induced hyperthermia in cervical cancer cells. Additionally, these studies suggest differential cytotoxicity between normal and transformed cells, conferring a possible favorable therapeutic index in patients [41].

The proposed mechanism of enhanced radiation response following HSP90 inhibition involves the selective degradation of several key proteins attributed to radiation resistance, including EGFR, ErbB2, Raf-1, and AKT [39–42]. Increased EGFR expression has been observed in a variety of tumors and strong correlation has been established between EGFR expression and radiation resistance [44, 45]. Additionally, preclinical studies demonstrate a strong link between EGFR inhibition and enhanced radiation response [46–48]. Similarly, differences in radiation sensitivity have been attributed to ErbB2 expression in prostate cancer cell lines [49]. The capacity of HSP90 inhibitors to downmodulate EGFR and ErbB2 expression, therefore, may represent a mechanism whereby the antitumor activity of radiation is enhanced. Other potential targets of HSP90 include AKT and RAF-1 signaling. In addition to residing downstream of the ErbB receptor family, these proteins play a central role in propagating pro-survival signals that confer resistance to various cytotoxic insults [16, 50–52]. Recent studies have shown a potential role for targeting both of these pathways in mediating radiation sensitivity [16, 50, 53, 54]. In light of the toxicity associated with current PI3K/AKT inhibitors and the still early clinical development of RAF-1 inhibitors, further examination of the capacity of HSP90 inhibitors to target these signaling pathways to enhance radiation response is warranted [53].

HDAC Inhibitors

Several HDAC inhibitors are progressing through clinical trials (Fig. 2) and have demonstrated promising preclinical interactions when combined with radiation [55–57]. The HDAC inhibitor mechanism of action suggests potential for enhancing radiation response by targeting multiple radiation resistance pathways. These include physical modifications of chromatin structure, thereby altering potential for radiation damage, and differential oncoprotein regulation following histone acetylation (Fig. 3) [58].

The primary mechanism of action of HDAC inhibitors involves the regulation of chromatin architecture through modification of histone tails. Histone proteins organize DNA into regular repeating structures of chromatin. The acetylation status of histones influences chromatin structure, which in turn regulates gene expression. Two classes of enzymes are known to affect the acetylation of histones – histone acetyltransferases (HATs) and HDACs, and alterations in their baseline activity have been identified in several human cancers. HDAC inhibitors promote hyperacetylation of histones, which in turn leads to chromatin relaxation and selective expression of genes involved in oncogenesis [55, 58].

The potential influence of chromatin structure and acetylation status on radiation-induced DNA damage and repair is well recognized [60–62]. Actively transcribed genes are generally more sensitive to the cytotoxic effects of radiation and compaction

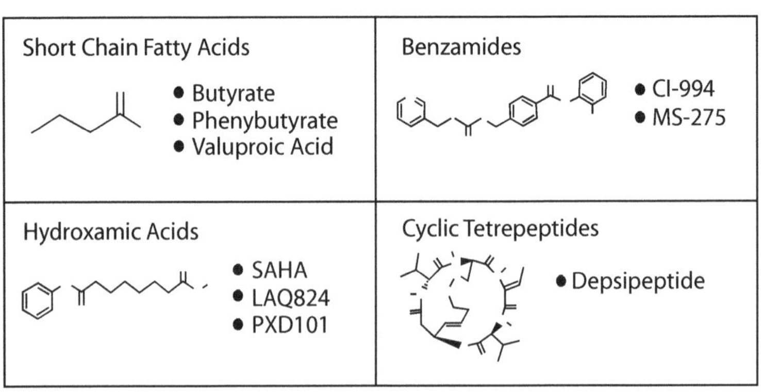

Fig. 2 HDAC inhibitor classes

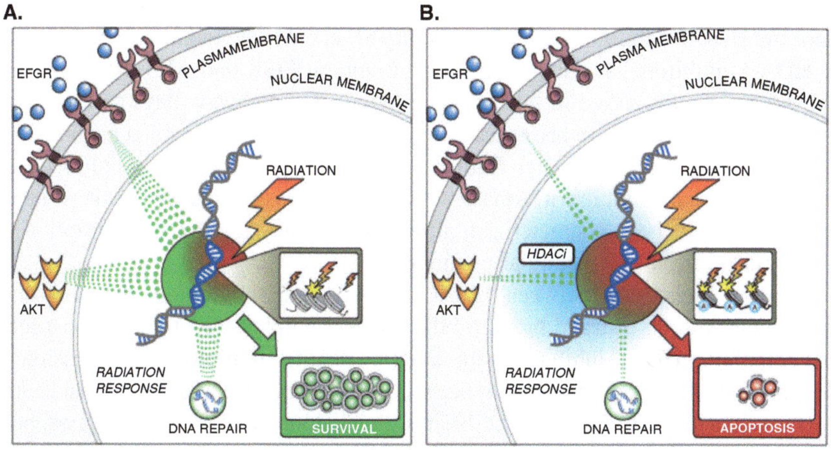

Fig. 3 HDAC inhibitor mechanisms. Potential mechanism of HDAC inhibitor interaction with radiation therapy. (**a**) Cancer cells possess a variety of mechanisms providing resistance to the cytotoxic effects of XRT, including chromatin compaction and increased pro-mitogenic/survival signaling (EGFR and AKT) and DNA repair processes. (**b**) HDAC inhibitors may act as potent XRT sensitizers by abrogating these pro-mitogenic/survival and DNA repair signaling pathways. Further, HDAC inhibition leads to chromatin relaxation, thereby increasing the DNA damaging effects of XRT. Reproduced with permission from [59]

of chromatin into higher-order structures appears to protect DNA against radiation-induced DSBs. Based on these findings, HDAC inhibitors, which facilitate both chromatin relaxation and gene transcription through histone acetylation, may potentiate cytotoxic effects of radiation through this physical modification of chromatin structure. These concepts are supported by the work of Camphausen et al. which demonstrated that histone hyperacetylation following HDAC inhibition was a marker for the degree of radiosensitization [63]. Additionally, specific genes differentially expressed or modified following HDAC inhibition may also impact radiation response. Potential targets include the pro-mitogenic and survival oncoproteins EGFR and AKT as well as proteins involved with DNA-dsb repair, including Rad51 and DNA-PK [64].

To date, much of the preclinical and clinical experience combining molecularly targeted agents with radiation has involved inhibiting EGFR signaling. Recent studies have determined the capacity of HDAC inhibitors to downmodulate the expression of EGFR and ErbB2, therefore representing another possible mechanism for HDAC inhibitors to enhance the antitumor activity of radiation [64–66]. Although mechanistically unclear, preliminary work has demonstrated the capacity of HDAC inhibitors to negatively regulate the ErbB promoter, leading to reduced expression of this family of oncoproteins [67]. In addition to histones, HDAC inhibitors may also acetylate other proteins leading to altered cellular function. Particular to ErbB signaling, HDAC inhibitors have been shown to acetylate

HSP90, thereby allowing disassociation of the client proteins EGFR and ErbB2 from the Hsp90 stabilizing complex, leading to receptor degradation [65, 66].

HDAC inhibitors have also been shown to inhibit PI3K and AKT signaling [64, 65]. As will be discussed in further detail below, this pathway plays an important role in conferring radiation resistance through pro-survival signaling and its inhibition increases radiation sensitivity. Rather than affecting AKT expression, HDAC inhibitors appear to inhibit its kinase activity. Mechanisms underlying these interactions have not been characterized, although they may involve the disruption of AKT translocation to the cellular membrane.

Another interaction between HDAC inhibitors and radiation response may involve DNA double strand break (DSB) repair. Camphausen et al. demonstrated that combining HDAC inhibitors with radiation resulted in prolonged expression of γH2AX [68]. γH2AX expression has been recently established as a sensitive indicator for radiation-induced DSBs. At DSB sites, the histone H2AX becomes phosphorylated rapidly (γH2AX), forming foci visible by immunoflourescent cytochemistry [69]. The dephosphorylation and dispersal of γH2AX in irradiated cells correlates with repair of the DNA DSBs [70, 71]. Prolonged expression of γH2AX when combining HDAC inhibitors with radiation therefore suggests HDAC inhibitors influence DNA repair processes. This may be mechanistically explained by the capacity of HDAC inhibitors to downmodulate RAD51 and DNA-PK expression, two critical proteins involved in HR and NHEJ repair.

Proteosome Inhibitors

The proteasome is a multisubunit protease complex that is involved in the turnover of cellular proteins via degradation and recycling (Fig. 4). In this ubiquitin (Ub)/ proteasome pathway, proteins are targeted for degradation by conjugation to polymers of the 8-kDa polypeptide, ubiquitin, and are degraded via an ATP-dependent process [72]. Over 80% of all cellular polyubiqitinylated proteins are recycled through the proteasome. The activation and conjugation of ubiquitin is, in part, mediated by E3 protein ligases. Examples of these include the BRCA1-BARD1 complex and the MDM2 protein which target the RAD51 and p53 proteins for proteasomal degradation, respectively [72].

Ubiquitin-mediated degradation of regulatory proteins may play an important role in the radioresponse of tumor and normal cells as they target proteins involved in cell cycle progression, signal transduction, transcriptional regulation, DNA repair and cell death including: histones, BAX, $p21^{WAF}$, $p27^{KIP}$, p53, RAD51, Cyclins (D,E,B), PARP and nuclear-factor kappa B (NF-kappaB).[72, 73]. NF-kappaB binds to its target sites (i.e., kappaB sites in the DNA) to initiate transcription following irradiation and along with antiapoptotic proteins, may be a critical target for chemical inhibitors of proteasome inhibition [72, 74]. Bortezomib (PS-341) is a dipeptide boronic acid that inhibits tumor cell or xenograft proliferation and is FDA approved for treatment of refractory multiple myeloma. PS-341 can radiosensitize

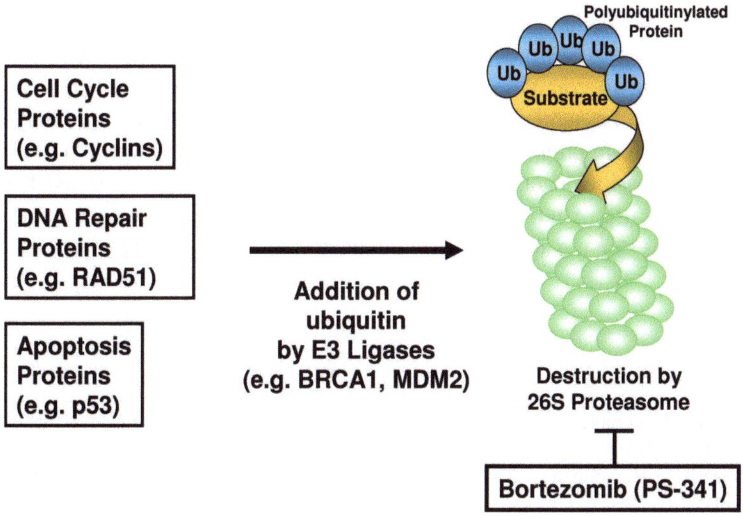

Fig. 4 Radiosensitization by inhibiting the proteasome. A number of proteins involved in the cellular radiotherapy response are degraded through the ubiquitin-mediated degradation pathway by the 26S proteasome. Proteins that are targeted for destruction become polyubiquitinylated by families of E3 ligases that include the BRCA1-BARD1 repair complex and the MDM2 protein involved in p53 stability. Preclinical studies have shown that PS-341 will also potentiate the cytotoxic effects of radiation therapy by altering the expression and function of proteins involved in cell cycle checkpoint control (e.g., cyclins, p53 and $p21^{WAF}$), DNA repair (RAD51) and/or cell death (e.g., p53, BAX) following exposure to ionizing radiation

a variety of tumor cell types in vitro and in vivo potentially by inhibiting NF-kappaB or BCL-2 [72, 75]. As an example, combined treatment with PS-341 and the bone seeking radionucleide 153-Sm-EDTMP more than doubled the survival of mice in a disseminated myeloma model as compared to treatment with either agent alone (A. Goel and S. Russell, submitted to Blood). On the basis of these promising results, multiple clinical trials are now in progress evaluating combinations of PS-341 with radiation and/or chemotherapy in multiple tumor types.

Conclusion

The increasing knowledge of molecular radiobiologic pathways will soon allow for both technical and biologic precision during clinical radiotherapy. Still required is a better understanding of the differences within the above molecular pathways between normal and malignant tissues within an irradiated volume to determine the therapeutic ratio for a given treatment. This approach supports the "molecular profiling" of patient responses to predict relevant side-effects and tumor response for a given patient.

It is likely that multiple molecular pathways will be targeted based on pretreatment biomarker studies. Additionally, the tumor microenvironment (e.g., hypoxia) must also be assessed to complete an accurate prediction of treatment response. This complexity may be achieved by the use of genomic and proteomic analyses of tissues derived from pretreatment biopsies or noninvasive techniques to track gene or protein expression during therapy. The use of biomarkers of tumor resistance, in addition to the use of novel agents designed to target these resistance pathways, will be a major step towards the individualization of cancer therapy.

References

1. Ward JF. The complexity of DNA damage: relevance to biological consequences. Int J Radiat Biol 1994; 66(5):427–432.
2. Hartwell LH, Kastan MB. Cell cycle control and cancer. Science 1994; 266(5192):1821–1828.
3. Lukas J, Lukas C, Bartek J. Mammalian cell cycle checkpoints: signalling pathways and their organization in space and time. DNA Repair (Amst) 2004; 3(8–9):997–1007.
4. Bradshaw PS, Stavropoulos DJ, Meyn MS. Human telomeric protein TRF2 associates with genomic double-strand breaks as an early response to DNA damage. Nat Genet 2005; 37(2):193–197.
5. Bristow RG, Harrington L. Genetic Instability and DNA Repair; Chapter 5. In: Tannock IF HR, Harrington L and Bristow RG, ed. The Basic Science of Oncology. 4th ed. New York: McGraw-Hill Ltd.; 2005:77–99.
6. Choudhury A, Cuddihy A, Bristow R. Radiation and Other New Molecular-Targeted Agents, Part I: Targeting ATM-p53, ATR-CHK1, DNA Repair and the Proteasome. Semin Radiat Oncol2006; 16:51–58.
7. Valerie K, Povirk LF. Regulation and mechanisms of mammalian double-strand break repair. Oncogene 2003; 22(37):5792–5812.
8. Powell SN, Kachnic LA. Roles of BRCA1 and BRCA2 in homologous recombination, DNA replication fidelity and the cellular response to ionizing radiation. Oncogene 2003; 22(37):5784–5791.
9. Jeggo PA. The fidelity of repair of radiation damage. Radiat Prot Dosimetry 2002; 99(1–4):117–122.
10. Kitada S, Krajewski S, Miyashita T, Krajewska M, Reed JC. Gamma-radiation induces upregulation of Bax protein and apoptosis in radiosensitive cells in vivo. Oncogene 1996; 12(1):187–192.
11. Kolesnick R, Fuks Z. Radiation and ceramide-induced apoptosis. Oncogene 2003; 22(37):5897–5906.
12. Ruiter GA, Zerp SF, Bartelink H, van Blitterswijk WJ, Verheij M. Alkyl-lysophospholipids activate the SAPK/JNK pathway and enhance radiation-induced apoptosis. Cancer Res 1999; 59(10):2457–2463.
13. Paris F, Fuks Z, Kang A, et al. Endothelial apoptosis as the primary lesion initiating intestinal radiation damage in mice. Science 2001; 293(5528):293–297.
14. Kasid U, Suy S, Dent P, Ray S, Whiteside TL, Sturgill TW. Activation of Raf by ionizing radiation. Nature 1996; 382(6594):813–816.
15. Gupta AK, Bakanauskas VJ, Cerniglia GJ, et al. The Ras radiation resistance pathway. Cancer Res 2001; 61(10):4278–4282.
16. Kasid U, Dritschilo A. RAF antisense oligonucleotide as a tumor radiosensitizer. Oncogene 2003; 22(37):5876–5884.

17. McKenna WG, Weiss MC, Endlich B, et al. Synergistic effect of the v-myc oncogene with H-ras on radioresistance. Cancer Res 1990; 50(1):97–102.
18. Bristow RG, Benchimol S, Hill RP. The p53 gene as a modifier of intrinsic radiosensitivity: implications for radiotherapy. Radiother Oncol 1996; 40(3):197–223.
19. Hahn SM, Bernhard EJ, Regine W, et al. A Phase I trial of the farnesyltransferase inhibitor L-778,123 and radiotherapy for locally advanced lung and head and neck cancer. Clin Cancer Res 2002; 8(5):1065–1072.
20. Nakamura S, Watanabe H, Miura M, Sasaki T. Effect of the insulin-like growth factor I receptor on ionizing radiation-induced cell death in mouse embryo fibroblasts. Exp Cell Res 1997; 235(1):287–294.
21. Perer ES, Madan AK, Shurin A, et al. Insulin-like growth factor I receptor antagonism augments response to chemoradiation therapy in colon cancer cells. J Surg Res 2000; 94(1):1–5.
22. Macaulay VM, Salisbury AJ, Bohula EA, Playford MP, Smorodinsky NI, Shiloh Y. Downregulation of the type 1 insulin-like growth factor receptor in mouse melanoma cells is associated with enhanced radiosensitivity and impaired activation of Atm kinase. Oncogene 2001; 20(30):4029–4040.
23. Allen GA, Armstrong E, Modhia F, Ludwig DL, Hicklin DJ, Harari PM. Inhibition of insulin-like growth factor-1 receptor signaling impairs proliferation of head and neck, lung, prostate and breast cancer cells. In: American Association of Cancer Research; 2005 April 9, 2005; Anaheim, CA; 2005.
24. Wen B, Deutsch E, Marangoni E, et al. Tyrphostin AG 1024 modulates radiosensitivity in human breast cancer cells. Br J Cancer 2001; 85(12):2017–2021.
25. Saucedo LJ, Gao X, Chiarelli DA, Li L, Pan D, Edgar BA. Rheb promotes cell growth as a component of the insulin/TOR signalling network. Nature Cell Biol 2003; 5(6):566–571 [erratum appears in Nat Cell Biol. 2003 Jul; 5(7):680].
26. Castro AF, Rebhun JF, Clark GJ, Quilliam LA. Rheb binds tuberous sclerosis complex 2 (TSC2) and promotes S6 kinase activation in a rapamycin- and farnesylation-dependent manner. J Biol Chem 2003; 278(35):32493–32496.
27. Garami A, Zwartkruis FJ, Nobukuni T, et al. Insulin activation of Rheb, a mediator of mTOR/S6K/4E-BP signaling, is inhibited by TSC1 and 2. Mol Cell 2003; 11(6):1457–1466.
28. Inoki K, Li Y, Xu T, Guan K-L. Rheb GTPase is a direct target of TSC2 GAP activity and regulates mTOR signaling. Genes Dev 2003; 17(15):1829–1834.
29. Shaw RJ, Bardeesy N, Manning BD, et al. The LKB1 tumor suppressor negatively regulates mTOR signaling. Cancer Cell 2004; 6(1):91–99.
30. Corradetti MN, Inoki K, Bardeesy N, DePinho RA, Guan KL. Regulation of the TSC pathway by LKB1: evidence of a molecular link between tuberous sclerosis complex and Peutz–Jeghers syndrome. Genes Dev 2004; 18(13):1533–1538.
31. Shi Y, Frankel A, Radvanyi LG, Penn LZ, Miller RG, Mills GB. Rapamycin enhances apoptosis and increases sensitivity to cisplatin in vitro. Cancer Res 1995; 55(9):1982–1988.
32. Wan X, Helman LJ. Effect of insulin-like growth factor II on protecting myoblast cells against cisplatin-induced apoptosis through p70 S6 kinase pathway. Neoplasia (New York) 2002; 4(5):400–408.
33. Geoerger B, Kerr K, Tang C-B, et al. Antitumor activity of the rapamycin analog CCI-779 in human primitive neuroectodermal tumor/medulloblastoma models as single agent and in combination chemotherapy. Cancer Res 2001; 61(4):1527–1532.
34. Beuvink I, Boulay A, Fumagalli S, et al. The mTOR inhibitor RAD001 sensitizes tumor cells to DNA-damaged induced apoptosis through inhibition of p21 translation. Cell 2005; 120(6):747–759.
35. Fowler JF. Biological factors influencing optimum fractionation in radiation therapy. Acta Oncol 2001; 40(6):712–717.
36. Bentzen SM. Repopulation in radiation oncology: perspectives of clinical research. Int J Radiat Biol 2003; 79(7):581–585.

37. Eshleman JS, Carlson BL, Mladek AC, Kastner BD, Shide KL, Sarkaria JN. Inhibition of the mammalian target of rapamycin sensitizes U87 xenografts to fractionated radiation therapy. Cancer Res 2002; 62(24):7291–7297.
38. Maloney A, Workman P. HSP90 as a new therapeutic target for cancer therapy: the story unfolds. Expert Opin Biol Ther 2002; 2(1):3–24.
39. Machida H, Matsumoto Y, Shirai M, Kubota N. Geldanamycin, an inhibitor of Hsp90, sensitizes human tumour cells to radiation. Int J Radiat Biol 2003; 79(12):973–980.
40. Russell JS, Burgan W, Oswald KA, Camphausen K, Tofilon PJ. Enhanced cell killing induced by the combination of radiation and the heat shock protein 90 inhibitor 17-allylamino-17- demethoxygeldanamycin: a multitarget approach to radiosensitization. Clin Cancer Res 2003; 9(10 Pt 1):3749–3755.
41. Bisht KS, Bradbury CM, Mattson D, et al. Geldanamycin and 17-allylamino-17-demethoxygeldanamycin potentiate the in vitro and in vivo radiation response of cervical tumor cells via the heat shock protein 90-mediated intracellular signaling and cytotoxicity. Cancer Res 2003; 63(24):8984–8995.
42. Bull EE, Dote H, Brady KJ, et al. Enhanced tumor cell radiosensitivity and abrogation of G2 and S phase arrest by the Hsp90 inhibitor 17-(dimethylaminoethylamino)-17-demethoxygeldanamycin. Clin Cancer Res 2004; 10(23):8077–8084.
43. Enmon R, Yang WH, Ballangrud AM, et al. Combination treatment with 17-N-allylamino-17-demethoxy geldanamycin and acute irradiation produces supra-additive growth suppression in human prostate carcinoma spheroids. Cancer Res 2003; 63(23):8393–8399.
44. Zhu A, Shaeffer J, Leslie S, Kolm P, El-Mahdi AM. Epidermal growth factor receptor: an independent predictor of survival in astrocytic tumors given definitive irradiation. Int J Radiat Oncol Biol Phys 1996; 34(4):809–815.
45. Sheridan MT, O'Dwyer T, Seymour CB, Mothersill CE. Potential indicators of radiosensitivity in squamous cell carcinoma of the head and neck. Radiat Oncol Invest 1997; 5(4):180–186.
46. Milas L, Fan Z, Andratschke NH, Ang KK. Epidermal growth factor receptor and tumor response to radiation: in vivo preclinical studies. Int J Radiat Oncol Biol Phys 2004; 58(3):966–971.
47. Huang SM, Bock JM, Harari PM. Epidermal growth factor receptor blockade with C225 modulates proliferation, apoptosis, and radiosensitivity in squamous cell carcinomas of the head and neck. Cancer Res 1999; 59(8):1935–1940.
48. Bianco C, Tortora G, Bianco R, et al. Enhancement of antitumor activity of ionizing radiation by combined treatment with the selective epidermal growth factor receptor-tyrosine kinase inhibitor ZD1839 (Iressa). Clin Cancer Res 2002; 8(10):3250–3258.
49. Agus DB, Scher HI, Higgins B, et al. Response of prostate cancer to anti-Her-2/neu antibody in androgen-dependent and -independent human xenograft models. Cancer Res 1999; 59(19):4761–4764.
50. Grana TM, Rusyn EV, Zhou H, Sartor CI, Cox AD. Ras mediates radioresistance through both phosphatidylinositol 3-kinase-dependent and Raf-dependent but mitogen-activated protein kinase/extracellular signal-regulated kinase kinase-independent signaling pathways. Cancer Res 2002; 62(14):4142–4150.
51. Kennedy SG, Wagner AJ, Conzen SD, et al. The PI 3-kinase/Akt signaling pathway delivers an anti-apoptotic signal. Genes Dev 1997; 11(6):701–713.
52. Vanhaesebroeck B, Leevers SJ, Panayotou G, Waterfield MD. Phosphoinositide 3-kinases: a conserved family of signal transducers. Trends Biochem Sci 1997; 22(7):267–272.
53. McKenna WG, Muschel RJ, Gupta AK, Hahn SM, Bernhard EJ. The RAS signal transduction pathway and its role in radiation sensitivity. Oncogene 2003; 22(37):5866–5875.
54. Gupta AK, Cerniglia GJ, Mick R, et al. Radiation sensitization of human cancer cells in vivo by inhibiting the activity of PI3K using LY294002. Int J Radiat Oncol Biol Phys 2003; 56(3):846–853.
55. Marks P, Rifkind RA, Richon VM, Breslow R, Miller T, Kelly WK. Histone deacetylases and cancer: causes and therapies. Nat Rev Cancer 2001; 1(3):194–202.

56. Marshall JL, Rizvi N, Kauh J, et al. A phase I trial of depsipeptide (FR901228) in patients with advanced cancer. J Exp Ther Oncol 2002; 2(6):325–332.
57. Kelly WK, Richon VM, O'Connor O, et al. Phase I clinical trial of histone deacetylase inhibitor: suberoylanilide hydroxamic acid administered intravenously. Clin Cancer Res 2003; 9(10 Pt 1): 3578–3588.
58. Johnstone RW. Histone-deacetylase inhibitors: novel drugs for the treatment of cancer. Nat Rev Drug Discov 2002; 1(4):287–299.
59. Chinnaiyan P, Allen G, Harari PM. Radiation and new molecular agents, Part II: Targeting HDAC, HSP90, IGF-1R, PI3K and Ras. Semin Radiat Oncol 2006; 16:59–65.
60. Ljungman M. The influence of chromatin structure on the frequency of radiation-induced DNA strand breaks: a study using nuclear and nucleoid monolayers. Radiat Res 1991; 126(1):58–64.
61. Nackerdien Z, Michie J, Bohm L. Chromatin decondensed by acetylation shows an elevated radiation response. Radiat Res 1989; 117(2):234–244.
62. Warters RL, Childers TJ. Radiation-induced thymine base damage in replicating chromatin. Radiat Res 1982; 90(3):564–574.
63. Camphausen K, Scott T, Sproull M, Tofilon PJ. Enhancement of xenograft tumor radiosensitivity by the histone deacetylase inhibitor MS-275 and correlation with histone hyperacetylation. Clin Cancer Res 2004; 10(18 Pt 1):6066–6071.
64. Chinnaiyan P, Valabhaneni G, Armstrong E, Huang S, Harari PM. Modulating radiation response with the histone deacetylase (HDAC) inhibitor SAHA in human carcinomas. Int J Radiat Oncol Biol Phys 2005; 62(1):223–229.
65. Fuino L, Bali P, Wittmann S, et al. Histone deacetylase inhibitor LAQ824 down-regulates Her-2 and sensitizes human breast cancer cells to trastuzumab, taxotere, gemcitabine, and epothilone B. Mol Cancer Ther 2003; 2(10):971–984.
66. Yu X, Guo ZS, Marcu MG, et al. Modulation of p53, ErbB1, ErbB2, and Raf-1 expression in lung cancer cells by depsipeptide FR901228. J Natl Cancer Inst 2002; 94(7):504–513.
67. Lippman ME, Benz C, Chinnaiyan A, et al. Consensus statement: expedition inspiration 2004 Breast Cancer Symposium 'Breast Cancer – the Development and Validation of New Therapeutics'. Breast Cancer Res Treat 2005; 90(1):1–3.
68. Camphausen K, Burgan W, Cerra M, et al. Enhanced radiation-induced cell killing and prolongation of gammaH2AX foci expression by the histone deacetylase inhibitor MS-275. Cancer Res 2004; 64(1):316–321.
69. Rogakou EP, Pilch DR, Orr AH, Ivanova VS, Bonner WM. DNA double-stranded breaks induce histone H2AX phosphorylation on serine 139. J Biol Chem 1998; 273(10):5858–5868.
70. Nazarov IB, Smirnova AN, Krutilina RI, et al. Dephosphorylation of histone gamma-H2AX during repair of DNA double-strand breaks in mammalian cells and its inhibition by calyculin A. Radiat Res 2003; 160(3):309–317.
71. Rothkamm K, Kruger I, Thompson LH, Lobrich M. Pathways of DNA double-strand break repair during the mammalian cell cycle. Mol Cell Biol 2003; 23(16):5706–5715.
72. McBride WH, Iwamoto KS, Syljuasen R, Pervan M, Pajonk F. The role of the ubiquitin/proteasome system in cellular responses to radiation. Oncogene 2003; 22(37):5755–5773.
73. Krogan NJ, Lam MH, Fillingham J, et al. Proteasome involvement in the repair of DNA double-strand breaks. Mol Cell 2004; 16(6):1027–1034.
74. Kurland JF, Meyn RE. Protease inhibitors restore radiation-induced apoptosis to Bcl-2-expressing lymphoma cells. Int J Cancer 2001; 96(6):327–333.
75. Teicher BA, Ara G, Herbst R, Palombella VJ, Adams J. The proteasome inhibitor PS-341 in cancer therapy. Clin Cancer Res 1999; 5(9):2638–2645.

7
Clinical Application of EGFR Inhibitors in Head and Neck Squamous Cell Cancer

Igor Astsaturov, Roger B. Cohen, and Paul M. Harari

Introduction

Epidermal growth factor receptor (EGFR) signaling inhibition represents a highly promising arena for the application of molecularly targeted cancer therapies. Evolving from several decades of systematic research in cancer cell biology, a series of EGFR inhibitors from both the monoclonal antibody (mAb) and tyrosine kinase inhibitor (TKI) class have been developed and entered the clinic. Four EGFR inhibitors have recently gained FDA approval for cancer therapy in the United States (and many other countries) including the mAbs cetuximab (Erbitux) and panitumumab (Vectibix), and the small molecule TKIs gefitinib (Iressa) and erlotinib (Tarceva). The rapidly expanding preclinical and clinical data supporting the FDA drug registrations validate a central role for the EGFR as an important molecular target in epithelial malignancies. In this report, we highlight the relevant aspects of EGFR biology and the translation of these observations into recent treatment advances in head and neck squamous cell cancer (HNSCC). Key recent clinical findings include a survival advantage for the addition of the anti-EGFR monoclonal antibody cetuximab to definitive radiation therapy in patients with locoregionally advanced HNSCC, and palliative benefits for the use of cetuximab in patients with incurable HNSCC. Small molecule EGFR TKIs also show considerable promise in this disease, alone and in combination with radiation and chemotherapy. Both classes of anti-EGFR agent are generally well-tolerated with side effects (notably skin rash) that are distinct from those of conventional chemotherapy. Recently completed and ongoing clinical trials will continue to refine the role for EGFR inhibitors in all treatment phases of HNSCC [1, 2].

Concurrent chemoradiation has emerged worldwide as a standard of care for many patients with locoregionally advanced HNSCC [3]. With state-of-the-art radiation (RT) and chemotherapy (along with nodal dissection and salvage surgery, when appropriate) multidisciplinary teams regularly achieve cure rates of approximately 40–50% for stage III and 30% for stage IV HNSCC patients [4] with recently published studies showing even better disease-free and overall

M.P. Mehta et al. (eds.), *Radiation Oncology Advances.*

survival outcomes [5, 6]. Data from individual studies are supported by the conclusions of a recent meta-analysis that showed a small but significant survival advantage with the addition of concurrent chemotherapy to definitive RT (8% survival gain at 5 years) [3, 7]. Chemotherapy can irreversibly damage the DNA of HNSCC cells, thereby sensitizing them to the effects of RT. High-dose cisplatin (100 mg/m^2 every 3 weeks) is the sensitizer used in most of the reported US and European clinical trials. Other cisplatin doses and schedules as well as other drugs, including carboplatin, 5-fluorouracil, and the taxanes, also have clinically useful radiosensitizing properties [5, 6, 8–11]. The price of improved locoregional control and a somewhat lower incidence of distant metastases in all of the studies of chemoradiation is an increase in treatment toxicity, especially acute effects such as grades 3 and 4 mucositis. Recently completed (RTOG-0129) and ongoing Cooperative Group trials continue to evaluate variations on the theme of cisplatin-based chemotherapy and altered RT fractionation schemes in order to improve cure and locoregional control rates. The current toxicity profile of comprehensive chemoradiation treatment regimens for HNSCC patients, however, suggests that we may find it difficult to intensify such therapy further. New agents with novel mechanisms of action and potentially non-overlapping toxicity profiles that can be integrated with or even substituted for some of the current treatments remain a high priority for clinical investigation.

EGFR Biology

The epidermal growth factor itself was isolated in 1965 [12] with receptor purification following in 1980 [13, 14]. Mendelsohn et al. were among the first to propose that "blockade" of the EGFR would have antitumor effects [15, 16]. The discovery that the v-erbB oncogene is a truncated EGF receptor solidified the link between EGFR signaling and oncogenesis [17]. Experiments reported by the Mendelsohn lab and others showed that EGFR inhibition enhanced the effects of chemotherapy in preclinical tumor models [18, 19]. Further experiments in the late 1990s demonstrated similar enhancement of radiation therapy by EGFR inhibitors [20, 21]. HNSCC represents a particularly promising focus for clinical investigation of EGFR inhibitors as the vast majority of these cancers are EGFR positive by immunohistochemistry (IHC) [22, 23].

Recent preclinical work has begun to elucidate the mechanism of EGFR-mediated radiosensitization (Fig. 1). EGFR signaling plays a vital role in cell survival and radiation-induced DNA damage repair [20, 21]. In addition, there is an inverse relationship in tumor model systems between the level of EGFR expression and response to radiation with high levels of EGFR expression associated with inferior response to radiation [24, 25]. Treatment of human tumor xenografts (many tumor histologies, not just HNSCC) with the

Preclinical Features Contributing to Favorable Impact of EGFR Inhibition Plus Radiation

Antiproliferative effects

Multiple cell cycle checkpoints

- Radiation:G2
- EGFR blockade:G1

Apoptosis induction

Inhibition of DNA damage repair

Anti-angiogenic effects

Fig. 1 Preclinical features contributing to favorable impact of EGFR inhibition plus radiation

chimeric anti-EGFR monoclonal antibody cetuximab (C225), for example, markedly enhances the cytotoxic response to RT, reflected in tumor growth delay and cure rates in animals [26, 27]. Serial injections of cetuximab in conjunction with radiation could suppress tumor growth of A431 tumor xenografts for as long as 4 weeks [28]. Mechanisms mediating these effects of cetuximab include enhancement of radiation induced apoptosis in vitro and arrest of cancer cells in the G1 phase of the cell cycle [29] (Fig. 1). Histologic changes in treated tumors, including central necrosis and heavy infiltration with granulocytes, suggest that angiogenesis inhibition and antibody-dependent cell-mediated cytotoxicity (ADCC) may contribute to the observed antitumor effects. Enhancement of response to RT is not limited to cetuximab; diverse EGFR inhibitors, including small molecule EGFR TKIs gefitinib and erlotinib, have similar effects in multiple model systems [21, 30, 31].

Empiric studies of archived human tumor specimens provide additional support for therapeutic EGFR targeting in the clinic. Thus, high EGFR levels (by IHC) correlate with radioresistance and inferior clinical outcome in HNSCC [24, 25, 32]. A retrospective analysis of archival specimens from HNSCC patients receiving definitive RT in a recent RTOG study, for example, clearly showed that HNSCC patients with high EGFR expression had worse overall ($p = 0.0006$) and disease-free survival ($p = 0.0016$), although EGFR expression level did not correlate with T and N stage or incidence of distant metastases. These observations suggest that there may be a specific role of the EGFR in the local tumor response to RT similar to observations from the preclinical experiments [24, 25]. In a multivariate analysis EGFR expression was an independent determinant of survival and a good independent predictor of locoregional relapse [33]. More recent clinical data have shown that patients with HNSCC with high EGFR expression appear to benefit more from hyperfractionated accelerated RT compared to patients with low levels of expression [34].

Anti-EGFR Monoclonal Antibodies

There are several anti-EGFR monoclonal antibodies in clinical trials for human epithelial cancers, including HNSCC, with multiple reports on clinical trials of at least five of these antibodies [2]. There are some differences in the structure of these antibodies as well as the EGFR epitope they target; these differences may have effects on efficacy and toxicity.

To date, the largest clinical database is on patients treated with the anti-EGFR antibody cetuximab (C225), a chimeric monoclonal antibody that is approximately 2/3 human and 1/3 mouse. Humanized antibodies (>95% human) such as matuzumab (EMD72000) [35] and nimotuzumab (h-R3) [36] are also under active clinical investigation. Panitumumab (ABX-EGF [37]) is a fully human antibody. The murine Ig component of the variable region of cetuximab might account for the low rate of infusional allergic reactions that have been described in the clinic with this drug. Such reactions have rarely been seen with humanized or fully human mAbs.

The original therapeutic hypothesis for use of these antibodies was that they would block receptor–ligand interactions, in this case interaction of the EGFR with its principal ligands EGF and TGF-α, causing inhibition of signal transduction. In fact, the effects of antibody–receptor interactions are extremely complex and varied. An antibody molecule that binds the EGFR may elicit an antitumor response via several mechanisms. Depending on the particular antibody, more than one mechanism may be operative. Cetuximab, matuzumab, and nimotuzumab are based on a human immunoglobulin IgG1 framework, for example, whereas panitumumab is constructed on an IgG2 framework. The potential therapeutic importance of this difference in Ig isotype is that IgG1 mediates ADCC by natural killer (NK) cells and macrophages whereas the IgG2 isotype does not [38, 39].

Radiation Plus Cetuximab For Locoregionally Advanced HNSCC

The USA FDA in March 2006 approved cetuximab for use in combination with radiation as an option in the treatment with curative intent of patients with locoregionally advanced HNSCC. This study was the first demonstration that administration of an anti-EGFR agent could provide a survival benefit for patients with an advanced solid malignancy [40]. The pivotal registration study was preceded by a phase I/II trial [41], showing that it was safe to administer weekly cetuximab with a course of definitive RT in the treatment of locally advanced HNSCC. In that study cetuximab was given as a loading dose of 100–500 mg/m^2 starting 1 week before RT, followed by weekly infusions of 100–250 mg/m^2 for 7–8 weeks, with the weekly schedule of cetuximab administration based on a plasma half-life of around 90 h [41, 42]. The rationale for a loading dose was to saturate all EGFR in the body, including EGFR receptors found in normal liver and skin [42]. Patients in the phase I study had locoregionally advanced HNSCC (oropharynx, larynx, and hypopharynx) not suitable for surgery. Most [12] received conventional once daily RT (70 Gy, 2 Gy/d) with the last three patients on the study receiving hyperfractionated RT (76.8 Gy, 1.2 Gy bid). The most common toxicities attributable to cetuximab were skin reactions in the radiation field; these were grade 3 (desquamating) in five patients. Infusion reactions occurred in four patients (one resulted in discontinuation of antibody therapy). Other than the one infusion reaction none of these toxicities was considered dose-limiting. In this small study the investigators noted that the rates and intensity of mucositis and odynophagia seemed no worse than those seen with radical RT alone. All patients who received cetuximab and radiation and were therefore evaluable responded well to this regimen with 13 CR and 2 PR. Prolonged follow-up of these patients has shown that these responses are durable. The investigators concluded that cetuximab could be safely combined with RT as a loading dose of 400–500 mg/m^2, followed by a weekly dose of 250 mg/m^2 [41]. In a separate study in patients with HNSCC investigators established that this dose and schedule of cetuximab gave a high percentage of EGFR binding in tumor tissue [43].

The multicenter, international phase III trial enrolled 424 patients and is one of the largest randomized studies conducted in HNSCC. In this study patients with locoregionally advanced HNSCC were randomized to definitive RT alone ($n = 213$), or the combination of definitive RT and weekly cetuximab (at a loading dose of 400 mg/m^2 followed by 250 mg/m^2 weekly for 8 weeks) ($n = 211$). The first dose of cetuximab was given 1 week before the initiation of RT. Stratification factors included performance status, tumor stage, nodal involvement, and RT fractionation regimen. At the time of the design of this study (1998–1999), RT alone without chemotherapy was considered by many experts to represent an appropriate standard of care in the treatment of patients with locoregionally advanced HNSCC. Reflecting prevailing practice patterns in the radiation oncology community, three RT fractionation schedules were permitted in the trial: once daily, twice daily or concomitant boost. Investigators had to specify the RT regimen prior to randomization. Distinct treatment delivery options regarding RT pertain to the current era as well (IMRT, IGRT, etc.) and inform contemporary trial designs in this disease (e.g., RTOG 0522). Most patients on this study were men (80%) in relatively good health (most had a Karnofsky score of 90–100). Tumor sites were oropharynx (60%), larynx (25%) and hypopharynx (15%) but not oral cavity (usually treated with surgery) or nasopharyngeal cancer. There was no requirement for EGFR testing of tumors as a study entry criterion [40].

The phase III study showed that cetuximab added to definitive radiation conferred a statistically significant improvement in the median duration of locoregional control from 14.9 to 24.4 months (log-rank $p = 0.005$), lowering the risk of locoregional failure by 32% (hazard ratio =0.68). Cetuximab also decreased the risk of death by 26% (HR = 0.74, $p = 0.03$) with a clinically significant improvement in median survival (29.3–49 months) [40]. This result validated the preclinical models that informed the clinical investigation program of cetuximab [44]. Toxicity in both arms of the trial was strikingly similar with the exception of skin rash that was more common in patients receiving cetuximab. In particular, the incidence of grades 3 and 4 mucositis was the same in both arms suggesting that the addition of cetuximab

Phase III Trial of Radiation plus Cetuximab in H&N Cancer*

- First phase III trial to demonstrate survival increase using molecular targeted agent combined with radiation
- Benefits achieved without notable increase in overall toxicity, including grades 3-4 mucositis
- Addition of cetuximab did not compromise delivery of full course radiation schedule

*Bonner J, Harari P, Giralt J, et al. N Engl J Med 2006;354:567–578

Fig. 2 Phase III trial of radiation plus Cetuximab in H&N Cancer*

to definitive RT did not exacerbate this important and often disabling side effect of therapy (Fig. 2). Several pertinent ad hoc subset analyses were performed. These showed that patients with oropharynx cancer had the greatest benefit from EGFR blockade, with a doubling in this subgroup in the median duration of locoregional control (23 months vs. 49 months). On the other hand, there was little improvement in outcome for patients with carcinomas of larynx and hypopharynx, although the rate of larynx sparing was better in the patients who received cetuximab. Thus, the rate of laryngeal preservation (absence of total laryngectomy) was 8% higher in the cetuximab arm and the hazard ratio for laryngeal preservation was 0.62 although neither result is statistically significant [45]. Patients with hypopharyngeal cancer had a generally poor outcome (~13.5 months median survival with or without cetuximab).

Concurrent chemoradiation, generally using platinum compounds as radiation enhancers, remains a standard of care for young, medically fit patients with locoregionally advanced unresectable (or not appropriate for resection) HNSCC being treated with curative intent. The pivotal trial did not compare cetuximab plus radiation to chemoradiation. Therefore, noninferiority with chemoradiation has not been established. The data in the pivotal study do support the use of cetuximab plus RT as a viable option that is superior to RT alone for those patients not suitable for chemoradiation.

Cetuximab, Cisplatin, and Radiation in Locoregionally Advanced HNSCC

Outcomes for patients with locoregionally advanced HNSCC have certainly improved with contemporary chemoradiation but treatment resistance and eventual local and distant failure remains a very important clinical problem. Several common acquired genetic abnormalities in HNSCC may contribute to this phenomenon, including mutations of p53 and other genes governing apoptosis [46]. EGFR blockade alone (or chemotherapy for that matter) may not be able to overcome these molecular lesions [25]. With this in mind the simultaneous application of two radiosensitizers such as cisplatin and cetuximab with complementary mechanisms of action, is a logical extension of the data in an attempt to provide additional improvements in locoregional control and survival over those seen with either agent alone. Pfister et al. [47] enrolled patients with locoregionally advanced HNSCC onto a small study (n=21) of cisplatin, cetuximab and RT in which patients received RT 70 Gy (concomitant boost) together with concurrent weekly cetuximab and high dose cisplatin (100 mg/m^2 on weeks 1 and 4). Enrollment was halted prematurely after two on-study deaths (one pneumonia, one cause unknown) and one occurrence each of myocardial infarction, bacteremia, and atrial fibrillation. At a median follow-up of 44 months with all survivors followed for a minimum of 31 months, the 3-year overall and progression free survivals were encouraging (76 and 59%, respectively). These long-term follow-up data prompted evaluation of a regimen similar to this as the experimental arm of the ongoing RTOG trial 0522, "A Randomized Phase III Trial of Concurrent Accelerated Radiation and Cisplatin vs. Concurrent Accelerated Radiation, Cisplatin, and Cetuximab (C225) for Stage III and IV Head and Neck Carcinomas." This trial will eventually enroll over 700 patients with primary endpoints of survival and locoregional control. It is clear, however, that the potential regimen-related toxicities observed in the Pfister study warrant continued caution until further clinical trials establish the safety and efficacy of a chemoradiotherapy plus cetuximab regimen.

Cetuximab ± Chemotherapy in Recurrent and/or Metastatic HNSCC

In March 2006, the FDA also approved cetuximab for use as monotherapy in patients with platin-refractory incurable HNSCC. The FDA indication for cetuximab is the first approval of a new agent in this setting in more than 30 years. Some patients with HNSCC (10%) are initially diagnosed with distant metastatic disease while others develop locoregional and systemic recurrence despite aggressive local treatment. Subsequent treatment options for these generally incurable patients remain inadequate. Indeed, there has been little tangible progress in chemotherapy despite the introduction of many new agents including the taxanes [48]. Aggressive surgical salvage therapy as well as reirradiation [49] are appropriate and helpful for selected patients, but most patients need effective palliation with agents that preserve or improve quality of life. Preliminary data are showing a survival advantage for anti-EGFR therapies in this setting, and these newer drugs offer patients a meaningful clinical benefit (tumor response) with a toxicity profile that compares favorably with cytotoxic chemotherapy [50].

The key study in the platin-refractory HNSCC population was a multicenter phase II study conducted in Europe [51]. Patients (n = 103) with metastatic or recurrent

HNSCC with documented radiographic evidence of disease progression after 2–6 cycles of standard platin-based chemotherapy received cetuximab weekly until disease progression. Patients who did not respond to cetuximab monotherapy could go on to receive a combination of cetuximab plus *cis*- or carboplatin (at the same dose and schedule of the platin received prior to study entry). The overall objective response rate was ~13% (all partial responses), with a disease control rate (response plus stable disease) of 46%. Median time-to-progression and survival was 85 and 175 days, respectively; this represents a 2.5-month increase in the median survival when compared with the survival of platinum-refractory historical controls receiving second-line chemotherapy. There were no responses in those patients failing to respond to cetuximab who crossed over to combination therapy, a result that stands in contrast to the ability of cetuximab to resensitize patients with metastatic colorectal cancer who are no longer responding to irinotecan [52, 53]. Cetuximab-related adverse events in the platin-refractory setting included the characteristic rash, paronychia, fatigue, fever, chills, and nausea. On the basis of this study the investigators concluded that single-agent cetuximab is biologically active in platin-refractory HNSCC with clinically meaningful responses and an acceptable toxicity profile.

At this time it is not clear if adding chemotherapy to cetuximab in patients with platin-refractory HNSCC offers additional benefit. Two studies, one in the USA and the other in Europe, enrolled patients progressing on platin-based therapy and added cetuximab to the platin regimen they were failing. The overall partial response rate in both trials [54, 55] was very similar to the response rate (~13%) seen with cetuximab monotherapy in this setting [51, 56].

Cetuximab with Chemotherapy in the First-Line Treatment of Patients with Recurrent and/or Metastatic HNSCC

There are emerging clinical data showing that cetuximab may be combined safely with chemotherapy in this setting and a suggestion that the response rate may also be superior to chemotherapy alone. Burtness et al. conducted a randomized phase III clinical trial through ECOG in which chemotherapy naïve patients with recurrent/metastatic HNSCC ($n = 117$) were enrolled and treated with cisplatin 100 mg/m^2 every 4 weeks with weekly cetuximab or placebo [57]. Progression-free survival (PFS) was the primary end-point of the study. Median PFS was somewhat better for patients receiving cetuximab (4.2 months) compared to those receiving placebo (2.7 months) but this result was not statistically significant and median overall survival was similar on both arms (9.2 months for cetuximab vs. 8.0 months for placebo). On the other hand, the response rate was significantly higher in patients who received cetuximab (26%) vs. placebo (10%) ($p = 0.03$). Interestingly, the response rate was higher in those patients with EGFR staining in less than 80% of tumor cells.

Several larger studies are underway to assess more definitively the combination of chemo- and anti-EGFR therapy in this setting. The EXTREME phase III clinical trial has completed enrollment and is assessing the efficacy of cisplatin (or carboplatin) and 5-FU with or without cetuximab in patients with recurrent and/or metastatic HNSCC who have not received palliative chemotherapy. The primary end-point of the study is overall survival. An earlier phase I trial by the same group demonstrated that carboplatin or cisplatin (both with 5-FU) in combination with cetuximab were reasonably well-tolerated with encouraging response rates. Carboplatin and 5-fluorouracil appeared to be the more tolerable doublet for combination with cetuximab [58].

EGFR Tyrosine Kinase Inhibitors (TKIs)

TKIs with activity in HNSCC are mostly quinazoline-derived, low molecular weight synthetic molecules that competitively inhibit the Mg-ATP-catalytic site of the intracellular tyrosine kinase domain. Gefitinib and erlotinib are relatively specific for the EGFR. As classic enzyme inhibitors, TKIs block ligand-induced receptor autophosphorylation thereby abrogating intracellular downstream signaling (Fig. 3). A number of second generation EGFR TKIs block more than one receptor in addition to the EGFR, such as Her2 and VEGF-R2 [59, 60]. EKB-659 is distinct as an irreversible inhibitor of the EGFR [61]. We do not know the optimal approach to EGFR inhibition: small molecules that are relatively selective with preferential activity against one tyrosine kinase vs. less specific agents that inhibit multiple kinases. Some of the relevant distinctions between TKIs and antibodies

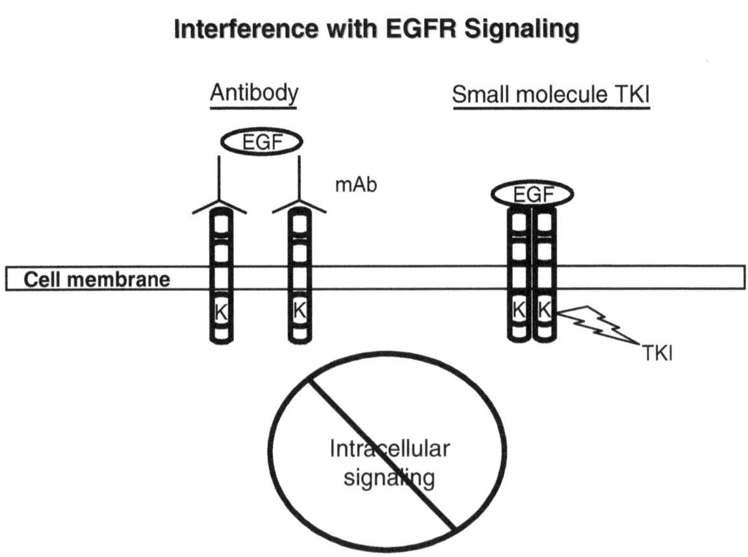

Fig. 3 Interference with EGFR signaling

include daily oral administration of TKIs vs. weekly (or less often) intravenous delivery of antibodies. TKIs cause GI side effects (nausea and diarrhea), which are occasionally dose-limiting. Infusion reactions can occur with monoclonal antibodies. TKIs and antibodies (other than nimotuzumab [36]) both cause the characteristic mechanism-based skin rash.

TKI Monotherapy in HNSCC

When gefitinib monotherapy is given to patients with incurable (metastatic, recurrent) HNSCC, the results are strikingly similar to those obtained in the same setting with antibodies such as cetuximab. Gefitinib at high dose (500mg orally daily) showed an overall response rate of ~11% and disease control rate of 53% in 47 evaluable patients [62]. Most patients in this study had received prior platin-containing therapy, but they probably were not a truly platin-refractory population. Time-to-progression (3.4 months) and median survival (8.1 months) were also encouraging and gefitinib was well-tolerated except for grade 3 diarrhea (three patients). The development of rash correlated with favorable response, progression, and survival. The observation that response appeared to be independent of prior chemotherapy exposure suggested that anti-EGFR agents may be non-crossresistant with agents such as *cis*- and carboplatin. Similar results for gefitinib at 500mg day were reported from a study in the UK ($n = 47$) with a response rate of 8% and a disease control rate of 36% [63]. A third study showed that gefitinib at a dose of 250mg daily (the FDA-approved dose for advanced NSCLC) was much less active in HNSCC with only one partial response in 70 patients (RR 1.4%) [64]. Why there is an apparent dose–response for gefitinib in HNSCC is not known.

Erlotinib in this type of refractory patient gives very similar response, disease control, and survival results. In a study of 115 patients with recurrent and/or metastatic HNSCC most of whom had received prior platin-based therapy, erlotinib at 150mg daily gave a partial response rate of 4.3% and approximately a third of patients (38%) had disease stabilization for a median duration of 16.1 weeks. The median PFS was 9.6 weeks and the median overall survival was 6.0 months [65].

TKIs in Combination with Radiation Therapy

Studies from the University of Chicago have shown that it is safe to integrate gefitinib into definitive chemoradiation delivered with curative intent to patients with loco-regionally advanced HNSCC. Among 69 subjects treated with their regimen THFX in which gefitinib 250mg by mouth (or PEG tube) was substituted for paclitaxel, they reported a CR rate of 88% with rates of grade 3 and 4 toxicities similar to those reported with chemoradiotherapy. Other investigators have presented similar data from a phase I/II study of erlotinib combined with cisplatin and radiotherapy. It is clear that chemoradiation regimens that include small molecule EGFR TKIs are feasible, tolerable, and worthy of further evaluation [66, 67].

TKIs with Dual Specificity

Lapatinib (GW572016) is an oral small molecule inhibitor of the EGFR and Her2 tyrosine kinase activities [59, 60] that was recently approved for use in advanced Her2 positive breast cancer in combination with capecitabine. There are preliminary data in HNSCC suggesting that mutations in Her2 may determine, in part, the response of HNSCC to agents such as gefitinib [68]. A pilot phase I clinical trial in which patients with locoregionally advanced HNSCC received escalating doses of daily lapatinib with concurrent cisplatin-sensitized chemoradiation showed good tolerability of lapatinib at a dose of 1,500 mg by mouth daily [69]. Whether lapatinib enhances chemoradiation is unknown. Of note, in metastatic and recurrent HNSCC single agent lapatinib had little objective antitumor activity [70]. The reasons for this lack of single agent activity are unclear.

Vandetanib (ZD6474) is an orally bioavailable inhibitor of the EGFR and VEGF-R2 tyrosine kinase activities [71]. AEE-788 is another oral agent that inhibits at least three receptor tyrosine kinases including EGFR, Her-2, and VEGFR and has antiproliferative and antiangiogenic effects in preclinical studies [72]. Both agents warrant further testing in HNSCC and are in early phase clinical trials.

Patient Selection

Currently, we do not have keen insight regarding how best to select patients for EGFR inhibitor therapies. Almost all HNSCC are EGFR positive, albeit to varying degrees. There is a suggestion from some of the studies that EGFR inhibitors may have greater benefits in patients bearing tumors with low to moderate EGFR expression compared to those with high EGFR expression [57]. But this finding may simply be a selection effect; we already know that patients with high-expressing EGFR tumors have an inferior outcome [33, 73]. It is conceivable that patients with high EGFR expression require higher doses of EGFR inhibitor therapy in order to achieve the best results. The superior response rate to high (500 mg) compared with low (250 mg) dose gefitinib in patients with advanced HNSCC reported by investigators at the University of Chicago provides some preliminary support for this notion [62].

Assessment of EGFR expression by IHC in tumor samples seems simple but is not at all straightforward with multiple technical and methodological issues confounding the analysis. The intensity of EGFR staining can vary depending on a number of factors that include tissue processing and storage procedures, as well as variability in the staining antibodies and the quantitative analysis and scoring methods used. Variation across institutions and laboratories is a major issue. In one study, for example, there was a correlation between the storage time of formalin-fixed tissue samples and a decrease in EGFR staining [74]. Primary tumors and metastatic deposits in HNSCC (and other cancers) are intrinsically heterogeneous. Analysis of small biopsy specimens may not be representative of most of the tumor [75].

Activating mutations of the EGFR tyrosine kinase domain in NSCLC predict for response to EGFR inhibitors. In NSCLC these somatic mutations cluster around the ATP binding cleft of the kinase and mediate enhanced ligand-dependent signaling and tenfold higher susceptibility to gefitinib inhibition [76–78]. The majority of these alterations are in-frame deletions of exon 19 or L858R point mutation in the exon 20, which result in increased signaling activity of the mutant EGFR [79, 80]. In HNSCC, by contrast, there is no strong evidence for somatic activating mutations of the EGFR [62, 68, 78, 81–83]. Studies screening small numbers of archived HNSCC continue [84] and there are some preliminary data suggesting that EGFR mutation in HNSCC may be higher in East Asia. Thus, Korean investigators recently presented data [85] showing the presence of an in-frame EGFR exon 19 deletion in three out of 41 unselected patients with HNSCC but there are no data linking any of these HNSCC EGFR mutations to response to TKI therapy. There is a single preclinical report that sensitivity to erlotinib in a panel of HNSCC cell lines correlated with the number of CA single sequence repeats in intron 1 of the EGFR [86]. To date, there are no published analyses correlating EGFR gene copy number in HNSCC to response, survival or clinical benefit, unlike reports of these relationships in mCRC [87] and NSCLC [88].

One recurrent correlation in multiple clinical studies of EGFR inhibitors (antibodies and TKIs) in patients with solid tumors is an apparent correlation between clinical benefit (survival) and the intensity of the characteristic skin rash caused by anti-EGFR therapy [40, 53, 57, 64, 89–92]. These observations require confirmation in other studies, ideally as a prospective endpoint. A mechanistic explanation for the correlation remains elusive; skin rash could be a surrogate marker for another global biologic factor (e.g., immune status) without any direct connection to response of tumor EGFR to the inhibitor [93].

Conclusions

The stepwise advancement of molecular targeted therapies from the laboratory to the clinic offers a new set of versatile tools that can be used effectively alone or in combination with conventional cancer treatment modalities. EGFR signaling inhibition represents one of the most mature emerging strategies within this new cancer treatment paradigm. Disruption of EGFR signaling has been amply validated as an anticancer strategy in preclinical tumor models and is now undergoing extensive clinical testing. Indeed, over the past several years, the clinical utility of EGFR inhibitors has been confirmed in nonsmall cell lung, pancreatic, and now HNSCC, reflected in rising patient use (Fig. 4). Over the next several years, there will be

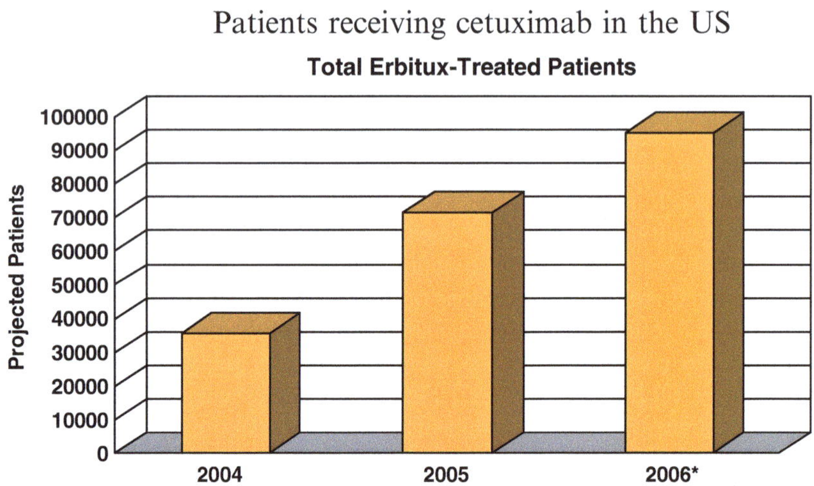

Fig. 4 Patients receiving cetuximab in the US

further integration of various EGFR inhibitors into established treatment regimens for HNSCC, including induction therapy, concurrent chemoradiation, adjuvant therapy, reirradiation, and palliative therapy. Studies will clarify whether EGFR inhibitors are best used in combination with chemoradiation or whether they may be substituted for chemotherapy in certain settings. Randomized clinical trials will evaluate their utility as maintenance therapy in the management of high-risk patients. It is conceivable that EGFR inhibitors may even be used in cancer prevention strategies in certain high-risk patients. Whether mAb EGFR inhibitors also work by immunological mechanisms in addition to signaling inhibition will be clarified. Novel EGFR inhibitors designed to enhance ADCC, inhibit multiple kinases, or mitigate skin and GI toxicity will expand the utility and tolerability of this therapeutic class. Improved understanding regarding patient selection factors, including predictors of response (including skin rash or better yet, simple and accurate molecular profiles), will further optimize the benefit to patients of these promising anticancer agents.

References

1. Astsaturov I, Cohen RB, Harari P. Targeting epidermal growth factor receptor signaling in the treatment of head and neck cancer. Expert Rev Anticancer Ther 2006; 6(9):1179–1193.
2. Astsaturov I, Cohen RB, Harari PM. EGFR-targeting monoclonal antibodies in head and neck cancer. Curr Cancer Drug Targets 2006; 6(8):691–710.
3. Bourhis J, Amand C, Pignon J. Update of MACH-NC (Meta-Analysis of Chemotherapy in Head and Neck Cancer) database focused on concomitant chemoradiotherapy.. J Clin Oncol (Meeting Abstracts), 2004; 22(14 suppl): 5505.

4. Kufe D, et al. Cancer Medicine 6. *6th ed.* Hamilton Ont. London (BC Decker), 2v (2003).
5. Calais G, Alfonsi M, Bardet E, et al. Randomized trial of radiation therapy versus concomitant chemotherapy and radiation therapy for advanced-stage oropharynx carcinoma. J Natl Cancer Inst 1999; 91(24):2081–2086.
6. Brizel DM, Albers ME, Fisher SR, et al. Hyperfractionated irradiation with or without concurrent chemotherapy for locally advanced head and neck cancer. N Engl J Med 1998; 338(25):1798–1804.
7. Pignon JP, Bourhis J, Domenge C, Designe L. Chemotherapy added to locoregional treatment for head and neck squamous-cell carcinoma: three meta-analyses of updated individual data. MACH-NC Collaborative Group. Meta-Analysis of Chemotherapy on Head and Neck Cancer. Lancet 2000; 355(9208):949–955.
8. Adelstein DJ, Li Y, Adams GL, et al. An intergroup phase III comparison of standard radiation therapy and two schedules of concurrent chemoradiotherapy in patients with unresectable squamous cell head and neck cancer. J Clin Oncol 2003; 21(1):92–98.
9. Forastiere AA, Goepfert H, Maor M, et al. Concurrent chemotherapy and radiotherapy for organ preservation in advanced laryngeal cancer. N Engl J Med 2003; 349(22): 2091–2098.
10. Bernier J, Domenge C, Ozsahin M, et al. Postoperative irradiation with or without concomitant chemotherapy for locally advanced head and neck cancer. N Engl J Med 2004; 350(19): 1945–1952.
11. Laramore GE, Scott CB, al-Sarraf M, et al. Adjuvant chemotherapy for resectable squamous cell carcinomas of the head and neck: report on Intergroup Study 0034. Int J Radiat Oncol Biol Phys 1992; 23(4):705–713.
12. Cohen S. The stimulation of epidermal proliferation by a specific protein (EGF). Dev Biol 1965; 12(3):394–407.
13. Cohen S, Carpenter G, King L Jr. Epidermal growth factor-receptor-protein kinase interactions. Co-purification of receptor and epidermal growth factor-enhanced phosphorylation activity. J Biol Chem 1980; 255(10):4834–4842.
14. Ushiro H, Cohen S. Identification of phosphotyrosine as a product of epidermal growth factor-activated protein kinase in A-431 cell membranes. J Biol Chem 1980; 255(18):8363–8365.
15. Masui H, Kawamoto T, Sato JD, Wolf B, Sato G, Mendelsohn J. Growth inhibition of human tumor cells in athymic mice by anti-epidermal growth factor receptor monoclonal antibodies. Cancer Res 1984; 44(3):1002–1007.
16. Mendelsohn J. Growth factor receptors as targets for antitumor therapy with monoclonal antibodies. Prog Allergy 1988; 45147–45160.
17. Downward J, Yarden Y, Mayes E, et al. Close similarity of epidermal growth factor receptor and v-erb-B oncogene protein sequences. Nature 1984; 307(5951):521–527.
18. Fan Z, Masui H, Altas I, Mendelsohn J. Blockade of epidermal growth factor receptor function by bivalent and monovalent fragments of 225 anti-epidermal growth factor receptor monoclonal antibodies. Cancer Res 1993; 53(18):4322–4328.
19. Baselga J, Norton L, Masui H, et al. Antitumor effects of doxorubicin in combination with anti-epidermal growth factor receptor monoclonal antibodies. J Natl Cancer Inst 1993; 85(16):1327–1333.
20. Balaban N, Moni J, Shannon M, Dang L, Murphy E, Goldkorn T. The effect of ionizing radiation on signal transduction: antibodies to EGF receptor sensitize A431 cells to radiation. Biochim Biophys Acta 1996; 1314(1–2):147–156.
21. Schmidt-Ullrich RK, Mikkelsen RB, Dent P, et al. Radiation-induced proliferation of the human A431 squamous carcinoma cells is dependent on EGFR tyrosine phosphorylation. Oncogene 1997; 15(10):1191–1197.
22. Rubin Grandis J, Melhem MF, Barnes EL, Tweardy DJ. Quantitative immunohistochemical analysis of transforming growth factor-alpha and epidermal growth factor receptor in patients with squamous cell carcinoma of the head and neck. Cancer 1996; 78(6):1284–1292.
23. Rubin Grandis J, Melhem MF, Gooding WE, et al. Levels of TGF-alpha and EGFR protein in head and neck squamous cell carcinoma and patient survival. J Natl Cancer Inst 1998; 90(11):824–832.

24. Sheridan MT, O'Dwyer T, Seymour CB, Mothersill CE. Potential indicators of radiosensitivity in squamous cell carcinoma of the head and neck. Radiat Oncol Investig 1997; 5(4):180–186.
25. Akimoto T, Hunter NR, Buchmiller L, Mason K, Ang KK, Milas L. Inverse relationship between epidermal growth factor receptor expression and radiocurability of murine carcinomas. Clin Cancer Res 1999; 5(10):2884–2890.
26. Saleh MN, Raisch KP, Stackhouse MA, et al. Combined modality therapy of A431 human epidermoid cancer using anti-EGFr antibody C225 and radiation. Cancer Biother Radiopharm 1999; 14(6):451–463.
27. Milas L, Fan Z, Andratschke NH, Ang KK. Epidermal growth factor receptor and tumor response to radiation: in vivo preclinical studies. Int J Radiat Oncol Biol Phys 2004; 58(3):966–971.
28. Milas L, Mason K, Hunter N, et al. In vivo enhancement of tumor radioresponse by C225 antiepidermal growth factor receptor antibody. Clin Cancer Res 2000; 6(2):701–708.
29. Huang SM, Bock JM, Harari PM. Epidermal growth factor receptor blockade with C225 modulates proliferation, apoptosis, and radiosensitivity in squamous cell carcinomas of the head and neck. Cancer Res 1999; 59(8):1935–1940.
30. Harari PM, Huang S. Radiation combined with EGFR signal inhibitors: head and neck cancer focus. Semin Radiat Oncol 2006; 16(1):38–44.
31. Zhou H, Kim YS, Peletier A, McCall W, Earp HS, Sartor CI. Effects of the EGFR/HER2 kinase inhibitor GW572016 on EGFR- and HER2-overexpressing breast cancer cell line proliferation, radiosensitization, and resistance. Int J Radiat Oncol Biol Phys 2004; 58(2):344–352.
32. Dassonville O, Formento JL, Francoual M, et al. Expression of epidermal growth factor receptor and survival in upper aerodigestive tract cancer. J Clin Oncol 1993 ; 11(10):1873–1878.
33. Ang KK, Berkey BA, Tu X, et al. Impact of epidermal growth factor receptor expression on survival and pattern of relapse in patients with advanced head and neck carcinoma. Cancer Res 2002; 62(24):7350–7356.
34. Bentzen SM, Atasoy BM, Daley FM, et al. Epidermal growth factor receptor expression in pretreatment biopsies from head and neck squamous cell carcinoma as a predictive factor for a benefit from accelerated radiation therapy in a randomized controlled trial. J Clin Oncol 2005; 23(24):5560–5567.
35. Vanhoefer U, Tewes M, Rojo F, et al. Phase I study of the humanized antiepidermal growth factor receptor monoclonal antibody EMD72000 in patients with advanced solid tumors that express the epidermal growth factor receptor. J Clin Oncol 2004; 22(1):175–184.
36. Crombet T, Osorio M, Cruz T, et al. Use of the humanized anti-epidermal growth factor receptor monoclonal antibody h-R3 in combination with radiotherapy in the treatment of locally advanced head and neck cancer patients. J Clin Oncol 2004; 22(9):1646–1654.
37. Tyagi P. Recent results and ongoing trials with panitumumab (ABX-EGF), a fully human anti-epidermal growth factor receptor antibody, in metastatic colorectal cancer. Clin Colorectal Cancer 2005; 5(1):21–23.
38. Cartron G, Dacheux L, Salles G, et al. Therapeutic activity of humanized anti-CD20 monoclonal antibody and polymorphism in IgG Fc receptor FcgammaRIIIa gene. Blood 2002; 99(3):754–758.
39. Weng WK, Levy R. Two immunoglobulin G fragment C receptor polymorphisms independently predict response to rituximab in patients with follicular lymphoma. J Clin Oncol 2003; 21(21):3940–3947.
40. Bonner JA, Harari PM, Giralt J, et al. Radiotherapy plus Cetuximab for Squamous-Cell Carcinoma of the Head and Neck. N Engl J Med 2006; 354(6):567–578.
41. Robert F, Ezekiel MP, Spencer SA, et al. Phase I study of anti-epidermal growth factor receptor antibody cetuximab in combination with radiation therapy in patients with advanced head and neck cancer. J Clin Oncol 2001; 19(13):3234–3243.
42. Baselga J, Pfister D, Cooper MR, et al. Phase I studies of anti-epidermal growth factor receptor chimeric antibody C225 alone and in combination with cisplatin. J Clin Oncol 2000; 18(4):904–914.

43. Shin DM, Donato NJ, Perez-Soler R, et al. Epidermal growth factor receptor-targeted therapy with C225 and cisplatin in patients with head and neck cancer. Clin Cancer Res 2001; 7(5):1204–1213.
44. Bonner JA, Raisch KP, Trummell HQ, et al. Enhanced apoptosis with combination C225/radiation treatment serves as the impetus for clinical investigation in head and neck cancers. J Clin Oncol 2000; 18(suppl1):47s–53s.
45. Bonner JA, Harari PM, Giralt J, et al. Cetuximab improves locoregional control and survival of locoregionally advanced head and neck cancer: independent review of mature data with a median followup of 45 months. AACR-NCI-EORTC International Conference. Mol Targets Cancer Ther Clin Cancer Res 2005; 11(24, part 2): 9058s.
46. Geisler SA, Olshan AF, Weissler MC, et al. p16 and p53 protein expression as prognostic indicators of survival and disease recurrence from head and neck cancer. Clin Cancer Res 2002; 8(11):3445–3453.
47. Pfister DG, Su YB, Kraus DH, et al. Concurrent cetuximab, cisplatin, and concomitant boost radiotherapy for locoregionally advanced, squamous cell head and neck cancer: a pilot phase II study of a new combined-modality paradigm. J Clin Oncol 2006; 24(7):1072–1078.
48. Diaz E, Sturgis E, Laramore G, Sabichi A, Lippman S, Clayman G. Neoplasms of the head and neck. Cancer 6 Medicine 2003; 21325–21371.
49. Benchalal M, Bachaud JM, Francois P, et al. Hyperfractionation in the reirradiation of head and neck cancers. Result of a pilot study. Radiother Oncol 1995; 36(3):203–210.
50. Cohen EE. Role of epidermal growth factor receptor pathway-targeted therapy in patients with recurrent and/or metastatic squamous cell carcinoma of the head and neck. J Clin Oncol 2006; 24(17):2659–2665.
51. Trigo R, Hitt P, Koralewski E, et al. Cetuximab monotherapy is active in patients (pts) with platinum-refractory recurrent/metastatic squamous cell carcinoma of the head and neck (SCCHN): results of a phase II study. ASCO Annual Meeting; 2004.
52. Saltz LB, Lenz H, Hochster H, et al. Randomized phase II trial of Cetuximab/Bevacizumab/Irinotecan (CBI) versus Cetuximab/Bevacizumab (CB) in Irinotecan-Refractory Colorectal Cancer. 2005 ASCO Annual Meeting, Abstract No: 3508 (2005).
53. Cunningham D, Humblet Y, Siena S, et al. Cetuximab monotherapy and cetuximab plus irinotecan in irinotecan-refractory metastatic colorectal cancer. N Engl J Med 2004; 351(4):337–345.
54. Baselga J, Trigo JM, Bourhis J, et al. Phase II multicenter study of the antiepidermal growth factor receptor monoclonal antibody cetuximab in combination with platinum-based chemotherapy in patients with platinum-refractory metastatic and/or recurrent squamous cell carcinoma of the head and neck. J Clin Oncol 2005; 23(24):5568–5577.
55. Herbst RS, Arquette M, Shin DM, et al. Phase II multicenter study of the epidermal growth factor receptor antibody cetuximab and cisplatin for recurrent and refractory squamous cell carcinoma of the head and neck. J Clin Oncol %R 10.1200/JCO.2005.07.120 2005; 23(24):5578–5587.
56. Vermorken J, et al. Cetuximab in recurrent/metastatic (R&M) squamous cell carcinoma of the head and neck (SCCHN) refractory to first-line platinum-based therapies. J Clin Oncol 2005; 23(16 suppl):5505.
57. Burtness B, Goldwasser MA, Flood W, Mattar B, Forastiere AA. Phase III randomized trial of cisplatin plus placebo compared with cisplatin plus cetuximab in metastatic/recurrent head and neck cancer: an Eastern Cooperative Oncology Group study. J Clin Oncol 2005; 23(34):8646–8654.
58. Vermorken JB, Mesia R, Vega-Villegas ME, Remenar E, Hitt R, Kawecki A. Cetuximab in combination with cisplain or carboplatin and 5-fluorouracil in the first-line treatment of patients with recurrent and/or metastatic squamous cell carcinoma of the head and neck. J Clin Oncol 2006; 24(18S):5537.
59. Burris HA III, Hurwitz HI, Dees EC, et al. Phase I safety, pharmacokinetics, and clinical activity study of lapatinib (GW572016), a reversible dual inhibitor of epidermal growth factor

receptor tyrosine kinases, in heavily pretreated patients with metastatic carcinomas. J Clin Oncol %R 10.1200/JCO.2005.16.584 2005; 23(23):5305–5313.
60. Spector NL, Xia W, Burris H III, et al. Study of the biologic effects of Lapatinib, a reversible inhibitor of ErbB1 and ErbB2 tyrosine kinases, on tumor growth and survival pathways in patients with advanced malignancies. J Clin Oncol %R 10.1200/JCO.2005.12.157 2005; 23(11):2502–2512.
61. Erlichman C, Hidalgo M, Boni JP, et al. Phase I study of EKB-569, an irreversible inhibitor of the epidermal growth factor receptor, in patients with advanced solid tumors. J Clin Oncol 2006; 24(15):2252–2260.
62. Cohen EE, Rosen F, Stadler WM, et al. Phase II trial of ZD1839 in recurrent or metastatic squamous cell carcinoma of the head and neck. J Clin Oncol 2003; 21(10):1980–1987.
63. Kirby AM, A'Hern RP, D'Ambrosio C, et al. Gefitinib (ZD1839, Iressa) as palliative treatment in recurrent or metastatic head and neck cancer. Br J Cancer 2006; 94(5):631–636.
64. Cohen EE, Kane MA, List MA, et al. Phase II trial of gefitinib 250 mg daily in patients with recurrent and/or metastatic squamous cell carcinoma of the head and neck. Clin Cancer Res 2005; 11(23):8418–8424.
65. Soulieres D, Senzer NN, Vokes EE, Hidalgo M, Agarwala SS, Siu LL. Multicenter phase II study of erlotinib, an oral epidermal growth factor receptor tyrosine kinase inhibitor, in patients with recurrent or metastatic squamous cell cancer of the head and neck. J Clin Oncol 2004; 22(1):77–85.
66. Doss H, Greco F, Meluch A, et al. Induction chemotherapy + gefitinib followed by concurrent chemotherapy/radiation therapy/gefitinib for patients (pts) with locally advanced squamous carcinoma of the head and neck: A phase I/II trial of the Minnie Pearl Cancer Research Network. ASCO Annual Meeting Proceedings 2006; 24(18S):290s.
67. Savvides P, Agarwala S, Greskovich J, et al. Phase I study of the EGFR tyrosine kinase inhibitor erlobtinib in combination with docetaxel and radiation in locally advanced squamous cell cancer of the head and neck (SCCHN). ASCO Annual Meeting Proceedings 2006; 24(18S):291s.
68. Cohen EE, Lingen MW, Martin LE, et al. Response of some head and neck cancers to epidermal growth factor receptor tyrosine kinase inhibitors may be linked to mutation of ERBB2 rather than EGFR. Clin Cancer Res 2005; 11(22):8105–8108.
69. Herrington KJ, Bourhis J, Nutting CM, Rosine D, Theodosiou AM, Gardiner S. A phase I, open-label study of lapatinib plus chemoradiation in patients with locally advanced squamous cell carcinoma of the head and neck. J Clin Oncol 2006; 24(18S):5553.
70. Abidoye OO, Cohen EE, Wong SJ, et al. A phase II study of lapatinb in recurrent/metastatic squamous carcinoma of the head and neck. J Clin Oncol 2006; 24(18S):5568.
71. Ryan AJ, Wedge SR. ZD6474–a novel inhibitor of VEGFR and EGFR tyrosine kinase activity. Br J Cancer 2005; 92(suppl): 1S6–13.
72. Traxler P, Allegrini PR, Brandt R, et al. AEE788: a dual family epidermal growth factor receptor/ErbB2 and vascular endothelial growth factor receptor tyrosine kinase inhibitor with antitumor and antiangiogenic activity. Cancer Res 2004; 64(14):4931–4941.
73. Milas L, Mason KA, Ang KK. Epidermal growth factor receptor and its inhibition in radiotherapy: in vivo findings. Int J Radiat Biol 2003; 79(7):539–545.
74. Atkins D, Reiffen KA, Tegtmeier CL, Winther H, Bonato MS, Storkel S. Immunohistochemical detection of EGFR in paraffin-embedded tumor tissues: variation in staining intensity due to choice of fixative and storage time of tissue sections. J Histochem Cytochem 2004; 52(7):893–901.
75. Johnson GA, Mannel R, Khalifa M, et al. Epidermal growth factor receptor in vulvar malignancies and its relationship to metastasis and patient survival. Gynecol Oncol 1997; 65(3):425–429.
76. Haber DA, Bell D, Sordella R, Lynch T, Settleman J. Activating mutations in the epidermal growth factor receptor underlie responsiveness of non-small cell lung cancer to the tyrosine kinase inhibitor Gefitinib. American Association for Cancer Research 96th Annual Meeting, April 17 (2005).

77. Price DK, Figg WD. Mutations in the EGFR: the importance of genotyping. Cancer Biol Ther 2004; 3(5):434–435.
78. Lynch TJ, Bell DW, Sordella R, et al. Activating mutations in the epidermal growth factor receptor underlying responsiveness of non-small-cell lung cancer to gefitinib. N Engl J Med 2004; 350(21):2129–2139.
79. Pao W, Miller VA. Epidermal growth factor receptor mutations, small-molecule kinase inhibitors, and non-small-cell lung cancer: current knowledge and future directions. J Clin Oncol 2005; 23(11):2556–2568.
80. Pao W, Miller V, Zakowski M, et al. EGF receptor gene mutations are common in lung cancers from "never smokers" and are associated with sensitivity of tumors to gefitinib and erlotinib. PNAS 2004; 101(36):13306–13311.
81. Loeffler-Ragg J, Witsch-Baumgartner M, Tzankov A, et al. Low incidence of mutations in EGFR kinase domain in Caucasian patients with head and neck squamous cell carcinoma. Eur J Cancer 2006; 42(1):109–111.
82. Pao W, Miller VA. Epidermal growth factor receptor mutations, small-molecule kinase inhibitors, and non-small-cell lung cancer: current knowledge and future directions. J Clin Oncol %R 10.1200/JCO.2005.07.799 2005; 23(11):2556–2568.
83. Paez J, et al.. EGFR mutations in lung cancer: correlation with clinical response to gefitinib therapy. Science 10.112/1099314 (2004).
84. Willmore-Payne C, Holden JA, Layfield LJ. Detection of EGFR- and HER2-activating mutations in squamous cell carcinoma involving the head and neck. Mod Pathol 2006; 19(5):634–640.
85. Lee JW, Soung YH, Kim SY, et al. Somatic mutations of EGFR gene in squamous cell carcinoma of the head and neck. Clin Cancer Res 2005; 11(8):2879–2882.
86. Amador ML, Oppenheimer D, Perea S, et al. An epidermal growth factor receptor intron 1 polymorphism mediates response to epidermal growth factor receptor inhibitors. Cancer Res 2004; 64(24):9139–9143.
87. Moroni M, Veronese S, Benvenuti S, et al. Gene copy number for epidermal growth factor receptor (EGFR) and clinical response to antiEGFR treatment in colorectal cancer: a cohort study. Lancet Oncol 2005; 6(5):279–286.
88. Hirsch FR, Varella-Garcia M, McCoy J, et al. Increased epidermal growth factor receptor gene copy number detected by fluorescence in situ hybridization associates with increased sensitivity to gefitinib in patients with bronchioloalveolar carcinoma subtypes: a Southwest Oncology Group Study. J Clin Oncol 2005; 23(28):6838–6845.
89. Gordon AN, Finkler N, Edwards RP, et al. Efficacy and safety of erlotinib HCl, an epidermal growth factor receptor (HER1/EGFR) tyrosine kinase inhibitor, in patients with advanced ovarian carcinoma: results from a phase II multicenter study. Int J Gynecol Cancer 2005; 15(5):785–792.
90. Tang PA, Tsao MS, Moore MJ. A review of erlotinib and its clinical use. Expert Opin Pharmacother 2006; 7(2):177–193.
91. Cohen EE, Haraf DJ, Stenson KM, et al. Integration of Gefitinib (G), into a Concurrent Chemoradiation (CRT) Regimen Followed by G Adjuvant Therapy in Patients with Locally Advanced Head and Neck Cancer (HNC) – a Phase II Trial. 2005 ASCO Annnual Meeting, Abstract No: 5506 (2005).
92. Herchenhorn D, Dias FL, Araujo CM, et al. Phase I/II study of erlotinib combined with cisplatin and radiotherapy for locally advanced squamous cell carcinoma of the head and neck (SCCHN). J Clin Oncol (Meeting Abstracts) 2005; 23(16_suppl)5596.
93. Perez-Soler R, Saltz L. Cutaneous adverse effects with HER1/EGFR-targeted agents: is there a silver lining? J Clin Oncol 2005; 23(22):5235–5246.

8
Advancement of Antiangiogenic and Vascular Disrupting Agents Combined with Radiation

Deborah Citrin and Kevin Camphausen

Introduction

Technologic advances in therapeutic radiation targeting and delivery have led to improved tumor cure and reduced normal tissue toxicity. While further progress in these areas is probable, it is evident that significant improvements in the therapeutic ratio may result from alterations in the biologic response of tumors and normal tissues to ionizing radiation. By selectively enhancing the lethality of radiation by targeting unique aspects of tumors, improved local control may be achieved without increasing normal tissue toxicity.

One area of ongoing research has focused on identifying potential targets specific to tumors that may be manipulated to enhance the response to ionizing radiation. These agents are diverse in their origin, action, and efficacy. Agents that target the established or proliferating vasculature of a tumor are one class of such agents. Agents that target tumor vasculature can be further classified as antiangiogenic agents, that primarily inhibit the formation of new blood vessels, and vascular disrupting agents (VDAs), that target established tumor vasculature. For the purpose of this chapter, antiangiogenic and VDAs will be discussed separately, however, several compounds have been found to exhibit both antiangiogenic and vascular disrupting properties.

Tumor Vasculature

The process of angiogenesis, the formation of new blood vessels, occurs in a limited number of physiologic processes, such as wound healing and in some reproductive processes. The lack of angiogenesis in most normal tissues is a reflection of a balanced expression of numerous endogenous pro- and antiangiogenic factors. In the event of wounding and in physiologic events requiring new blood vessel growth, this normal balance is disrupted in favor of the elaboration of pro-angiogenic factors. This event has been described as the angiogenic switch [1].

The organized expression of a variety of pro- and antiangiogenic factors in physiologic processes results in the ordered recruitment, migration, and proliferation

M.P. Mehta et al. (eds.), *Radiation Oncology Advances.*

of components of the vessel wall. The final result of this complex process in physiologic processes is a well-organized, functional network of vessels that perfuses the parent tissue.

Numerous pro-angiogenic factors and enzymes are known to be involved in the formation of new blood vessels including the vascular endothelial growth factor (VEGF) family, platelet derived growth factor (PDGF), matrix metalloproteinases (MMPs), hepatocyte growth factor (HGF), and basic fibroblast growth factor (bFGF). Initiation of angiogenesis often occurs in response to stressors, such as hypoxia. Activation of hypoxia inducible transcription factors (HIFs) results in the expression of a number of proangiogenic molecules, including VEGF [2–4].

In order for tumors to grow beyond a microscopic stage, they must also establish a network of vessels to provide nutrients and oxygen. A tumor can use several methods to increase its blood supply including co-option of existing vessels, recruitment of bone marrow progenitor cells into existing vasculature (vasculogenesis), intussusception of preexisting vessels, and vessel sprouting (angiogenesis) [5]. While each of these processes can be used to create vasculature, angiogenesis is the predominant method of vessel growth in tumors [5].

Angiogenesis in tumors results in an anatomically and functionally abnormal networks of vasculature (reviewed in [6]). Tumor vessels are often tortuous and lack the normal hierarchy of vessels that promotes homogenous distribution of oxygen and nutrients [6]. Shunts, blind loops, dilated regions, and excessive branching result in disorganized flow.

In addition to abnormal architecture, the composition of tumor vessels appears to be distinct from normal vasculature. Endothelial cells in normal vasculature are arranged in a monolayer with tight junctions that limit vessel permeability. In capillaries and venules, the endothelial monolayer is closely associated with pericytes, cells that play an important role in vascular stabilization [6, 7]. The endothelial monolayer and associated pericytes in normal vasculature are enclosed in the organized, uniform acellular matrix known as the vascular basement membrane.

The components of the vessel wall are disordered in tumor vessels compared to normal capillaries. The endothelium is irregularly arranged with interendothelial gaps, regions of absent and disorganized basement membrane, with portions of endothelial vessel wall replaced by tumor cells [8]. Pericytes are present in tumor vessels, however, they appear very different from their normal capillary counterparts. Tumor pericytes are only loosely associated with endothelial cells, have abnormal cytoplasmic projections toward tumor cells, and abnormally express surface markers compared to normal capillaries [9].

Not only do tumor vessels appear abnormal from an organizational and structural standpoint, but they also appear to have abnormal function as well. Tumor vessels are often maximally dilated and exhibit little response to physiologic stressors [10]. The result of this structurally and functionally abnormal tumor vascular network is heterogeneity in tumor perfusion with areas of chronic hypoxia, intermittent hypoxia, and necrosis [11–13]. These characteristics interfere with delivery and penetration of cytotoxic agents into the tumor and with the effectiveness of radiotherapy.

Targeting the Tumor Vasculature

Tumor vasculature is an attractive target for anticancer therapy for a variety of reasons. While the biologic characteristics and sensitivities of tumor cells vary within and between tumors, the tumor vasculature should provide a more homogenous and stable target as tumor endothelium is thought to lack the varying sensitivities and acquired resistance to anticancer agents commonly associated with tumor cells [14, 15]. While tumor endothelial cells are thought to be genetically stable, they proliferate at rapid rates in tumors, resulting in expression of markers not found on mature endothelial cells of the normal vasculature (reviewed in [16]). This differential expression allows the development of inhibitors specific to the rapidly proliferating endothelium that is limited to the tumor vasculature and a few physiologic processes.

Additionally, the tumor vasculature is in direct contact with the bloodstream allowing uncomplicated delivery of agents to the target cells [17], whereas delivery of cytotoxic agents to tumor cells is complicated by perfusion, interstitial pressure, vessel permeability, and other aspects of the tumor microenvironment. Disrupting flow though a single tumor vessel may result in the death of numerous tumor cells fed by that vessel [17], amplifying the effect of the treatment. As the tumor vasculature is a pathway of metastases disruption of this pathway may reduce a tumor's metastatic capacity.

Methods of targeting tumor vasculature can be broadly classified as direct vascular targeting (antivascular or vascular disrupting therapy) or as targeting the formation of new tumor blood vessels (antiangiogenic therapy). As tumors at the macroscopic stage contain a combination of mature and newly forming blood vessels, each of these agents may play a role in targeting tumor vasculature. While the targets of these agents are seemingly similar, their mechanisms of action and the result of therapy are distinct.

Antiangiogenic Agents

Angiogenesis inhibitors prevent the growth of new blood vessels in tumors, and can be expected to prevent further tumor growth through this mechanism of action. Additionally, prolonged VEGF inhibition decreases tumor vascularity and normalizes the structure and architecture of remaining tumor vessels [18]. The result of these changes is a more organized network of tumor vessels which appears more similar to normal tissue vasculature [19]. This normalization in tumor vasculature may explain the observed improvement in oxygenation after treatment with antiangiogenic therapy [20].

A variety of agents with antiangiogenic activity have been discovered or developed (Table 1). Angiogenesis inhibitors can be broadly classified as synthetic agents and naturally occurring inhibitors. Synthetic agents include antibodies to pro-angiogenic receptors, scavengers of pro-angiogenic ligands,

Table 1 Representative antiangiogenic agents

Category	Representative agents	Mechanism of action
Endogenous inhibitors		
Matrix derived	Endostatin	Blocks endothelial cell motility and VEGF signaling, induces endothelial cell apoptosis, down regulates proangiogenic genes
	Arresten	Inhibits binding of $\alpha_1\beta_1$ integrin and type I collagen, inhibits endothelial cell tube formation
	Endorepellin	Inhibits endothelial cell migration and tube formation
	Thrombospondins	Pro-apoptotic for endothelial cells, may inhibit VEGF-induced endothelial cell migration and tube formation
Nonmatrix derived	Angiostatin	Inhibits pH regulation and upregulates apoptosis in endothelial cells, inhibits endothelial cell migration and tube formation
	Interleukins	Can inhibit angiogenic activity of bFGF (IL-4), FGF (IL-1β, IL-18). Induces downstream antiangiogenic cytokines
	Tissue inhibitors of matrix metalloproteinases	Inhibit MMP activity, inhibit extracellular matrix turnover, inhibit endothelial cell proliferation caused by several pro-angiogenic factors
	Vasostatin	Inhibits endothelial cell proliferation in response to pro-angiogenic signals such as bFGF
Scavengers		
Scavengers of VEGF	Soluble VEGFR1	Sink for VEGF
	Soluble neuropilin-1	Sink for VEGF
	muAb VEGFA.4.6.1 (Bevacizumab)	Monoclonal antibody specific for VEGFA
Tyrosine kinase inhibitors		
EGFR (ErbB1) inhibitors	Gefitinib (Iressa)	Selective EGFR (ErbB1) tyrosine kinase inhibitor
	Erlotinib (Tarceva)	Reversible and selective inhibitor of EGFR (ErbB1)
VEGFR inhibitors		Inhibit endothelial cell migration, inhibit tube formation, upregulate apoptosis
	SU5416 (Semaxinib)	Nonselective inhibitor of VEGFR-2, c-KIT and FLT3
	PTK787/ZK 222584 (Vatalanib)	Selective inhibitor of VEGFR-1 and VEGFR-2

(continued)

Table 1 (continued)

Category	Representative agents	Mechanism of action
	SU11248 (Sutent)	Inhibitor of VEGFR, PDGFR, c-KIT and FLT-3
	BAY-43–9006 (Sorafinib)	Inhibitor of C-Raf, B-Raf, VEGFR-2, platelet-derived growth factor receptor-ß, CKIT, and FLT3 kinase
	DC101	Inhibitor of VEGFR-2
Fumagillin analogs	TNP-40	Upregulates apoptosis in endothelial cells through targeting protein myristolation
	TNP-470	
COX-2 inhibitors		Inhibit prostaglandin sythesis and the production of VEGF in tumor cells, upregulates apoptosis in tumor and endothelial cells
Thalidomide and analogs	Thalidomide	Supresses NF-κB activity, decreases expression of cytokines and angiogenic factors

inhibitors of pro-angiogenic enzymes, and inhibitors of tyrosine kinase activity of pro-angiogenic receptors. Naturally occurring antiangiogenic agents can be further classified as matrix derived and nonmatrix derived endogenous angiogenesis inhibitors [21]. Matrix-derived agents are components of the basement membrane and extracellular matrix which have inhibitory effects on endothelial cells or other components of angiogenesis. Endostatin, endorepellin, and thrombospondin-1 and -2 are examples of matrix-derived endogenous angiogenesis inhibitors. Nonmatrix derived agents include a variety of peptides, metabolites, cytokines, and other molecules such as angiostatin, vasostatin, interferons, and interleukins [21].

Numerous synthetic agents have been developed as antiangiogenic therapies and many are now in use in clinical trials and as standard therapies for patient with cancer. Inhibitors of VEGF, such as anti-VEGF antibodies (Bevacizumab) and soluble VEGF receptors, act in a fashion to reduce levels of VEGF, thus reducing an angiogenic stimulus. Inhibitors of pro-angiogenic receptor signaling include inhibitors of VEGF receptors, inhibitors of endothelial growth factor receptor (EGFR), inhibitors of fibroblast growth factor (FGF) receptor, and inhibitors of platelet derived growth factor receptors (PDGFR). These receptor inhibitors may inhibit signaling through a single receptor or multiple receptors. Additionally, these agents may block ligand binding or inhibit the tyrosine kinase activity of the receptor.

A variety of other synthetic inhibitors of angiogenesis have been developed with a range of targets. Other synthetic inhibitors of angiogenesis, such as cyclooxygenase-2 (COX-2) inhibitors, can inhibit the production of VEGF and other pro-angiogenic molecules. Thalidomide exhibits antiangiogenic properties through inhibition of FGF-2 and VEGF. Antibodies and inhibitors of $\alpha_v\beta_3$ integrin, a membrane-bound molecule preferentially expressed by proliferating endothelium, have also been evaluated as angiogenesis inhibitors.

Recently, interest in continuous delivery of low doses of cytotoxic chemotherapy, also known as metronomic dosing, has been evaluated as an antiangiogenic therapy [22]. The target of the chemotherapeutic agent in this method of drug delivery is the tumor endothelial cells undergoing division [22]. It is thought that metronomic dosing of chemotherapy can circumvent issues such as multidrug resistance that develops in tumor cells as they are no longer the therapeutic target. Additionally, the toxicity of chemotherapy delivered in this fashion may be less than when the same agent is delivered in cytotoxic doses [23].

Vascular Disrupting Agents

Disruption of existing vessels provides another means to target tumor vasculature. While antiangiogenic agents inhibit the formation of new blood vessels, VDAs target all vessels within a tumor. These agents take advantage of differences between normal host vasculature and tumor vasculature to selectively target tumor vasculature, although the reasons for this selectivity are not entirely clear. Possible differences between normal and tumor vasculature which may explain this selectivity include altered permeability of tumor vessels, differences in tumor vessel structure, and aspects of the tumor microenvironment [24].

Numerous VDAs have been described, including tubulin binding agents (colchicine, vincristine, vinblastine, combretostatins, ZD6216) and agents with multiple antivascular actions (flavone acetic acid (FAA) and 5,6-dimethylxanthenone-4-acetic acid) [24] (Table 2). The tubulin binding agents appear to alter the endothelial cytoskeleton which results in an increase in vascular permeability, a disruption of tumor blood flow with stagnation, and eventual coagulation and complete vascular disruption [24]. The endothelial cells in tumors appear to be

Table 2 Representative antivascular agents

Category	Representative agents	Mechanism of action
Flavenoids	5,6-Dimethylxanthone-4-acetic acid (DMXAA) flavone acetic acid (FAA)	Induction of cytokines, especially TNF-α. May have direct effects on vessel permeability
Combretastatins	Combretastatin A-4 phosphate (CA4P)	Tubulin binding, microtubule depolymerizing resulting in alterations in the cytoskeleton of endothelial cells and vascular disruption
	ZD 6126	
	AVE8062	

particularly sensitive to tubulin binding agents as they are highly dependent on the tubulin cytoskeleton to maintain their cell shape [25, 26], while normal endothelial cells have more mature interactions with the surrounding basement membrane and pericytes which prevent conformational changes as a result of tubulin disruption [27, 28].

Flavenoids, such as FAA and its derivative DMXAA, appear to act by inducing tumor necrosis factor-α (TNF-α) expression by macrophages [29, 30]. However, it appears that TNF-α is not the only mediator of the vascular disrupting effect of DMXAA as tumor cure can be obtained in TNF-α knockout mice, albeit at higher doses of the agent [31]. In these TNF-α knockout mice, DMXAA has been found to directly and indirectly increase tumor vessel permeability [32].

While extensive tumor necrosis results from the rapid vascular disruption that occurs in response to the delivery of these agents, single dose therapy often results in a rim of viable tissue on the surface of the tumor [24] (Fig. 1). The remaining

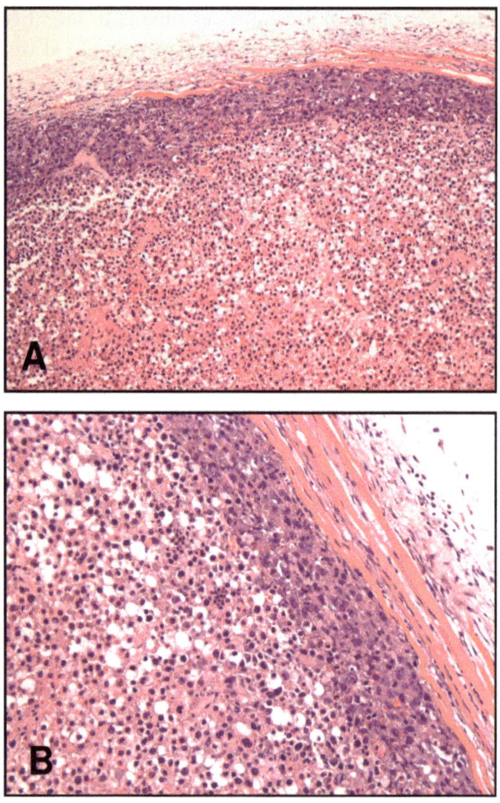

Fig. 1 Histologic effects of vascular disrupting agents. H&E stained sections from Caki tumors (renal cell) in nude mice, treated with 100 mg/kg CA4DP. Original magnification 100× (**a**) and 200× (**b**). The sections illustrate the extensive necrosis induced by CA4DP with a persistent, viable peripheral rim, typically ranging from 3 to 6 cell layers. Adjacent skeletal muscle, soft tissue and vessels are undamaged. Photographs courtesy of Dr. Amyn Rojiani

viable tissue at the periphery of a tumor after treatment with VDAs may be a result of the ability of the tissue to receive oxygen and nutrients through diffusion from nearby surrounding tissues that are unaffected by the agent. Additionally, there may be factors related to the tumor microenvironment or tumor microvasculature in the most peripheral regions of a tumor compared to the center of the tumor which would result in different sensitivity to these agents.

Combining Antiangiogenic and Vascular Disrupting Agents with Radiation

Because antiangiogenic agents and VDAs target tumor vasculature, altering the delivery of oxygen and nutrients, it is a significant concern that these agents may alter the efficacy of radiation. Oxygen is critical to maximal effectiveness of radiation. Hypoxic tumor cells exhibit a reduced sensitivity to ionizing radiation due to a lack of stabilization of radiation induced DNA damage. Therefore, the use of antiangiogenic agents and VDAs with radiation would seem a poor choice as decreasing new blood vessel formation and the destruction of existing vasculature should leave a tumor hypoxic and less sensitive to radiation. The use of antiangiogenic agents and VDAs in combination with radiation has proved more complex and appears to be related to the complex changes in the tumor environment that occur with the use of these agents.

Antiangiogenic Agents and Radiation in the Laboratory

While antiangiogenic agents inhibit new vessel growth and can result in regression of existing vessels, the administration of angiogenesis inhibitors improves tumor oxygenation and the response of tumors to radiation *in vivo* [20]. This observation has been duplicated in numerous preclinical models [33].

The mechanism of this increase in tumor oxygenation is unclear but may be related to improved nutrient delivery through tumor vessel stabilization and normalization [34, 35] and a decrease in interstitial fluid pressure [34, 36] leading to improved perfusion. The increase in radiation response may be due to the improved oxygen delivery to tumor tissues or to increased endothelial cell radiosensitivity after delivery of antiangiogenic agents [37, 38].

An additional factor that may partially explain the enhanced tumor response when antiangiogenic agents are combined with radiation is the finding that angiogenic factors are upregulated in response to radiation [38, 39]. Expression of these pro-angiogenic survival factors may play a role in radiation resistance [40], which may be mitigated through blocking their effects with antiangiogenic agents [38]. The hypothesis that pro-angiogenic factors can enhance radiation resistance is supported by clinical studies in which increased tumor and serum VEGF expression has been correlated with worse outcome following radiation therapy [41–44], although it remains unclear if expression of pro-angiogenic factors is reflective of radiation resistance in these patient subsets or merely a poor prognostic factor regardless of treatment employed.

Regardless of the mechanism of the effect, a clear enhancement in preclinical outcomes has been demonstrated with combination radiotherapy and antiangiogenic therapy compared to either treatment alone. This effect has been demonstrated *in vivo* in a variety of tumor cell lines with numerous antiangiogenic agents (reviewed in [33]. Furthermore, these observations have been seen in both single fraction and fractionated radiation regimens [33]).

Several tumor characteristics appear to influence the magnitude of additional tumor regrowth delay obtained when these agents are delivered in combination with radiation. Tumor size at the time of treatment has important implications for response to both radiation [45] and angiogenesis inhibitors. Tumors appear to be maximally sensitive to both radiation [33] and angiogenesis inhibitors [46] during the rapid phase of tumor growth. The causes for this differential response are likely due to characteristics of larger tumors, such as lower oxygen tension, decreased nutrient supply, and lowered pH (reviewed in [33]).

Based on the mechanism of action of these agents, it is reasonable to assume that the timing of drug delivery in relation to radiation is important. Delivery of the antiangiogenic agent prior to radiation may normalize the tumor vasculature, thus reducing hypoxia and improving radiation response. Delivery of the agent following radiation may decrease the local concentration or signaling of pro-angiogenic molecules which may act as a survival factor following radiation. Only a thorough preclinical evaluation of each agent will determine the appropriate timing of the delivery of angiogenesis inhibitors in relation to radiation.

Tumor growth rate may also impact on the responsiveness of a tumor to angiogenesis inhibitors. Tumors with rapid growth rates and rapidly proliferating vasculature are likely to be more sensitive to the effects of angiogenesis inhibitors. It is possible that evaluation of angiogenesis inhibitors alone or in combination with radiation in large, slow growing tumors with extensive necrosis and hypoxic regions may result in an underestimation of their efficacy [33].

An additional concern when evaluating these agents is the timing of drug delivery in relation to radiation. Vessel normalization after prolonged delivery of some angiogenesis inhibitors may allow improved perfusion and oxygenation, thus increasing the efficacy of radiotherapy. This observation would support the delivery of angiogenesis inhibitors for a prolonged period prior to the delivery of radiotherapy. Importantly, angiogenesis inhibitors may also enhance the effect of radiotherapy by reducing the angiogenic response that follows radiation. It is possible that these issues vary from one angiogenesis inhibitor to another based on their principal mechanism of action, and these factors should be considered when evaluating these agents in preclinical and clinical experiments.

Because antiangiogenic agents alter the structure and hierarchy of existing vessels and prevent new vessel growth, they are expected to act in a cytostatic fashion when delivered as a single agent. This has significant implications for both preclinical experiment design and evaluation. While antiangiogenic therapy alone would be expected to prevent progression of tumors, it is not expected to cause vascular regression significant enough to result in tumor response unless the agent also exhibits vascular disrupting activity.

Angiogenesis Inhibitors and Radiation in the Clinic

Angiogenesis inhibitors have been tested as single agent therapy or in combination with chemotherapy in Phase I, Phase II, and Phase III trials. Based on the preclinical data that angiogenesis inhibitors enhance radiotherapy, they have also been combined with radiation. Completed and reported trials that have evaluated the combination of radiation and angiogenesis inhibitors are few in number, however several studies are ongoing.

Initial Phase I studies evaluated the toxicity of these agents, which is expected to be low based on the few physiologic processes that require angiogenesis. As expected, the toxicities observed in many of these early Phase I studies was mild. When angiogenesis inhibitors have been studied in combination with chemotherapy, occasional unexpected severe toxicity has been appreciated [47, 48]. It is important to consider that this may also occur when these agents are combined with radiotherapy or to standard regimens of combined chemotherapy and radiotherapy.

At this time, few studies have been reported that have evaluated the toxicity and efficacy of regimens that combine angiogenesis inhibitors with radiotherapy. One of the few reported series is a single center Phase I study of rhAngiostatin in combination with radiation in patients with solid tumors [33]. In this trial, patients with various histologies and primary sites received a treatment regimen of daily rhAngiostatin infusions prior to radiotherapy. Toxicity appeared mild with no added toxicity appreciated within the radiation treatment port, however, three of the 23 evaluable patients in this study experienced a mild skin rash. Because of the heterogeneity of the study population, conclusions regarding efficacy are not possible, however the authors report that 90% of patients enrolled in the study with measurable disease sustained responses.

A series of six patients with locally advanced adenocarcinoma of the rectum treated with radiation, 5-fluorouracil, and bevacizumab was reported by Willet et al. [49, 50]. The patients evaluated in this study received an initial course of bevacizumab followed by reevaluation with sigmoidoscopy with biopsies and functional CT to evaluate perfusion. At this initial reevaluation after single agent bevacizumab, one patient had a significant tumor regression, and several patients' tumors were found to have a significant reduction in tumor blood volume, tumor perfusion, and microvessel density. Following the completion of induction therapy and combined therapy with radiation, 5-fluorouracil, and bevacizumab, the patients underwent surgical resection at which time a marked response was observed in all patients with only microscopic disease identified in five of the six patients.

Another agent which has been tested extensively in clinical trials alone or in combination with chemoradiotherapy is Thalidomide. A Phase II trial was recently reported in which Thalidomide was evaluated in combination with radiation and temozolomide in patients with glioblastoma multiforme [51]. The toxicity of the combined treatment did not appear to be more severe or frequent than that observed with single agent temozolomide in combination with radiation.

Recent evidence supports the use of EGFR inhibitors as antiangiogenic therapy through a reduction in microvascular endothelial cell stimulation and decreased expression of pro-angiogenic ligands such as VEGF (reviewed in [52]). The EGFR inhibitor cetuximab has been tested alone and in combination with many chemotherapy agents. A Phase I study has been reported in which patients with locally advanced head and neck cancers received a combination of cetuximab with conventional radiation therapy [53]. Toxicity in this series included fever, asthenia, liver function test abnormalities, nausea, rash, and allergic reaction. All patients treated with this regimen developed an objective response with 13 complete remissions and two partial remissions of the 16 patients included in the study.

In addition, a Phase III international trial was recently reported in abstract form that evaluated radiation alone or in combination with cetuximab in patients with locally advanced head and neck cancer [54]. The 424 patients included in this study received once daily or concomitant boost radiotherapy alone or in combination with weekly cetuximab. The median survival of patients treated on the cetuximab arm was significantly improved compared to the radiation alone arm (28 months vs. 54 months, $p = 0.02$). Excess toxicity due to cetuximab appeared to be limited to infusion site reactions and grade 3/4 skin reaction (18% vs. 34%, $p = 0.0003$), while no significant difference in grade 3/4 mucositis was appreciated ($p = 0.50$).

Many trials evaluating angiogenesis inhibitors in combination with radiation are ongoing. While no regimen containing an angiogenesis inhibitor in combination with radiation is currently considered standard of care, the success of these agents when delivered in combination with chemotherapy suggests that angiogenesis inhibitors may eventually play an established role in combination with radiation.

Vascular Disrupting Agents and Radiation in the Laboratory

The use of VDAs results in rapid vascular collapse and coagulation with extensive tumor necrosis, however a small rim of viable tissue at the peripheral regions of the tumor is often appreciated. The area of residual tumor is thought to be well oxygenated, perhaps as a result of increased blood flow to surrounding tissues, making it an attractive target for radiotherapy [33]. This is the rational for combining radiotherapy and anti-VDAs, a combination which has now been found in numerous models to achieve an antitumor effect greater than that obtained with either agent alone.

Agents such as combretastatin A-4-disodium phosphate (CA4P) [55], ZD6126 [56], and 5,6-dimethylxanthenone-4-acetic acid (DMXAA) [57] have been tested in combination with radiation in murine tumor models where they have been found to enhance tumor regrowth delay following radiation. One concern when combining these agents with radiation is the optimal scheduling of the drug in relation to radiation.

Intuitively, it would seem best to deliver radiation after sufficient time has past for regions that were not rendered necrotic to recover some blood supply so that they may become better oxygenated and hence more sensitive to radiation.

The preclinical data seem to support this approach. In one study administration of ZD6126 at multiple timepoints before, immediately after, and up to 4 h following a radiotherapy in a KHT sarcoma model was found to enhance tumor cell killing compared to that obtained with radiation alone, with the best results achieved when ZD6126 was delivered within 0.5–1 h after radiation [56]. However, when ZD6126 was given 1 h before the 10 Gy dose there was no reduction in tumor cell survival compared to radiation alone. The authors concluded that the lack of reduction in tumor cell survival when ZD6126 was delivered 1 h before radiation was due to areas rendered hypoxic and thus resistant to radiation by transient decreased perfusion but not significantly hypoxic to result in ischemia and cell death.

Similarly, other studies have shown a protective effect when VDAs are delivered just prior to radiation. Waschberger et al. [58] described the effects of ZD6216 in the U87 glioblastoma tumor model. Delivery of ZD6126 1 h prior to radiation resulted in faster tumor regrowth compared to tumors that received radiation alone, which the authors attributed to hypoxia induced by ZD6126. This effect was noted at multiple radiation doses in both small and large tumors.

Another variable that appears to be important when combining VDAs with radiation is the size of the tumor. Siemann et al. [59] reported that large KHT tumors treated with ZD6216 and radiation had smaller percentages of tumor vessels that remained patent and a higher percentage of necrosis compared to smaller tumors. Additionally, *in vivo* to *in vitro* clonogenic survival curves revealed a decrease in surviving fraction as the size of the tumor increased. This finding may be attributable to the fact that larger tumors may be expected to be composed of a larger population of hypoxic cells, which appear to be more sensitive to the combination of VDAs combined with radiation based on *in vivo* to *in vitro* cell survival curve assays [56]. The authors concluded that these differences in efficacy based on tumor size may be due to an increased reliance on vessels from surrounding normal tissues in smaller tumors, vessels which would not be sensitive to disruption by ZD6216 [59]. They also suggest that the increased interstitial fluid pressure characteristic of larger tumors may facilitate the vascular collapse that occurs as a result of treatment with ZD6216.

Toxicity of VDAs would be expected to be minimal based on their mechanism of action. Preclinical studies have suggested that the delivery of CA4P in combination with radiation does not result in increased normal tissue toxicity [60].

Vascular Disrupting Agents with Radiation in the Clinic

Anti-VDAs have been successfully introduced into the clinic as anticancer therapies in the context of Phase I, Phase Ib, and Phase II trials. CA4P has been evaluated in various dosing schedules as a single agent in Phase I trials attempting to define toxicity and pharmacokinetics [61–65]. The toxicity observed in these studies included dyspnea, myocardial ischemia, neurologic events, and tumor pain [66]. Surprisingly, significant responses, including a complete pathologic response in a patient with anaplastic thyroid cancer, were seen when the drug was delivered as single agent therapy in some patients with advanced solid tumors.

CA4P has now moved into Phase Ib and II trials in combination with chemotherapy, radiation, and radioisotopes. A Phase Ib trial of the agent in combination with radiation in patients with locally advanced non-small cell lung cancer and prostate cancer was recently reported in abstract form [67]. In this study CA4P was delivered in a weekly schedule concurrently with hypofractionated radiation. Toxicity in this early report included grade I hypertension, postural syncope, lymphopenia, neutropenia, and tumor pain. The efficacy of the combination of CA4P was not described in this early report. Currently, CA4P delivered concurrently with radiation following chemotherapy is being evaluated in patients with anaplastic thyroid cancer in a Phase II study.

Other VDAs, such as DMXAA, have now entered Phase I trials alone and in combination with chemotherapy. Results from these studies are pending. Additional agents have been evaluated in the preclinical setting including ZD6216. As the mechanism of action of these agents are better characterized, it is likely that additional agents with may be developed for clinical use.

Future Directions

Angiogenesis inhibitors and anti-VDAs are now being evaluated in combination with radiation in numerous clinical trials, and many additional agents are undergoing preclinical evaluation. There are numerous factors that must be addressed when designing clinical trials to assess the efficacy of these agents alone or in combination with radiation or chemotherapy. The timing of drug delivery in relation to other therapeutics, the schedule of drug delivery, optimal dosing, and appropriate measures of response must be determined for each of these agents.

Historically, tumor response has been measured by longitudinal physical examination or tumor measurements obtained radiographically. Because these angiogenesis inhibitors and VDAs are expected to result in rapid and potentially dramatic changes in tumor physiology without a correspondingly rapid reduction in tumor size, standard tumor measurements may not provide an accurate measure of tumor response. Numerous biologic and functional endpoints have been evaluated in the context of treatment with these agents and may provide surrogate markers of response.

Tumor biopsies may be used to determine alterations in microvessel density, endothelial cell apoptosis, tumor hypoxia, gene expression, and other histologic and molecular characteristics of tumors following antiangiogenic therapy. While these methods provide valuable information regarding tumor response, these investigations require an invasive procedure to obtain tumor tissue, which complicates a longitudinal evaluation of tumor response. Additionally, sampling error may reduce the quality of information gathered with this approach.

Surrogate markers of VDA efficacy, such as functional computerized tomography (CT) and dynamic contrast enhanced magnetic resonance imaging (DCE-MRI), may provide a useful measure of drug efficacy. The noninvasive nature of these modalities provides the option of longitudinal evaluation, while allowing an evaluation of response within specific areas of a heterogenous tumor. These methods have been employed to evaluate the functional changes associated with antiangiogenic [68–70] and VDA [62, 65] therapies in clinical trials.

Other surrogate markers of disease status, drug efficacy, or the overall angiogenic state of a patient may provide indirect evidence of drug efficacy which may not be obvious based on measurements of tumor size. Circulating growth factors [44], circulating endothelial surface markers [71, 72], circulating endothelial cells and endothelial precursor cells [73], and circulating cytokines [74] are candidate surrogate biomarkers for antiangiogenic response. These biologic surrogates are more thoroughly explored in the context of angiogenesis inhibitors, although it is probable that similar measures of VDA efficacy may be developed. For example, serum TNF-α may provide a surrogate marker of VDA efficacy.

By using these novel noninvasive markers, further information may be gathered regarding the optimal timing and delivery schedule of these agents in relation to chemotherapy and radiation. These methods provide the opportunity to gather significantly more information regarding drug effect by thoroughly studying fewer patients in a serial fashion.

In addition to the complexities of assessing response, patient selection for protocols including these agents is important in maximizing the potential benefit. As discussed earlier, the activity of these agents may be affected by tumor size, hypoxia, and other microenvironmental factors. In addition, tumor histology and degree of differentiation have been shown to influence the efficacy of antiangiogenic therapy [75–78]. For these reasons, patients with large bulky tumors may be more appropriate for enrollment on trials assessing VDA strategies, while patients with smaller tumors with a propensity for metastasizing may be expected to experience a greater response in trials assessing an antiangiogenic strategy. These are simply examples, as the optimal patients to select for evaluation for each of these strategies in combination with radiation remains largely unknown at this time.

Conclusion

Solid tumors require the development of vasculature for tumor progression. Angiogenesis inhibitors and VDAs provide a highly selective strategy for targeting tumor vasculature. These agents also provide a nonselective method of therapy, largely resulting in antitumor efficacy in a broad range of tumor types. The complex physiologic alterations induced by these agents have important implications for their use in combination with radiation therapy. Dosing and timing of these agents in relation to radiation appears to be important in maximizing the benefit of the combination. Additionally, appropriate selection of the tumor stage and histology may be important to realizing a potential benefit.

Multiple angiogenesis inhibitors and VDAs have been found to enhance the tumor regrowth delay obtained with radiotherapy when delivered in combination. Additionally, several of these agents have been found to enhance the antitumor effects of chemotherapy and radiotherapy in clinical trials. The toxicity of these agents appears to be mild with a few notable exceptions. Numerous clinical trials are ongoing to determine the safety and efficacy of these agents alone and in combination with other cytotoxic therapies.

Acknowledgment This research was supported by the Intramural Research Program of the NIH, National Cancer Institute, Center for Cancer Research.

References

1. Hanahan D, Folkman J. Patterns and emerging mechanisms of the angiogenic switch during tumorigenesis. Cell 1996; 86:353–364.
2. Liu Y, Cox SR, Morita T, Kourembanas S. Hypoxia regulates vascular endothelial growth factor gene expression in endothelial cells. Identification of a 5′′ enhancer. Circ Res 1995; 77:638–643.
3. Levy AP, Levy NS, Wegner S, Goldberg MA. Transcriptional regulation of the rat vascular endothelial growth factor gene by hypoxia. J Biol Chem 1995; 270:13333–13340.
4. Shweiki D, Neeman M, Itin A, Keshet E. Induction of vascular endothelial growth factor expression by hypoxia and by glucose deficiency in multicell spheroids: implications for tumor angiogenesis. Proc Natl Acad Sci USA 1995; 92:768–772.
5. Carmeliet P, Jain RK. Angiogenesis in cancer and other diseases. Nature 2000; 407:249–257.
6. Baluk P, Hashizume H, McDonald DM. Cellular abnormalities of blood vessels as targets in cancer. Curr Opin Genet Dev 2005; 15:102–111.
7. Gerhardt H, Betsholtz C. Endothelial–pericyte interactions in angiogenesis. Cell Tissue Res 2003; 314:15–23.
8. Chang YS, di Tomaso E, McDonald DM, Jones R, Jain RK, Munn LL. Mosaic blood vessels in tumors: frequency of cancer cells in contact with flowing blood. PNAS 2000; 97:14608–14613.
9. Morikawa S, Baluk P, Kaidoh T, Haskell A, Jain RK, McDonald DM. Abnormalities in pericytes on blood vessels and endothelial sprouts in tumors. Am J Pathol 2002; 160:985–1000.
10. Chan RC, Babbs CF, Vetter RJ, Lamar CH. Abnormal response of tumor vasculature to vasoactive drugs. J Natl Cancer Inst 1984; 72:145–150.
11. Chaplin DJ, Durand RE, Olive PL. Acute hypoxia in tumors: implications for modifiers of radiation effects. Int J Radiat Oncol Biol Phys 1986; 12:1279–1282.
12. Chaplin DJ, Olive PL, Durand RE. Intermittent blood flow in a murine tumor: radiobiological effects. Cancer Res 1987; 47:597–601.
13. Helmlinger G, Yuan F, Dellian M, Jain RK. Interstitial pH and pO2 gradients in solid tumors in vivo: high-resolution measurements reveal a lack of correlation. Nat Med 1997; 3:177–182.
14. Boehm T, Folkman J, Browder T, O'Reilly MS. Antiangiogenic therapy of experimental cancer does not induce acquired drug resistance. Nature 1997; 390:404–407.
15. Drevs J, Laus C, Mendinger M, Schmidt-Gersbach C, Unger C. Antiangiogenesis: current clinical data and future perspectives. Onkologie 2002; 25:520–527.
16. Nanda A, St Croix B. Tumor endothelial markers: new targets for cancer therapy. Curr Opin Oncol 2004; 16:44–49.

17. Ruegg C, Meuwly JY, Driscoll R, Werffeli P, Zaman K, Stupp R. The quest for surrogate markers of angiogenesis: a paradigm for translational research in tumor angiogenesis and anti-angiogenesis trials. Curr Mol Med 2003; 3:673–691.
18. Benjamin LE, Golijanin D, Itin A, Pode D, Keshet E. Selective ablation of immature blood vessels in established human tumors follows vascular endothelial growth factor withdrawal. J Clin Invest 1999; 103:159–165.
19. Jain RK. Normalizing tumor vasculature with anti-angiogenic therapy: a new paradigm for combination therapy. Nat Med 2001; 7:987–989.
20. Teicher BA, Holden SA, Ara G, et al. Influence of an anti-angiogenic treatment on 9L gliosarcoma: oxygenation and response to cytotoxic therapy. Int J Cancer 1995; 61:732–737.
21. Nyberg P, Xie L, Kalluri R. Endogenous inhibitors of angiogenesis. Cancer Res 2005; 65:3967–3979.
22. Browder T, Butterfield CE, Kraling BM, et al. Antiangiogenic scheduling of chemotherapy improves efficacy against experimental drug-resistant cancer. Cancer Res 2000; 60:1878–1886.
23. Colleoni M, Rocca A, Sandri MT, et al. Low-dose oral methotrexate and cyclophosphamide in metastatic breast cancer: antitumor activity and correlation with vascular endothelial growth factor levels. Ann Oncol 2002; 13:73–80.
24. Tozer GM, Kanthou C, Baguley BC. Disrupting tumour blood vessels. Nat Rev Cancer 2005; 5:423–435.
25. Galbraith SM, Chaplin DJ, Lee F, et al. Effects of combretastatin A4 phosphate on endothelial cell morphology in vitro and relationship to tumour vascular targeting activity in vivo. Anticancer Res 2001; 21:93–102.
26. Kanthou C, Tozer GM. The tumor vascular targeting agent combretastatin A-4-phosphate induces reorganization of the actin cytoskeleton and early membrane blebbing in human endothelial cells. Blood 2002; 99:2060–2069.
27. Micheletti G, Poli M, Borsotti P, et al. Vascular-targeting activity of ZD6126, a novel tubulin-binding agent. Cancer Res 2003; 63:1534–1537.
28. Davis PD, Dougherty GJ, Blakey DC, et al. ZD6126: a novel vascular-targeting agent that causes selective destruction of tumor vasculature. Cancer Res 2002; 62:7247–7253.
29. Philpott M, Ching LM, Baguley BC. The antitumour agent 5,6-dimethylxanthenone-4-acetic acid acts in vitro on human mononuclear cells as a co-stimulator with other inducers of tumour necrosis factor. Eur J Cancer 2001; 37:1930–1937.
30. Philpott M, Joseph WR, Crosier KE, Baguley BC, Ching LM. Production of tumour necrosis factor-alpha by cultured human peripheral blood leucocytes in response to the anti-tumour agent 5,6-dimethylxanthenone-4-acetic acid (NSC 640488). Br J Cancer 1997; 76:1586–1591.
31. Zhao L, Ching LM, Kestell P, Baguley BC. The antitumour activity of 5,6-dimethylxanthenone-4-acetic acid (DMXAA) in TNF receptor-1 knockout mice. Br J Cancer 2002; 87:465–470.
32. Zhao L, Ching LM, Kestell P, Kelland LR, Baguley BC. Mechanisms of tumor vascular shutdown induced by 5,6-dimethylxanthenone-4-acetic acid (DMXAA): increased tumor vascular permeability. Int J Cancer 2005; 116:322–326.
33. Wachsberger P, Burd R, Dicker AP. Tumor response to ionizing radiation combined with antiangiogenesis or vascular targeting agents: exploring mechanisms of interaction. Clin Cancer Res 2003; 9:1957–1971.
34. Lee CG, Heijn M, di Tomaso E, et al. Anti-Vascular endothelial growth factor treatment augments tumor radiation response under normoxic or hypoxic conditions. Cancer Res 2000; 60:5565–5570.
35. Tong RT, Boucher Y, Kozin SV, Winkler F, Hicklin DJ, Jain RK. Vascular normalization by vascular endothelial growth factor receptor 2 blockade induces a pressure gradient across the vasculature and improves drug penetration in tumors. Cancer Res 2004; 64:3731–3736.
36. Yuan F, Chen Y, Dellian M, Safabakhsh N, Ferrara N, Jain RK. Time-dependent vascular regression and permeability changes in established human tumor xenografts induced by an

anti-vascular endothelial growth factor/vascular permeability factor antibody. Proc Natl Acad Sci USA 1996; 93:14765–14770.
37. Folkman J, Camphausen K. Cancer. What does radiotherapy do to endothelial cells? Science 2001; 293:227–228.
38. Gorski DH, Beckett MA, Jaskowiak NT, et al. Blockage of the vascular endothelial growth factor stress response increases the antitumor effects of ionizing radiation. Cancer Res 1999; 59:3374–3378.
39. Koukourakis MI, Giatromanolaki A, Sivridis E, et al. Squamous cell head and neck cancer: evidence of angiogenic regeneration during radiotherapy. Anticancer Res 2001; 21:4301–4309.
40. Gupta VK, Jaskowiak NT, Beckett MA, et al. Vascular endothelial growth factor enhances endothelial cell survival and tumor radioresistance. Cancer J 2002; 8:47–54.
41. Smith BD, Smith GL, Carter D, Sasaki CT, Haffty BG. Prognostic significance of vascular endothelial growth factor protein levels in oral and oropharyngeal squamous cell carcinoma. J Clin Oncol 2000; 18:2046–2052.
42. Kang JO, Hong SE. The prognostic effect of VEGF expression in squamous cell carcinoma of the cervix treated with radiation therapy alone. J Korean Med Sci 2004; 19:693–697.
43. Nam DH, Park K, Suh YL, Kim JH. Expression of VEGF and brain specific angiogenesis inhibitor-1 in glioblastoma: prognostic significance. Oncol Rep 2004; 11:863–869.
44. Chan LW, Moses MA, Goley E, et al. Urinary VEGF and MMP levels as predictive markers of 1-year progression-free survival in cancer patients treated with radiation therapy: a longitudinal study of protein kinetics throughout tumor progression and therapy. J Clin Oncol 2004; 22:499–506.
45. Shipley WU, Stanley JA, Steel GG. Tumor size dependency in the radiation response of the Lewis lung carcinoma. Cancer Res 1975; 35:2488–2493.
46. Bergers G, Javaherian K, Lo KM, Folkman J, Hanahan D. Effects of angiogenesis inhibitors on multistage carcinogenesis in mice. Science 1999; 284:808–812.
47. Kuenen BC, Rosen L, Smit EF, et al. Dose-finding and pharmacokinetic study of cisplatin, gemcitabine, and SU5416 in patients with solid tumors. J Clin Oncol 2002; 20:1657–1667.
48. Marx GM, Steer CB, Harper P, Pavlakis N, Rixe O, Khayat D. Unexpected serious toxicity with chemotherapy and antiangiogenic combinations: time to take stock! J Clin Oncol 2002; 20:1446–1448.
49. Willett CG, Boucher Y, di Tomaso E, et al. Direct evidence that the VEGF-specific antibody bevacizumab has antivascular effects in human rectal cancer. Nat Med 2004; 10:145–147.
50. Willett CG, Boucher Y, Duda DG, et al. Surrogate markers for antiangiogenic therapy and dose-limiting toxicities for bevacizumab with radiation and chemotherapy: continued experience of a Phase I trial in rectal cancer patients. J Clin Oncol 2005; 23:8136–8139.
51. Chang SM, Lamborn KR, Malec M, et al. Phase II study of temozolomide and thalidomide with radiation therapy for newly diagnosed glioblastoma multiforme. Int J Radiat Oncol Biol Phys 2004; 60:353–357.
52. van Cruijsen H, Giaccone G, Hoekman K. Epidermal growth factor receptor and angiogenesis: opportunities for combined anticancer strategies. Int J Cancer 2005; 117:883–888.
53. Robert F, Ezekiel MP, Spencer SA, et al. Phase I study of anti–epidermal growth factor receptor antibody cetuximab in combination with radiation therapy in patients with advanced head and neck cancer. J Clin Oncol 2001; 19:3234–3243.
54. Bonner JA, Harari PM, Giralt J, et al. Cetuximab prolongs survival in patients with locoregionally advanced squamous cell carcinoma of head and neck: a phase III study of high dose radiation therapy with or without cetuximab. J Clin Oncol (meeting abstracts) 2004; 22:5507.
55. Li L, Rojiani A, Siemann DW. Targeting the tumor vasculature with combretastatin A-4 disodium phosphate: effects on radiation therapy. Int J Radiat Oncol Biol Phys 1998; 42:899–903.
56. Siemann DW, Rojiani AM. Enhancement of radiation therapy by the novel vascular targeting agent ZD6126. Int J Radiat Oncol Biol Phys 2002; 53:164–171.

57. Wilson WR, Li AE, Cowan DS, Siim BG. Enhancement of tumor radiation response by the antivascular agent 5,6-dimethylxanthenone-4-acetic acid. Int J Radiat Oncol Biol Phys 1998; 42:905–908.
58. Wachsberger PR, Burd R, Marero N, et al. Effect of the tumor vascular-damaging agent, ZD6126, on the radioresponse of U87 glioblastoma. Clin Cancer Res 2005; 11:835–842.
59. Siemann DW, Rojiani AM. The vascular disrupting agent ZD6126 shows increased antitumor efficacy and enhanced radiation response in large, advanced tumors. Int J Radiat Oncol Biol Phys 2005; 62:846–853.
60. Murata R, Overgaard J, Horsman MR. Combretastatin A-4 disodium phosphate: a vascular targeting agent that improves that improves the anti-tumor effects of hyperthermia, radiation, and mild thermoradiotherapy. Int J Radiat Oncol Biol Phys 2001; 51:1018–1024.
61. Cooney MM, Radivoyevitch T, Dowlati A, et al. Cardiovascular safety profile of Combretastatin A4 phosphate in a single-dose phase I study in patients with advanced cancer. Clin Cancer Res 2004; 10:96–100.
62. Stevenson JP, Rosen M, Sun W, et al. Phase I trial of the antivascular agent Combretastatin A4 phosphate on a 5-Day schedule to patients with cancer: magnetic resonance imaging evidence for altered tumor blood flow. J Clin Oncol 2003; 21:4428–4438.
63. Anderson HL, Yap JT, Miller MP, Robbins A, Jones T, Price PM. Assessment of pharmacodynamic vascular response in a Phase I trial of Combretastatin A4 Phosphate. J Clin Oncol 2003; 21:2823–2830.
64. Rustin GJS, Galbraith SM, Anderson H, et al. Phase I clinical trial of weekly Combretastatin A4 Phosphate: clinical and pharmacokinetic results. J Clin Oncol 2003; 21:2815–2822.
65. Dowlati A, Robertson K, Cooney M, et al. A Phase I pharmacokinetic and translational study of the novel vascular targeting agent combretastatin A-4 phosphate on a single-dose intravenous schedule in patients with advanced cancer. Cancer Res 2002; 62:3408–3416.
66. Young SL, Chaplin DJ. Combretastatin A4 phosphate: background and current clinical status. Expert Opin Investig Drugs 2004; 13:1171–1182.
67. Ng QS, Carnell D, Milner J, Meer K, Saunders MI, Hoskin PJ. Phase Ib trial of Combretastatin A4 Phosphate (CA4P) in combination with radiotherapy (RT): initial clinical results. J Clin Oncol (Meeting Abstracts) 2005; 23:3117.
68. Peterson AC, Swiger S, Stadler WM, Medved M, Karczmar G, Gajewski TF. Phase II Study of the Flk-1 Tyrosine Kinase Inhibitor SU5416 in advanced melanoma. Clin Cancer Res 2004; 10:4048–4054.
69. Eder JP Jr, Supko JG, Clark JW, et al. Phase I clinical trial of recombinant human endostatin administered as a short intravenous infusion repeated daily. J Clin Oncol 2002; 20:3772–3784.
70. Thomas JP, Arzoomanian RZ, Alberti D, et al. Phase I pharmacokinetic and pharmacodynamic study of recombinant human endostatin in patients with advanced solid tumors. J Clin Oncol 2003; 21:223–231.
71. Bewick M, Conlon M, Lee H, et al. Evaluation of sICAM-1, sVCAM-1, and sE-selectin levels in patients with metastatic breast cancer receiving high-dose chemotherapy. Stem Cells Dev 2004; 13:281–294.
72. Pasieka Z, Stepien H, Komorowski J, Kolomecki K, Kuzdak K. Evaluation of the levels of bFGF, VEGF, sICAM-1, and sVCAM-1 in serum of patients with thyroid cancer. Recent Results Cancer Res 2003; 162:189–194.
73. Mancuso P, Calleri A, Cassi C, et al. Circulating endothelial cells as a novel marker of angiogenesis. Adv Exp Med Biol 2003; 522:83–97.
74. Negrier S, Perol D, Menetrier-Caux C, et al. Interleukin-6, interleukin-10, and vascular endothelial growth factor in metastatic renal cell carcinoma: prognostic value of interleukin-6–from the Groupe Francais d'Immunotherapie. J Clin Oncol 2004; 22:2371–2378.
75. Bussink J, Kaanders JH, van der Kogel AJ. Tumor hypoxia at the micro-regional level: clinical relevance and predictive value of exogenous and endogenous hypoxic cell markers. Radiother Oncol 2003; 67:3–15.

76. Bernsen HJ, Rijken PF, Oostendorp T, van der Kogel AJ. Vascularity and perfusion of human gliomas xenografted in the athymic nude mouse. Br J Cancer 1995; 71:721–726.
77. Takada K, Yamada S, Teramoto A. Correlation between tumor vascularity and clinical findings in patients with pituitary adenomas. Endocr Pathol 2004; 15:131–139.
78. Tan G, Cioc AM, Perez-Montiel D, Ellison EC, Frankel WL. Microvascular density does not correlate with histopathology and outcome in neuroendocrine tumors of the pancreas. Appl Immunohistochem Mol Morphol 2004; 12:31–35.

9
Overcoming Therapeutic Resistance in Malignant Gliomas: Current Practices and Future Directions

Arnab Chakravarti and Kamalakannan Palanichamy

Introduction

Malignant gliomas are comprised of World Health Organization (WHO) Grade III and IV gliomas. Median survival times for patients with Grade IV tumors, also known as glioblastoma multiforme (GBM), is noted to be especially poor, remaining just over one year with current therapeutic regimens [1–4]. The treatment regimen for malignant glioma patients has traditionally involved maximal surgical debulking, followed by radiation +/– chemotherapy. Cooperative group trials over the past several decades have demonstrated that adjuvant radiation significantly prolongs survival compared to surgery alone in malignant glioma patients [2, 3]. The role of upfront chemotherapy with radiation for malignant gliomas has been less well defined until more recently. Newer generation chemotherapeutic agents such as temozolomide (TMZ) have demonstrated activity in malignant gliomas, both when used as single agents as well as in combination with radiotherapy. Further, targeted therapies have been developed which inhibit specific molecular pathways required for tumor-specific survival, proliferation, migration, and angiogenesis. This review will detail the possible mechanisms of treatment resistance in malignant gliomas and the roles of chemotherapeutic and biotherapeutic modifiers of radiation response in patients with malignant gliomas.

Signal Transduction Pathways Involved in Treatment Resistance

Molecular pathways that are important for cellular proliferation and survival in gliomas are becoming better understood, yet far from complete. It is known that certain genetic events are common in gliomagenesis. In secondary GBMs, which arise from lower-grade gliomas, initial events involve TP53 loss or mutation combined with RB and PTEN mutations as tumors progress in grade. Primary GBMs do not have clear histories of arising from lower-grade tumors, and have certain molecular features that distinguish them from secondary GBMs, although morphologically

M.P. Mehta et al. (eds.), *Radiation Oncology Advances.*

identical. For instance, amplification of the epidermal growth factor receptor (EGFR) and overexpression of the EGFR protein are relatively common events in primary GBMs, occurring in upward of 50% of cases. Often, along with enhanced signaling through EGFR, there is concommitant loss of the INK4 gene, which codes for both p16 and p14^{ARF} in primary GBMs. Many primary GBMs express the constitutively active EGFRvIII mutant that lacks the extracellular binding domain and is essentially constitutively active. The prognostic value of EGFR in GBM has been a controversial issue. Wild-type EGFR expression, as determined by immunohistochemical analysis does not appear to be of prognostic value in GBMs. There are reports that the constitutively active EGFRvIII mutant has prognostic value in selected series; however, it has yet to be rigorously confirmed in a prospective manner.

Loss of heterozygosity of chromosome 10 is a common event in GBMs, occurring in upward of 90% of cases. PTEN (phosphatase and tensin homology gene), which is a 3′ phosphoinositol phosphatase is located on chromosome 10q23.3 and is commonly lost in both primary and secondary GBMs. Loss of PTEN results in constitutive activation of downstream mediators of the phosphatidyl 3-inositol kinase (PI3K) pathway, including AKT, which is a potent pro-survival molecule in many human tumors including gliomas. Fig. 1 illustrates this pathway as well as upstream regulators (e.g., EGFR). PI3K is a lipid kinase that promotes diverse biological functions including cellular proliferation, survival, and motility [5]. The PI3K signaling pathways is frequently deregulated in glioblastoma [6, 7], often in combination with the ERK pathway, and mouse genetic studies suggest a causal role of this pattern [8]. The PI3K pathway (and RAS/ERK pathway) can become deregulated on the basis of oncogene activation and tumor suppressor gene losses that are commonly seen in glioblastoma. Up to 40% of glioblastomas harbor alterations of the PTEN tumor suppressor gene, a negative regulator of PI3K signaling that results in constitutive activation of the PI3K pathway [7]. Upstream of PI3K, the epidermal growth factor receptor (EGFR) is commonly over-expressed, frequently in association with its constitutively activated EGFRvIII variant (and other variants), which may lead to deregulated PI3K and RAS/ERK signaling [9–15]. Other receptor tyrosine kinases such as PDGFR and c-MET are also commonly over-expressed in glioblastomas, and may deregulate these same pathways [9–17]. The PI3K and RAS/ERK pathways connect richly to other signaling cascades, thereby integrating signals associated with other cell surface events, stress activation pathways, and extracellular matrix proteins. RAC1 is one such protein that links PI3K and RAS signaling with integrin-linked signaling, potentially playing a key role in promoting glioblastoma growth and survival [18].

Therefore, the PI3K and ERK signaling pathways, and associated molecules, provide important therapeutic targets. Figure 1 also illustrates various points within this pathway that can be targeted. The connectivity of the PI3K signaling pathway in GBM has recently been demonstrated by Mischel et al. It was demonstrated that PTEN loss was tightly linked to AKT activation, which in turn was linked to mTor and FHKR phosphorylation. The correlation between PTEN expression and activation of molecules downstream of AKT was found to diminish, suggesting the presence

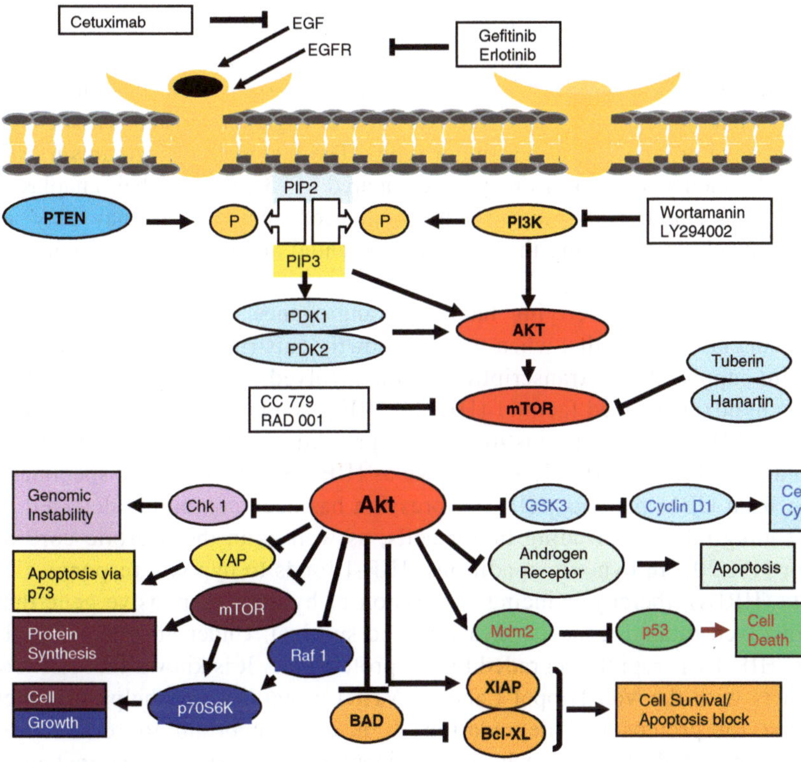

Fig. 1 Illustrates the PI3K signaling pathway. In GBMs, many tumors have deregulation of this pathway either through enhanced activation from upstream pathways (e.g., EGFR) or constitutive activation via PTEN loss or mutation

of other inputs into this pathway. There was also strong evidence of the link between EGFR expression with ERK activation and EGFRvIII expression with activation of downstream AKT targets. In a separate study, it was found that activation of key PI3K signaling molecules is associated with increasing tumor grade and adverse clinical outcome in glioma patients on multivariate analysis. Further, it was determined that in a subset of glioblastoma patients treated by radiation alone, activation of PI3K pathway members was associated with adverse clinical outcome providing direct clinical evidence of the role of PI3K signaling in radiation resistance in GBMs.

Angiogenesis Pathways

There is ample evidence that angiogenesis plays an important role in the pathogenesis and treatment resistance in gliomas. It is known that GBMs are distinguished from anaplastic astrocytomas by the presence of microvascular hyperplasia and necrosis. Vascular hyperplasia is characterized by proliferating endothelial cells that form a tufted micro-aggregate front at the leading edge of host blood vessels. The most extreme form of microvascular proliferation is termed glomeruloid bodies which may signify an accelerated course of angiogenesis and is associated with adverse prognosis in other tumor types. The fact that the median survival of GBM patients is just over one year, compared to ~3 years for their anaplastic astrocytoma counterparts, suggests that enhanced angiogenesis may play an important role in enhancing the malignant potential and treatment resistance in gliomas.

One of the key underlying factors of angiogenesis may be the hypoxic environment that results when tumor growth outstrips blood and, hence, nutrient supply. A key transcription factor involved in angiogenesis in gliomas is hypoxia-induced factor 1 (HIF-1). HIF-1 is a heterodimer protein consisting of HIF-1α and a constitutively expressed aryl hydrocarbon receptor nuclear translocator (ARNT, also known as HIF-1β). In pathologic specimens taken from GBM patients, HIF-1 expression has been commonly detected in the leading edge of invading tumor cells, as well as in the necrotic core of tumor [19, 20]. In hypoxic conditions, HIF-1 binds to hypoxia response elements (HREs), thereby inducing expression of hypoxia-responsive gene that are involved in angiogenesis, invasion, and survival. Under normoxic conditions, HIF-1α is rapidly degraded by the proteosome. It is known that HIF-1α interacts with the Von Hippel Landau (VHL) protein, which helps to target HIF-1α for proteosomal degradation. It is also important to realize that hypoxia-independent factors may serve to increase HIF-1^{α} expression, including loss of PTEN [21].

The vascular endothelial growth factor (VEGF) has also been found to play an important role in angiogenesis in malignant gliomas. VEGF is a highly specific endothelial mitogen. In addition to VEGF (VEGF-A), there are other important family members of this pathway including VEGF-B, VEGF-C, VEGF-D, VEGF-E, and placenta growth factor (PGF). There appears to be an accumulation of VEGF that increases with tumor grade and tumor size in gliomas [22]. Extracellular VEGF is known to bind to its tyrosine kinase receptors, VEGFR1 and VEGFR2, which are strongly expressed on endothelial cells present in high-grade gliomas but absent in normal brain. Hypoxia serves to increase VEGF expression levels via the HIF family. It has been found that VEGF-A and VEGF-B mRNA are commonly overexpressed in GBMs [22]. One report suggests that expression of VEGF family members is tightly linked to EGFR expression levels [23]. Further, it has been found that PI3K pathway activation serves to increase VEGF mRNA expression levels independent of hypoxia. Given the potential importance of angiogenic pathways in mediating radiation resistance, these molecules present themselves as being attractive targets in GBMs. Figure 2 illustrates various strategies of antiangiogenic targeting and their possible mechanisms of action.

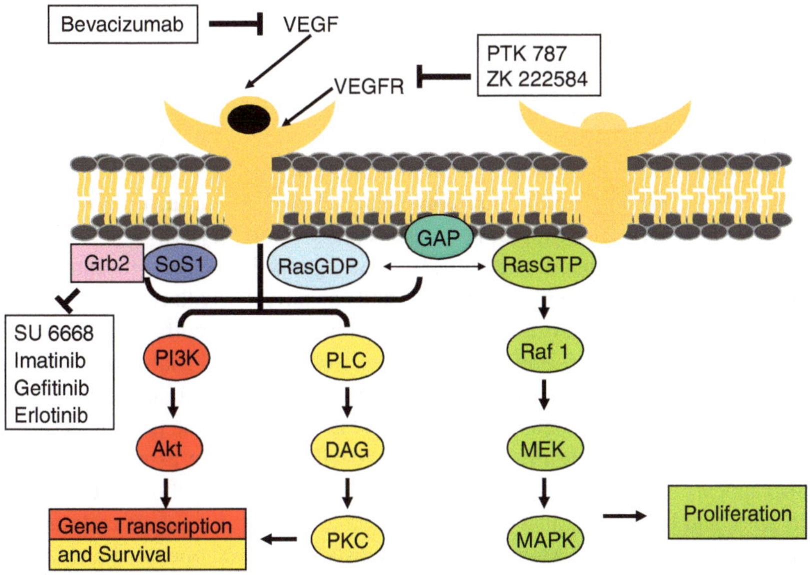

Fig. 2 Illustrates the VEGF signaling cascade, which serves to enhance tumor cell angiogenesis, and also highlights possible therapeutic strategies to inhibit this critical angiogenic pathway

Conventional Chemotherapeutic Agents in Malignant Gliomas

The indications for chemotherapy in the management of newly diagnosed malignant gliomas has been under active investigation for several decades. BCNU (1,3 bis (2-chloroethyl)-1-nitrosurea or carmustine) and CCNU (1-(2-chloroethyl)-3-cyclohexyl-1-nitrosurea or lomustine) have long been considered the standard chemotherapy for CNS tumors. BCNU and CCNU are members of the nitrosurea family of alkylating agents, which are known to have a high degree of lipid solubility and CNS penetration. BCNU is commonly administered intravenously at doses ranging upward of 200 mg/m^2 every 6–8 weeks. The primary toxicities include nausea, vomiting, and hematologic effects. CCNU is an orally administered nitrosurea, which is used most commonly with procarbazine and vincristine (PCV regimen). Procarbazine is another orally administered alkylating agent that is commonly used for CNS tumors. The microtubule inhibitor vincristine is commonly administered intravenously as part of the PCV regimen, with its primary toxicity being severe neuropathy.

Temozolomide (TMZ) is an alkylating agent that has close similarities to dacarbazine. It dissociates to form the active alkylating agent methyltriazeno-imidazole-arboxamide (MTIC) at physiologic pH, which methylates the O-6 position of guanylic acid in DNA. In contrast, MTIC is formed from dacarbazine only after metabolism by the liver. As hepatic metabolism can be influenced by agents such as anticonvulsant drugs and corticosteroids commonly taken by brain tumor patients, it is thought that bioavailability of MTIC may be more consistent with TMZ than with dacarbazine. With repeat dosing, TMZ can enter the CSF quite rapidly without accumulation. The normal dose of TMZ when administered alone is 150–200 mg/m^2 orally for 5 days, administered in 4-week cycles. TMZ is taken orally and is absorbed rapidly and completely after oral administration. The primary toxicities are myelosuppression, nausea, and vomiting [24].

These above-mentioned chemotherapeutic agents have been investigated in several settings: neoadjuvantly, adjuvantly, and concurrently with radiation. The first randomized trial to support a role for nitrosurea-based chemotherapy was BTSG 69–01 [2]. Fine et al. performed a meta-analysis of 17 clinical trials and found both 1- and 2-year survival advantages for patients treated with a combination of radiation and chemotherapy (nitrosurea-based) compared to radiation alone [25]. This survival advantage was most insignificant in patients with anaplastic astrocytoma (AA). It also appears that a distinct subset of GBM patients, especially those with relatively high KPS, and limited residual disease appeared to benefit. A separate meta-analysis performed by the Glioma Meta-Analysis Trialists Group demonstrated a significant improvement in survival with nitrosurea-based chemotherapy with a 15% decrease in the relative risk of death (hazard ratio 0.85; 95% confidence interval 0.78–0.91) [26]. Therefore, until more recently (see TMZ data below), adjuvant BCNU-based chemotherapy has been standardly used in clinical practice. Other nitrosurea-based chemotherapies have not appeared as promising as BCNU in clinical trials. There was a Phase III randomized clinical trial from the United Kingdom comparing radiation alone vs. radiation followed by PCV chemotherapy [27]. There were no survival differences found in this study, even stratified based on grade of tumor.

TMZ represents a newer class of chemotherapeutic agents that has demonstrated activity in the setting of high-grade gliomas. The antitumor activity of TMZ has been attributed primarily to the methylation of DNA, which is highly dependent upon the formation of a reactive methydiazonium cation [24]. Figure 3 illustrates mechanisms of action of TMZ, as well as potential mechanisms of resistance. Nearly 70% of total DNA methylation by TMZ occurs at the N^7-guanine, and ~9% and ~5% of adducts are formed at the N^3-adenine and O^6-guanine, respectively. The cytotoxicity of TMZ is influenced by three DNA repair activities in particular. The first is O^6-alkylguanine-DNA alkyltransferase (AGT). There is accumulating evidence that the cytotoxicity of TMZ is highly dependent on the formation of O^6-methylguanine, despite the fact that this lesion accounts for only a small percentage of the total DNA adducts formed. Adducts produced at the O^6-position of guanine have been found to be especially mutagenic and cytotoxic. Methyl adducts at the O^6-guanine in DNA are repaired by the cytoprotective DNA repair protein, AGT (also referred to as MGMT), which transfers the methyl group to an internal cysteine acceptor residue. This reaction results in an irreversible inactivation of AGT, requiring increased de novo protein synthesis to restore repair activity. Depletion of AGT via pretreatment with substrate analogs such as O^6-benzylguanine (O^6-BG) has been investigated. It has been demonstrated in preclinical models that

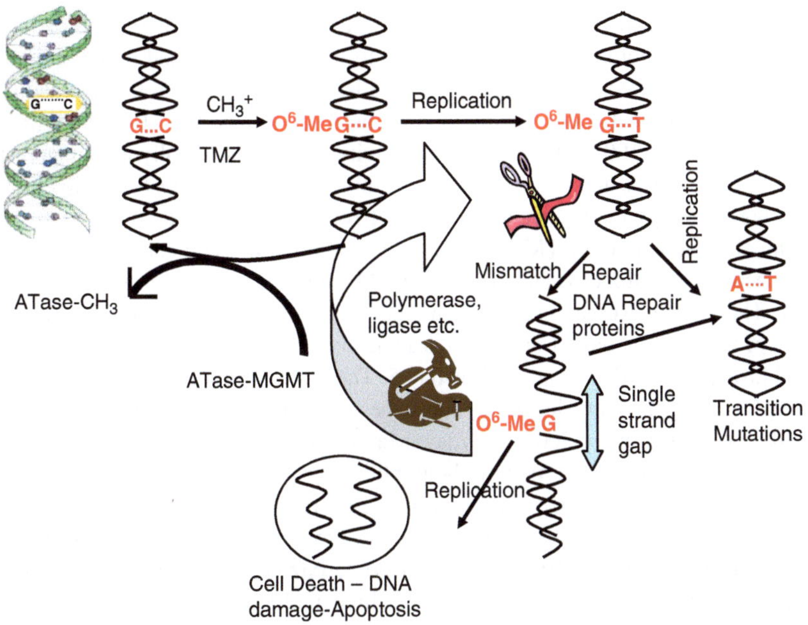

Fig. 3 Illustrates possible mechanisms of action of temozolomide, as well as potential resistance mechanisms to this drug

O^6-BG can increase the cytotoxicity of TMZ by several fold. It has been found that continuous administration of O^6-BG is more effective than intermittent dosing, indicating that regeneration of ACT activity following AGT inhibitor may be of clinical significance. The second mechanism of resistance to TMZ involves DNA mismatch repair pathways. One mechanism involves binding by a heterodimer complex consisting of hMSH2 and GTBP/p160 proteins and subsequent DNA incision following recruitment of an additional heterodimer consisting of hPMS2 and hMLH1 proteins. A section of DNA is then removed between the incision and the mismatch, and replaced by resynthesis and ligation. When this pathway is targeted to the strand directly opposite O^6-MG, its unsuccessful attempt to find a complementary base results in continued excision/insertion that produces persistent damage to the DNA. The resulting interruptions in the daughter strands prevent replication in the subsequent S-phase and may account for two cell divisions being required before the emergence of TMZ toxicity. Since the cytotoxicity of TMZ is dependent upon a functional DNA mismatch repair pathway, resistance may be conferred by a mutation in any of the genes encoding for a protein involved in mismatch recognition/incision (e.g., germline mutations in hereditary nonpolyposis colorectal cancer). Such abnormalities result in a TMZ "tolerant" phenotype which is unaffected by AGT activity. The third mechanism of TMZ resistance involves base excision repair and poly(ADP-ribose) polymerase. Methyl adducts produced at N^7-guanine and N^3-adenine by TMZ may also hinder DNA replication, as enzymatic or spontaneous depurination will ultimately result in DNA strand breakage.

Preclinical data also suggest that TMZ has at least additive activity with radiation in human glioblastoma cells [28]. It was determined that TMZ and radiation had at least an additive effect. In U373MG GBM cells, it was determined that the addition of 10 μM of TMZ to 1–2 Gy of radiation increased cell kill by 2.5–3.0-fold. However, in a cell line with 100-fold greater AGT activity, there was actually an antagonistic effect observed. This antagonistic effect was mitigated by co-incubation with O^6-BG, revealing a strategy to enhance the additive effect of TMZ and radiation.

The clinical activity of TMZ was initially examined in the recurrent setting. The pharmacokinetics, toxicity, and efficacy of TMZ has been studied in several phase I trials. The Cancer Research Campaign studies found that upon examining plasma levels of the drug on days 1 and 5, no drug accumulation was found [29]. The AUC was 34.8 mg/h/L on day 1 and 23.1 on day 5. The most common adverse events were nausea/vomiting and myelosuppression. The maximum tolerated dose was established at 1,000 mg/m^2 or 200 mg/m^2/day. Major clinical improvement was observed in 6/10 treated patients and major radiographic improvement in 5/10 patients.

A prospective randomized study compared temozolomide to procarbazine for recurrent GBM patients [30]. In this study, the 225 enrolled patients received either TMZ at doses of 200 or 150 mg/m^2/day or procarbazine at doses of 150 or 125 mg/m^2/day. The response rate in this study (which included either stable disease or partial response) was 45% for the TMZ arm compared to 32% for the procarbazine arm. The progression-free survival times were also found to be significantly improved with TMZ vs. procarbazine ($p = 0.008$). The overall 6-month survival times were also found to be improved in the TMZ group vs. the procarbazine group (60 weeks vs. 44 weeks, $p = 0.019$). It is also noteworthy that TMZ was associated with improved quality of life compared to procarbazine.

In a Phase II study reported by Stupp et al., the efficacy of TMZ in combination with radiation was demonstrated [31]. Sixty-four GBM patients were entered into this Phase II study. The subjects received TMZ (75 mg/m^2/day for 6–7 weeks) in a fasting state, 1 h before radiation and in the morning on days without radiation. Radiation was delivered to a total dose of 60 Gy administered at 2 Gy/fraction over 30 fractions. Four weeks after radiation, patients received TMZ (200 mg/m^2/day for 6 cycles). During the concomitant RT + TMZ phase, grade 3 or 4 neutropenia occurred in 6% of patients as did grade 3 or 4 thrombocytopenia. Grade 3 or 4 lymphocytopenia occurred in 79% of patients. Of the 62 patients treated by concurrent RT + TMZ, TMZ was discontinued early in four patients because of toxicity. All but four patients received the full radiation dose of 60 Gy. Adjuvant TMZ was administered to 49 patients. The median number of adjuvant cycles per patient was 5.5. Adjuvant TMZ was discontinued in 24 patients (39%) because of progressive disease. Twenty-four patients received all-planned cycles of TMZ concomitantly and adjuvantly (39%).

In the landmark EORTC 26981-22981/NCIC CE3 Phase III study of concomitant and adjuvant temozolomide and radiotherapy for newly diagnosed glioblastoma, 573 patients were randomized to receive either radiation alone or radiation in combination with TMZ, followed by adjuvant TMZ [1]. TMZ was administered at a dose of 75 mg/m^2 PO for 6 weeks during radiation, followed by 150–200 mg/m^2

PO QD d1–5 every 28 days for 6 cycles. In the radiation only group, 16% received biopsy and 84% underwent debulking surgery. Similarly, in the radiation + TMZ group, 17% underwent biopsy and 83% underwent debulking surgery. Of note, concurrent TMZ was tolerated well, with 85% of patients completing both RT and TMZ as planned. Hematologic toxicity was more common in the combined RT/TMZ group compared to RT alone. The rate of Grade I/II anemia was 51% in the RT/TMZ group compared to 27% in the RT only group. In contrast, Grade I/II Leukopenia was 27% in the RT/TMZ group compared to 5% to the RT only group; Grade I/II neutropenia was 14% in the RT/TMZ group compared to 1% in the RT only group. Grade III/IV toxicity was more uncommon, with less than 1%, 3%, 4%, and 3% of the patients in the RT/TMZ group experiencing anemia, leukopenia, neutropenia, or thrombocytopenia, respectively. None of the RT only patients experienced these hematologic Grade III/IV toxicities. Of the nonhematologic toxicities, nausea and vomiting were more common in the RT/TMZ at 37% vs. 17% in the RT only group. After radiotherapy, 223 patients in the RT + TMZ group (78%) started adjuvant TMZ and received a median of 3 cycles, with 47% of patients completing all 6 planned cycles. The primary reason for not beginning or completing adjuvant TMZ was disease progression. Only 8% of patients discontinued adjuvant TMZ due to toxic effects. Starting with cycle 2, the TMZ dose was escalated to 200 mg/m^2 in 67% of patients; only 9% of patients did not receive the higher dose to hematologic toxicity.

The median progression-free survival (PFS) was 6.9 months in the TMZ/RT group, compared with 5 months in the RT only group. The one- and two-year PFSs were 9% and 2%, respectively, in the RT only group, compared with 27% and 11%, respectively, in the RT+TMZ group (p<0.0001). The median survival was also significantly improved in the RT+TMZ group at 14.6 months, compared to 12.1 months in the RT only group (p<0.0001). The 2-year survival time likewise was significantly improved in the RT+TMZ group (26%) compared to the RT only group (10%). This represents one of the most significant improvements in survival found in any Phase III clinical study in newly diagnosed GBM patients within the past several decades. Of note, 72% of patients in the RT-only group received salvage chemotherapy after progression, which consisted of TMZ in 60% of these patients. Therefore, there is some uncertainty whether the benefit of TMZ is realized from its concurrent vs. adjuvant administration.

The encouraging results from this EORTC 26981-22981/NCIC CE3 Phase III trial raised the question of which patients would serve to derive greatest benefit from combining TMZ with RT. In an accompanying correlative study, Hegi et al. examined the potential role of MGMT (O^6-alkylguanine-DNA alkyltransferase) methylation in outcomes of these patients [32]. The MGMT gene, located on chromosome 10q26, encodes for a DNA repair protein that removes alkyl groups from the O^6 position of guanine, a critical site for DNA alkylation. Left unrepaired, lesions at this site commonly lead to cytotoxicity and apoptosis. As epigenetic silencing of the MGMT gene by promoter methylation is associated with loss of MGMT expression, it was hypothesized that TMZ-treated GBM patients with MGMT methylation would have improved outcomes compared to those with unmethylated promoters. In this study, methylation-specific PCR was performed on 307 out of 573 GBM specimens (53.6%); 266 patients did not have adequate paraffin tissue for analysis. MGMT methylation status could be determined in 206 out of 307 tumors (67.1%), representing 36% of tumors from the overall study population. Of the 206 tumors, 92 (44%) had appreciable MGMT promoter methylation. It was determined for these patients considered as a whole that there was a significant survival advantage for patients with MGMT promoter methylation (18.2 months vs. 12.2 months, respectively, $p < 0.001$). When both treatment assignment and MGMT promoter methylation status were considered, the longest median survival of 21.7 was observed among patients with promoter methylation who were randomized to receive both TMZ + RT. Of note, the 2-year survival in this group was 46%, compared to 22.7% among those with MGMT promoter methylation who were randomized to RT alone. In contrast, among patients with unmethylated MGMT promoters, the benefit of adding TMZ to RT was considerably more marginal. The median survival was 12.7 months in the RT + TMZ arm, compared to 11.8 months for those assigned to the RT only arm ($p = 0.06$). On multivariate analysis with the use of the Cox proportional-hazards model, stratified according to treatment group and including known clinical prognostic factors, the methylation status of the MGMT promoter ($p < 0.001$) and the score on the mini-mental status examination ($p < 0.007$) emerged as significant independent prognostic factors. An important follow-up study to the EORTC 26981-22981/NCIC CE3 trial will be the joint EORTC-RTOG 0525 Phase III clinical study which will be comparing TMZ administered using the Stupp regimen described above with a dose-dense regimen of TMZ administration. The hypothesis here is that a dose-dense TMZ schedule will prove to be more effective at depleting intracellular concentrations of MGMT, which will enhance tumor response.

Biotherapeutic Strategies

Antiepidermal Growth Factor Receptor (EGFR) Strategies

EGFR is a 170 kDa receptor tyrosine kinase (RTK) that is comprised of an extracellular binding domain, a transmembrane lipophilic segment, and an intracellular domain that has protein kinase activity [33–35]. There are four known family members of the EGFR family (erbB1-B4). ErbB1 (EGFR) is thought to be the critical player in GBMs. It has been observed that EGFR gene amplification is quite common in GBMs, occurring in ~50% of cases [4]. Many GBMs also express EGFRvIII, which is a mutant isoform of EGFR that lacks the extracellular binding domain and is essentially constitutively active, signaling through critical signal transduction cascades such as PI3K and ERK, among others. EGFR pathway activation has been demonstrated in preclinical models to enhance the malignant phenotype by increasing cellular proliferation, survival, migration/invasion, and angiogenesis [36–47].

Correlative studies have suggested a mixed picture, with regard to the prognostic value of EGFR status in human gliomas [46–53]. Generally, it has been observed that wild-type EGFR, as detected immunohistochemically, does not appear to have convincing prognostic value in GBM patients. Studies that have examined the prognostic values of EGFR gene amplification, EGFRvIII expression, and/or activation of downstream EGFR pathway members have more frequently been positive. One study suggests that EGFRvIII may have greater prognostic value in the setting of anaplastic astrocytoma than glioblastoma [54]. Therefore, the cumulative preclinical and correlative clinical data would appear to suggest that EGFR pathway antagonism may be a promising strategy for at least a subset of human gliomas.

Phase I/II studies on the safety and efficacy of anti-EGFR agents in the setting of GBM suggest modest activity in the recurrent setting. In a recently reported Phase I trial of gefitinib in the setting of recurrent GBM from the NABTC, it was determined that Iressa was well tolerated with skin rash, transaminase elevations, fatigue, and diarrhea representing the most common toxicities [55]. Doses up to 1,500 mg were found to be well tolerated. Seven out of the 55 patients were found to have objective radiographic responses to gefitinib in this study. In a recently reported Phase II study from Duke, the efficacy of gefitinib was prospectively examined in 53 patients with recurrent GBM [56]. The 6-month survival approached 60%, with a one-year survival of 37%. Interestingly, EGFR status, either measured by levels of IHC-detected EGFRwt or EGFRvIII or EGFR gene amplification, was not associated with outcome as measured by overall survival. Interestingly, gefitinib-treated GBM patients who developed diarrhea had improved survival times compared to those who did not. In a separate Phase II study of another EGFR tyrosine kinase inhibitor, erlotinib (OSI-774) in the setting of recurrent high-grade gliomas was examined [57]. In this study, 25 out of 37 patients were evaluated radiographically for response to erlotinib. Patients in this study were eligible to receive concurrent TMZ. Of the 25 radiographically evaluable patients, six demonstrated partial responses, two with minor responses, and three with prolonged disease stabilization. In a separate study investigating erlotinib alone in the setting of recurrent GBM, there was only one response out of 30 patients examined. Therefore, the emerging clinical data suggest that there is a subset of patients with malignant gliomas who are responsive to anti-EGFR therapies.

As response to anti-EGFR therapies when used as single agents in the recurrent setting appears to be independent of EGFR status, the role of downstream signaling pathways must be more carefully scrutinized. In one report, activation of phosphatidylinositol 3-kinase members (PI3K, AKT, $p70^{s6k}$) was associated with significantly worse survival times in glioma patients as a whole [58]. More specifically, in GBM patients treated with radiation as the primary adjuvant therapy without chemotherapy, activation of these critical PI3K pathway members was associated with adverse survival, indicating a direct role for this pathway in treatment resistance. As more evidence that activation of downstream pathways may mediate resistance to anti-EGFR agents, in a study of two primary GBM cell lines with equivalent expression of EGFR, the two cell lines were found to have very different sensitivities to the anti-EGFR agent AG1478 [59]. Further investigation revealed that upregulation of the insulin-like growth factor receptor 1 (IGFR1) contributed to resistance to AG1478. Downstream, it was determined that IGFR1-mediated activation of the PI3K/AKT signaling axis negated the effects of antagonizing EGFR in GBM cells. Upon dual inhibition of IGFR1 and EGFR, it was possible to more significantly downregulate activity of PI3K/AKT and reduce cellular survival as well as sensitivity to radiotherapy. These data suggest that GBMs can have redundant pathways that can compensate for loss of a given upstream signaling pathway. In a correlative study on patients with recurrent GBMs treated by anti-EGFR agents, it was determined that patients most responsive to anti-EGFR therapies are those with expression of EGFRvIII and PTEN. Tumors that were PTEN-deficient were found to be resistant to anti-EGFR agents as a rule. It can be conceptualized that EGFRvIII drives signaling through PI3K in tumors with intact PTEN and would therefore be responsive to anti-EGFR therapies. In contrast, tumors with PTEN deficiency have constitutive signaling through PI3K/AKT. Since neither EGFR nor EGFRvIII is driving PI3K pathway activation in PTEN-deficient tumors, it stands to reason that anti-EGFR agents would have limited efficacy in suppressing pro-survival signaling through PI3K/AKT. Strategies that would appear to be most effective in PTEN-deficient tumors would simultaneously involve co-targeting multiple pathways or would target critical survival pathways downstream of AKT.

The Radiation Therapy Oncology Group (RTOG) has investigated the safety and efficacy of Gefitinib, an EGFR tyrosine kinase inhibitor, in combination with radiation for newly diagnosed GBM patients (RTOG 0211) [60]. The Phase I portion of the study has been recently reported. Patients on RTOG 0211 were stratified based on whether they were on enzyme-inducing anticonvulsant drugs (EIACDs: Group I) or not (non-EIACDs: Group II). Gefitinib dose escalation during radiation was from 250 to 750 mg in Group I and 250 to 500 mg in Group II. A standard 3+3 design was used to evaluate dose-limiting toxicities (DLTs) which were defined as acute (<90 days) events. A total of 18 patients in Group I (16 eligible and analyzable) and 13 patients in Group II (12 eligible and analyzable) were included. In Group I, doses up to 750 mg were well tolerated and not associated with DLTs. Two patients experienced late (>90 days) grade 3 diarrhea and elevated SGOT values, respectively. At the 500-mg dose level in Group II, one patient had late grade 3 elevation of SGOT and one patient had acute grade 4 elevation of SGOT. As of this writing, Phase II data from RTOG 0211 have not yet matured.

mTor Pathway Inhibition: CCI-779

Targeting downstream signaling transduction pathways represents another promising strategy for the treatment of GBM patients. Preclinical data suggest that the mammalian target of rapamycin (mTor) pathway, which is downstream of EGFR and PI3K/AKT, represents an attractive therapeutic target. CCI-779 is a small molecule inhibitor (Rapamycin analog) of mTor, which represents a potent pro-survival pathway in many tumor types. In a recently reported NCCTG Phase II trial of CCI-779 in recurrent GBM, 41 patients with recurrent GBM were treated by CCI-779 at a dose of 250 mg IV per week [61]. The treatment was generally well tolerated, with grade 3 + hematologic toxicity observed in 12% and grade 3 nonhematologic toxicity observed in 51%, and consisted of hypercholesterolemia (15%), hypertriglceridemia (12%), hyperglycemia (10%), rash (5%), stomatitis (5%), and fatigue (2%). Assessment of tumor Akt and $p70^{s6k}$ kinase phosphorylation pretreatment demonstrated activation of Akt and $p70^{s6k}$ in the majority of patients (14/17 and 11/17 patients, respectively). Posttreatment, an analysis of peripheral blood mononuclear cell phosphorylation of $p70^{s6k}$ showed posttreatment inhibition in 7/10 patients. There were signs of some activity, with a significant decrease in T2 abnormality in five patients and a significant decrease in T1 gadolinium enhancement in three patients, which fell short of partial response. Investigation of mTor inhibitors in combination with radiation is presently ongoing.

Antiangiogenic Strategies

Given the promise of antiangiogenic strategies in human tumors, studies have been conducted in the setting of recurrent GBM. Vascular Endothelial Growth Factor-mediated signaling has been found to be important in GBM neovascularization in preclinical models. PTK 787/ZK 222584 is a drug that has been found to inhibit all known VEGF receptors and therefore inhibits signaling by VEGFs (A-D). In a study from M.D. Anderson and Duke University, 55 patients with recurrent GBM were treated by PTK-787 once daily as oral monotherapy starting at doses of 150 mg/day [62]. It was determined that doses up to 1,500 mg were well tolerated with side-effects including deep-vein thrombosis, cerebral edema, and fatigue occurring in a minority of patients. Among 47 evaluable patients, best responses were 2 (4%) partial responses, 31 (56%) stable disease, and 14 (25%) disease progression. Median duration of stable disease was 12.1 weeks. Dynamic contrast-enhanced (DCE) and dynamic susceptibility change (DSC) MRI revealed decreases in vascular permeability and cerebral blood volume, respectively, at days 2 and 30 of treatment. In a separate study from the same group, PTK-787 was combined with either TMZ or CCNU [63]. In this study, the starting dose of PTK787 was 500 mg/day, escalating to 1,000, 1,250, and 1,500 mg/day in cohorts of three to six patients. Concurrently, patients received either TMZ (200 mg/m^2/day for 5 days every 28 days) or CCNU (130 mg/m^2 every 6 weeks). In the 37 patients treated with PTK-787 + TMZ, 1 DLT (grade 3 dizziness) was reported at 1,500 mg/day, and the MTD was not reached. Among the 23 patients treated by PTK-787 + CCNU, DLTs included grade 3 febrile neutropenia in one patient each at the 500 and 1,000 mg levels and grade 4 transaminase elevation in one patient treated at the 1,000 mg level. Among 51 patients evaluable for response, four had a partial response (3 with PTK-787 + TMZ and 1 with PTK-787+CCNU) and 27 patients had stable disease (19 with PTK-787 + TMZ and 8 with PTK-787+CCNU) as best response. The median time to progression was

15.7 weeks (95% CI=8.6, 17.3 weeks) for the PTK-787+TMZ arm and 10.4 weeks for the PTK-787+CCNU arm. The investigators noted that the median TTP for the PTK-787+TMZ arm compared favorably with historical reports with TMZ alone. Phase I/II studies are currently planned investigating PTK-787+TMZ in combination with radiotherapy for newly diagnosed GBM patients.

Summary

Malignant gliomas remain among the most treatment-refractory tumors. Traditional upfront treatment regimens have incorporated nitrosurea-based chemotherapy. This strategy has evolved to include temozolomide-based approaches. Promising Phase I/II data with TMZ in the recurrent setting prompted a Phase III EORTC study of TMZ in combination with RT for patients with newly diagnosed GBM. The landmark EORTC 26981-22981/NCIC CE3 study demonstrated a significant improvement in not only median survival, but also in terms of 2-year survival. Given that over one-quarter of the patients enrolled on the TMZ + RT arm survived beyond 2-years, there appears to be a finite percentage of patients who derive long-term benefit from this treatment regimen. Given that the EORTC-based regimen represents an incremental improvement in the standard of care, rather than a truly curative solution for most patients, further efforts must be expended to identify novel therapeutic approaches. To this end, targeted therapies have emerged as an attractive option. Accumulating evidence suggests that certain molecular pathways are selectively upregulated in tumor vs. normal cells. Some of these pathways have been shown to be instrumental in proliferation, migration, invasion, angiogenesis, and/or survival in preclinical models. These would appear to represent ideal therapeutic targets, as their antagonism may lead to an improvement in the therapeutic ratio of radiation. Emerging data from clinical studies on "first generation" targeted therapies appear to demonstrate benefit for select patients. Further molecular/genetic profiling must be undertaken to identify exactly which patients benefit.

References

1. Stupp R, et al. Radiotherapy plus concomitant and adjuvant temozolomide for glioblastoma. N Engl J Med 2005; 352:987–996.
2. Walker MD, Alexander E, Hunt WE. *Evaluation of BCNU and/or radiotherapy in the treatment of anaplastic gliomas*. J Neurosurg 1978; 49:333–343.
3. Walker MD, Green SB, Byar DP. Randomized comparisons of radiotherapy and nitrosureas for the treatment of malignant gliomas after surgery. N Engl J Med 1980; 303:1323–1329.
4. Maher EA, et al. Malignant glioma: genetics and biology of a grave matter. Genes and Dev 2001; 15:1311–1333.
5. Vivanco I, Sawyers CL. The phosphatidylinositol 3-Kinase AKT pathway in human cancer. Nat Rev Cancer 2002; 2(7):489–501.

6. Choe G, Horvath S, Cloughesy TF, Crosby K, Seligson D, Palotie A, Inge L, Smith B, Sawyers CL, Mischel PS. Analysis of the Phosphatidyl 3′-Kinase Signaling Pathway in Glioblastoma Patients in Vivo. Cancer Res 2003; 63(11):2742–2746.
7. Ermoian RP, et al. Dysregulation of PTEN and protein kinase B is associated with glioma histology and patient survival. Clin Cancer Res 2002; 8(5):1100–1106.
8. Holland EC, et al. Combined activation of Ras and Akt in neural progenitors induce glioblastoma formation in mice. Nat Genet 2000; 25(1):55–57.
9. Frederick L, et al. Analysis of genomic rearrangements associated with EGRFvIII expression suggests involvement of Alu repeat elements. Neuro-oncol 2000; 2(3):159–163.
10. Kleihues P, et al. The WHO classification of tumors of the nervous system. J Neuropathol Exp Neurol 2002; 61(3):215–225; discussion 226–229.
11. Kleihues, P, Ohgaki H. *Primary and secondary glioblastomas: from concept to clinical diagnosis*. Neurooncol 1999; 1(1):44–51.
12. Mischel PS, Cloughesy TF. Targeted molecular therapy of GBM. Brain Pathol 2003; 13(1):52–61.
13. Rao RD, et al. Genetic and signaling pathway alterations in glioblastoma: relevance to novel targeted therapies. Front Biosci 2003; 8:E270–E280.
14. von Deimling A, et al. Subsets of glioblastoma multiforme defined by molecular genetic analysis. Brain Pathol 1993; 3(1):19–26.
15. Watanabe K, et al. Overexpression of the EGF receptor and p53 mutations are mutually exclusive in the evolution of primary and secondary glioblastomas. Brain Pathol 1996; 6(3):217–223; discussion 23–24.
16. Abounader R, et al. In vivo targeting of SF/HGF and c-met expression via U1snRNA/ribozymes inhibits glioma growth and angiogenesis and promotes apoptosis. Faseb J 2002; 16(1):108–110.
17. Abounader R, et al. Signaling pathways in the induction of c-met receptor expression by its ligand scatter factor/hepatocyte growth factor in human glioblastoma. J Neurochem 2001; 76(5):1497–1508.
18. Senger DL, et al. Suppression of Rac activity induces apoptosis of human glioma cells but not normal human astrocytes. Cancer Res 2002; 62(7):2131–2140.
19. Zagzag D, et al. Vascular apoptosis and involution in gliomas precede neovascularization: a novel concept for glioma growth and angiogenesis. Lab Invest 2000; 80(6):837–849.
20. Zagzag D, Capo V. Angiogenesis in the central nervous system: a role for vascular endothelial growth factor/vascular permeability factor and tenascin-C. Common molecular effectors in cerebral neoplastic and non-neoplastic “angiogenic diseases”. Histol Histopathol 2002; 17(1):301–321.
21. Zundel W, et al. Loss of PTEN facilitates HIF-1-mediated gene expression. Genes Dev 2000; 14(4):391–396.
22. Gollmer J, et al. Expression of vascular endothelial growth factor-b in human astrocytoma. Neurooncol 2000; 2(2):80–86.
23. Mischel PS, Shai R, Shi T, Horvath S, Lu KV, Choe G, Seligson D, Kremen TJ, Palotie A, Liau LM, Cloughesy TF, Nelson SF. Identification of Molecular Subtypes of Glioblastoma By Gene Expression Profiling. Oncogene 2003; 22(15):2361–2373.
24. Newlands ES, et al. Temozolomide: a review of its discovery, chemical properties, pre-clinical development, and clinical trials. Cancer Treat Rev 1997; 23:35–61.
25. Fine H, et al. Meta-analysis of radiation therapy with and without adjuvant chemotherapy for malignant gliomas in adults. Cancer 1993; 71(8):2585–2597.
26. Stewart LA. Chemotherapy in adult high-grade glioma: a systematic review and meta-analysis of individual patient data from 12 randomised trials. Lancet 2002; 359(9311):1011–1018.
27. Party MRCBTW. Randomized trial of procarbazine, lomustine, and vincristine in the adjuvant treatment of high-grade astrocytoma: a Medical Research Council trial. J Clin Oncol 2001; 19(2):509–518.
28. Wedge SR, et al. In vitro evaluation of temozolomide combined with X-irradiation. Anticancer Drugs 1997; 8(1):92–97.

29. Newlands ES, Blackledge G, Slack RS. Phase I trial of temozolomide (CCRG 81045: M&B 39831:NSC 362856). Br J Cancer 1992; 65:287–291.
30. Yung WK, et al. A phase II study of temozolomide vs. procarbazine in patients with glioblastoma at first relapse. Br J Cancer 2000; 83(5):588–593.
31. Stupp R, et al. Promising survival for patients with newly-diagnosed glioblastoma multiforme treated with concomitant radiation plus temozolomide followed by adjuvant temozolomide. J Clin Oncol 2002; 20(5):1375–1382.
32. Hegi ME, et al. MGMT gene silencing and benefit from temozolomide in glioblastoma. N Engl J Med 2005; 352:997–1003.
33. Hackel PO, et al. Epidermal growth factor receptors: critical mediators of multiple receptor pathways. Curr Opinion in Cell Biol 1999; 11:184–189.
34. Woodburn JR. The epidermal growth factor receptor and its inhibition in cancer therapy. Pharmacol Ther 1999; 82(2–3): 241–250.
35. Zwick E, et al. The EGF receptor as central transducer of heterologous signalling systems. Trends Pharmacol Sci 1999; 20:408–412.
36. Ang K, et al. Impact of Epidermal Growth Fatcor Receptor Expression on Survival and Pattern of Relapse in Patients with Advanced Head and Neck Carcinoma. Cancer Res 2002; 62:7350–7356.
37. Baselga J, Albanell J. Targeting epidermal growth factor receptor in lung cancer. Curr Oncol Rep 2002; 4(4):317–324.
38. Baselga J. Why the epidermal growth factor receptor? The rationale for cancer therapy. Oncologist 2002; 7 Suppl 4:2–8.
39. Balaban N, et al. The effect of ionizing radiation on signal transduction: antibodies to EGF receptor sensitize A431 cells to radiation. Biochim Biophys Acta 1996; 1314(1–2):147–156.
40. Chakravarti A, Dicker A, Mehta M. The contribution of EGFR signaling in human gliomas: a review of preclinical and correlative data. Int J Radiat Oncol Biol Phys 2004; 58(3):927–931.
41. Chakravarti A, Loeffler JS, Dyson NJ. Insulin-like growth factor receptor I mediates resistance to anti-epidermal growth factor receptor therapy in primary human glioblastoma cells through the continued activation of phosphoinositide 3-kinase signaling. Cancer Res 2002; 62(1):200–207.
42. Chakravarti A, et al. The epidermal growth factor receptor pathway mediates resistance to sequential administration of radiation and chemotherapy in primary human glioblastoma cells in a ras-dependent manner. Cancer Res 2002; 62(15):4307–4315.
43. Ciardiello F, et al. Antiangiogenic and antitumor activity of anti-epidermal growth factor receptor C225 monoclonal antibody in combination with vascular endothelial growth factor antisense oligonucleotide in human GEO colon cancer cells. Clin Cancer Res 2000; 6(9):3739–3747.
44. Ciardiello F. Epidermal growth factor receptor tyrosine kinase inhibitors as anticancer agents. Drugs 2000; 60 Suppl 1:25–32; discussion 41–42.
45. Dent P, et al. Radiation-induced release of transforming growth factor alpha activates the epidermal growth factor receptor and mitogen-activated protein kinase pathway in carcinoma cells, leading to increased proliferation and protection from radiation-induced cell death. Mol Biol Cell 1999; 10:2493–2506.
46. Barker FG, et al. EGFR overexpression and radiation response in glioblastoma multiforme. Int J Radiat Oncol Biol Phys 2001; 51(2):410–418.
47. Shinojima N, et al. Prognostic value of epidermal growth factor receptor in patients with Glioblastoma Multiforme. Cancer Res 2003; 63:6962–6970.
48. Chakravarti A, et al. Prognostic and Pathologic Significance of Quantitative Protein Expression Profiling in Human Gliomas. Clin Cancer Res 2001; 7:2387–2395.
49. Etienne M-C, et al. Epidermal growth factor receptor and labeling index are independent prognostic factors in glial turmor outcome. Clin Cancer Res 1998; 4(10):2383–2390.
50. Feldkamp MM, et al. Expression of activated epidermal growth factor receptors, Ras-guanosine triphosphate, and mitogen-activated protein kinase in human glioblastoma multiforme specimens. Neurosurgery 1999; 45(6):1442–1453.

51. Smith JS, et al. PTEN mutation, EGFR amplification, and outcome in patients with anaplastic astrocytoma and glioblastoma multiforme. J Nat Cancer Inst 2001; 93(16):1246–1256.
52. Rainov NG, Dobberstein KU, Bahn H. Prognostic factors in malignant glioma: Influence of the overexpression of oncogene and tumor-suppressor gene products on survival. J Neurooncol 1997; 35:13–28.
53. Chakravarti A, et al. Immunohistochemically determined total epidermal growth factor receptor (EGFR) levels are not of prognostic value in newly diagnosed glioblastoma multiforme (GBM): A Report from the Radiation Therapy Oncology Group (RTOG). Int J Radiat Oncol Biol Phys 2005; 62(2):318–327.
54. Buckner JC, et al. Immunohistochemical detection of EGFRvIII and prognostic significance in patinets with malignant glioma enrolled in NCCTG clinical trials. J Clin Oncol 2004; 22(14S):1508.
55. Prados M, et al. Phase I study of ZD1839 plus temozolomide in patients with malignant glioma. J Clin Oncol 2004; 22(14s):1504.
56. Rich J, et al. Phase II trial of gefitinib in recurrent glioblastoma. J Clin Oncol 2004; 22(1):133–142.
57. Prados M, et al. Phase I study of OSI-774 alone or with temozolamide in patients with malignant glioma. Proc Am Soc Clin Oncol 2003; 22:99.
58. Chakravarti A, et al. The Prognostic Significance of Phosphatidylinositol 3-Kinase Pathway Activation in Human Gliomas. J Clin Oncol 2004; 22(10):1926–1933.
59. Chakravarti A, Loeffler JS, Dyson NJ. Insulin-like growth factor receptor I mediates resistance to anti-epidermal growth factor receptor therapy in primary human glioblastoma cells through continued activation of physphoinositide 3-kinase signaling. Cancer Res 2002; 62(1):200–207.
60. Chakravarti A, et al. An update of phase I data from RTOG 0211: A phase I/II clinical study of gefitinib + radiation for newly-diagnosed GBM patients. J Clin Oncol 2004; 22(14S):1571.
61. Galanis E, et al. NCCTG phase II trial of CCI-779 in recurrent glioblastoma multiforme (GBM). J Clin Oncol 2004; 22(14S):1503.
62. Conrad C, et al. A phase I/II trial of single-agent PTK 787/ZK 222584 (PTK/ZK), a novel, oral angiogenesis inhibitor, in patients with recurrent GBM. J Clin Oncol 2004; 22(14S):1512.
63. Reardon DA, et al. A phase I/II trial of PTK-787/ZK 222584 (PTK/ZK), a novel, oral angiogenesis inhibitor, in combination with either temozolomide or lomustine for patients with recurrent GBM. J Clin Oncol 2004; 22(14S):1513.

Section III
Advances in Treatment Delivery and Planning

10 Advances in Intensity-Modulated Radiotherapy Delivery

John D. Fenwick, Stephen W. Riley, and Alison J.D. Scott

Introduction

Fixed-field radiation treatments delivered using conventional clinical linear accelerators (linacs) fitted with multileaf collimators have rapidly become the most common form of intensity-modulated radiotherapy (IMRT). Several alternative innovative IMRT planning and delivery systems are also now commercially available, and three are reviewed here – tomotherapy, highly manoeuvrable robotic linear accelerators, and conventional linear accelerators modulated by their jaws alone.

The evolution of these innovative IMRT technologies is placed in the context of the development of conventional linac-plus-multileaf IMRT systems. The rationales of the different IMRT approaches are discussed and their methods of dose delivery are described. Differences between the dose distributions delivered using the innovative technologies and the conventional fixed-field approach are outlined. Because conventional linear accelerator design has been finely honed over the years, innovative design enhancement of one aspect of system performance often limits another facet of machine capability. Consequently, the various delivery systems may prove optimal for different types of treatment, specific systems excelling for disease sites with specific target volume and normal structure topologies.

Background

IMRT has its origins in work published in 1982 by Brahme and colleagues [1], who studied a problem involving a rotational (arc-based) delivery, leading to further exploration [2, 3] of analytic connections between dose distributions and intensity-modulated coplanar radiation beams delivered from a continuum of gantry angles over the range 0° through to 360°. These analytic connections are similar to the mathematical links between emission computed tomography images and the projection data from which the images are reconstructed [4, 5]. The analytic approach is also closely related to earlier work of Birkhoff, which shows how drawings can be created by superposing multiple straight lines oriented at a range of angles [6]. Its direct application to radiotherapy is hindered by the mathematically reasonable

M.P. Mehta et al. (eds.), *Radiation Oncology Advances*.

but physically unachievable requirement for negative radiation fluence to be delivered by some beamlets in order to generate ideal distributions depositing zero dose outside target regions. Nonetheless, the analytical work has had a significant impact by seeding the idea of rotational IMRT.

Subsequently, numerical IMRT optimisation algorithms were developed in the late 1980s and early 1990s [7–11]. These algorithms iteratively search spaces of physically realisable (non-negative fluence) IMRT deliveries, to find dose distributions that conform most closely to the physically unachievable ideal distributions. A range of criteria can be used to judge how closely dose distributions conform to the ideal; specific criteria are selected whenever optimisation algorithms are run, and vary from treatment-site to treatment-site and potentially from patient to patient. To simplify the optimisation and delivery processes, the delivery search space can be restricted, for instance by specifying that treatments consist of just a few fields arranged at particular predefined angles – the fixed-field IMRT approach.

Fixed-field IMRT was first clinically implemented in 1995 [12, 13] and can generate highly conformal radiotherapy dose distributions using just a few fixed-angle radiation fields delivered by standard clinical linear accelerators (linacs) and modulated by conventional multileaf collimators operated in either dynamic [14] or step-and-shoot [15] mode. It is the most common form of IMRT, making the conventional linac-plus-multileaf combination the standard IMRT delivery system. Further refinements will occur, but the essential features of the fixed-field approach are established [13].

Alternative options, delivering other forms of IMRT, include axial tomotherapy [16, 17] which pre-dates fixed-field IMRT, and helical tomotherapy [18, 19] and CyberKnife robotic linac treatments [20–23] (Accuray Inc., Sunnyvale, CA) which have only become widely available since the introduction of the fixed-field approach. The development of direct aperture optimisation (DAO) [24] has also made it more practical to deliver IMRT using linacs modulated by their jaws alone rather than by a multileaf. These non-standard forms of IMRT have divergent rationales. Tomotherapy and CyberKnife systems have been purposefully engineered to have different geometric degrees of freedom, beam dimensions and modulation techniques than those of conventional linacs – differences which may in certain circumstances allow these systems to deliver superior treatments. On the other hand, jaws-only linac IMRT is being developed pragmatically, simply to facilitate IMRT delivery without the need for expensive multileaves. The various delivery systems are mutually contrasted in Table 1, adapted from a summary presented by Battista and Bauman [25].

Fixed-Field IMRT

Details of the standard fixed-field form of IMRT delivery have been extensively reviewed elsewhere [13, 16, 17, 26–28]. Here we describe the approach only in broad outline, conveying its general methodology and providing a backdrop against which the reader can pick out the distinctive rationale and features of each of the non-standard IMRT options.

Table 1 IMRT delivery systems

System	Gantry type	Beam geometry and beam angle degrees of freedom	Collimated by	Modulated by	Imaging	Gating potential
Conventional linac plus multileaf	C-arm	Cone-beam, non-coplanar	Jaws + conventional multileaf	Jaws + conventional multileaf	Portal image, fluoroscopy, kvCT, infra-red reflectors	Breath-hold, beam trigger or multileaf tracking
Conventional linac minus multileaf	C-arm	Cone-beam, non-coplanar	Jaws	Jaws	Portal image, fluoroscopy, kvCT, infra-red reflectors	Breath-hold, beam trigger or jaw tracking
Serial tomotherapy (conventional linac plus binary multileaf)	C-arm	Fan beam, coplanar – indexed slice-by-slice through planes	Jaws + binary multileaf	Binary multileaf	Portal image, fluoroscopy, kvCT, infra-red reflectors	Breath-hold during each slice
Helical tomotherapy (Hi-Art)	Ring	Fan beam, coplanar – taking helical trajectory through planes	Jaws + binary multileaf	Binary multileaf	MVCT, infra-red reflectors	Delivery synchronised with breathing cycle
Robotic linac (CyberKnife)	Robotic arm	Pencil-beam, non-coplanar	Circular collimator	Superposition of pencil-beams by robotic arm movement	Biplanar radiography, infra-red reflectors	Beam trigger or robotic tracking

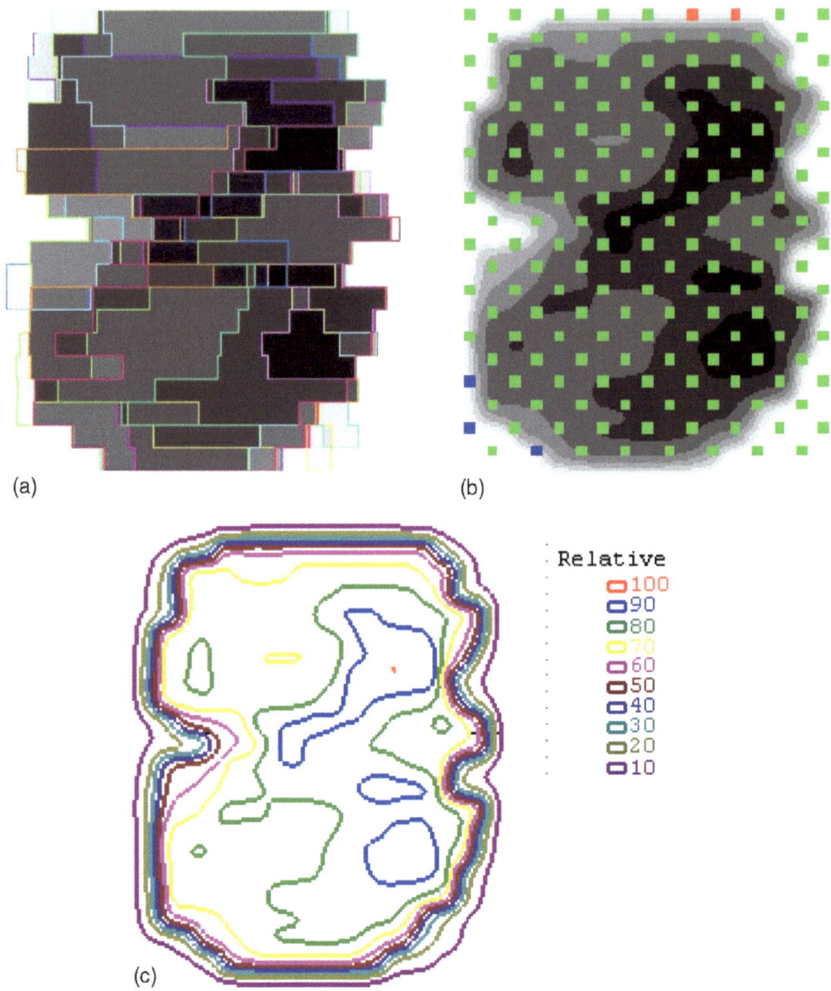

Fig. 1 (**a**) An intensity-modulated radiation field delivered using a step-and-shoot multileaf sequence. Segment edges are shown in a range of colours. The *underlying greyscale* represents the total number of monitor units with which each point in the field is irradiated.(**b**) A MapCHECK (Sun Nuclear Corp, Melbourne, FL) test of fluence delivery accuracy. *Green dots* mark the locations of diode detectors measuring expected doses (3% or 3 mm distance-to-agreement criterion) while *red and blue dots* mark points where doses are greater or less than expected. The detectors are separated by diagonal distances of 7 mm. The *underlying greyscale* represents the dose distribution calculated for the field. (**c**) An isodose map showing percentage (of maximum) doses across the field, calculated in the isocentric plane at 2 cm deep in water-equivalent plastic by the Pinnacle [3] treatment planning system (Philips Medical Systems, Madison, WI)

Figure 1 shows one of five intensity-modulated non-coplanar fields used to construct the first phase of a fixed-field IMRT treatment of an ethmoid sinus neuroendocrine carcinoma. The radiation fluence across the field is modulated by a multileaf collimator, in this case operated in step-and-shoot mode. This approach is a logical extension of modern 3D conformal radiotherapy techniques, which use multileaf collimators simply to shape radiation fields (their original purpose) rather than also to modulate them, the field-shaping excluding some normal tissue from the radiation fields without compromising target coverage (Fig. 2).

Planning studies from several centres including the University of Wisconsin have shown that intensity modulation improves unmodulated 3D conformal dose distributions, to a clinically meaningful extent for treatments of targets with complex shapes. In one study, fixed-field IMRT and 3D conformal 76 Gy prostate plans were compared [29], a feature of the work being the use of a rectal balloon for immobilisation and displacement of the posterior wall of the rectum. Volumes of rectal wall receiving doses in excess of 60 and 70 Gy (which have been shown to correlate with the risk of late complications [30, 31]) were substantially reduced using the balloon, and further reduced by intensity modulation. In another study comparing 60 Gy tomotherapy IMRT with 3D conformal therapy for patients with stage III inoperable non-small cell lung cancer, considerably lower lung dose–volume measures were calculated for tomotherapy than for 3D conformal plans (Fig. 3) [32]. Planned oesophageal and cord tomotherapy doses were also lower.

Step-and-shoot intensity-modulated radiation fields are built up out of simple unmodulated field segments shaped by multileaves, as illustrated in Fig. 1a. Historically, spatial patterns of radiation fluence intensity have been optimised for each field by a primary optimisation algorithm, and then passed to a secondary algorithm which converts them into step-and-shoot sequences of multileaf segment shapes and monitor unit settings. These step-and-shoot sequences deliver good, although discretised, approximations to the continuously varying fluence intensity patterns calculated by the primary optimiser. The number of segments used is a compromise between the over-coarse discretisation of fields made up of too few segments and the possibly excessive times taken to deliver fields comprising too many segments – overly long delivery times potentially being more of an issue for non-gridded gun linacs whose waveguide microwave power has to be run up between each segment.

Intensity-modulated fields can also be constructed using a sliding-window approach, which works by sliding leaf pairs dynamically across a field while the beam remains continuously on, varying leaf velocities to control the lengths of time for which different points lie within the irradiated gap between the leaves and thus controlling the pattern of intensity modulation. Compared to step-and-shoot, this technique has the advantage of delivering continuously varying non-discretised fluence patterns and the disadvantage that both the velocities and positions of multileaves need to be controlled accurately to ensure correct dose delivery, whereas step-and-shoot requires only positional accuracy. In practice, however, these differences are surprisingly fine: sufficient segments can usually be delivered in short enough times for the discretisation of step-and-shoot deliveries to be unproblematic; and leaf velocity accuracy during sliding-window deliveries is verified by checking that leaves pass through fixed control points after delivery of specific numbers of monitor units – not very different from the confirmation of leaf arrival at control points used to initiate monitor unit delivery at the start of each segment of step-and-shoot sequences.

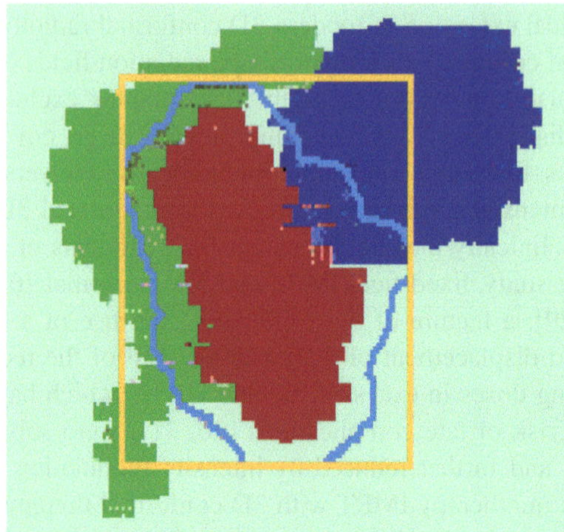

Fig. 2 The classic conformal paradigm: shaping of the lateral prostate field reduces high-dose volumes of rectal wall and bladder. The figure shows the prostate target (*red*) together with bladder (*blue*) and rectum (*green*), and contours of the shaped conformal field (*light blue*) and the rectangular field used historically (*gold*)

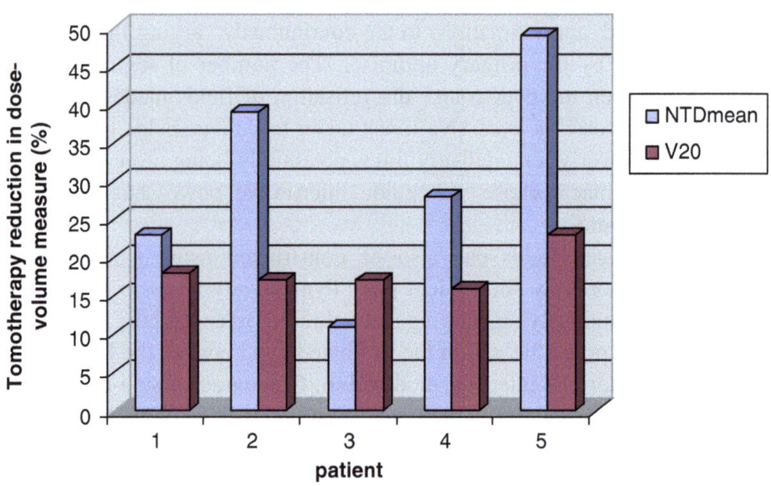

Fig. 3 Percentage reductions in planned lung NTD_{mean} and V_{20} dose–volume measures obtained by using helical tomotherapy IMRT rather than 3D conformal radiotherapy, calculated for five stage III non-small cell lung cancer patients

Direct Aperture Optimisation and Jaws-Only Linear Accelerator IMRT

Step-and-shoot intensity-modulated fields can be constructed entirely from rectangular-shaped segments collimated by linac jaws alone, rather than from the more irregularly shaped segments which can be created using multileaves. While equipment costs are cut by avoiding the need for multileaves, the reduction in field-shaping flexibility inevitably increases the number of segments required to construct modulated fields, and consequently jaws-only IMRT takes longer to deliver. This issue was first studied in 1999 by Dai and Hu [33] who found that the jaws-only approach lengthened delivery times by factors in the range 2–5.

More recently, DAO has been developed for step-and-shoot IMRT planning [24]. Whereas IMRT dose distributions are classically generated by optimising fluence intensities and then calculating sequences of segments which deliver discretised approximations to these optimised intensities, DAO algorithms instead directly optimise field segment shapes and weights. The number of segments per field is specified before the optimisation process begins. Dose distributions generated using direct aperture optimisation are just as good as those produced by classic IMRT optimisation, but can generally be delivered using fewer segments.

The fusion of jaws-only modulation and DAO techniques is quite powerful. Earl and colleagues [34] have compared jaws-only and multileaf-based direct aperture-optimised delivery times for abdomen, prostate and head-and-neck IMRT plans: multileaf-based plans can be delivered in 7–12 min using an Elekta Precise linac, with equally conformal jaws-only plans taking just about twice as long. A jaws-only IMRT planning algorithm has recently been commercialised (Prowess Inc, Chico, CA).

Tomotherapy

Using a conventional linac-plus-multileaf system, delivery of plans comprising many modulated fields can take a long time, a difficulty caused primarily by the rather inefficient nature of cone-beam modulation using a conventional multileaf. Larger numbers of monitor units are used when modulated fields are constructed from multiple smaller multileaf-collimated segments than when modulation is achieved using physical compensators or, of course, when fields are delivered unmodulated. Additionally, the multileaves have to move between each segment and for non-gridded-gun linacs, the waveguide microwave power has to be run up. Ideally, fixed-field IMRT would be delivered using an efficient physical metal compensator whose shape could somehow rapidly be changed between beams. But, although several researchers have designed modulator systems which come closer to this ideal [35–38], their work has not yet led to a commercial product.

However, early in the evolution of IMRT, it was appreciated that narrow fan beams of radiation could potentially be modulated efficiently using ‘binary’ multileaf collimators, with leaves designed to lie either totally across or completely outside the beam, and thus to either wholly obscure short lengths of the fan beam or leave them open. By rapidly driving leaves from one position to the other, modulation can be achieved along the length of the fan beam simply by varying the fraction of beam on time for which each leaf obscures the field. This efficient form of modulation opened up the possibility of realising the rotational IMRT contemplated in the initial analytic intensity-modulation studies, by irradiating patients slice-by-slice and treating each slice using a large number of coplanar-modulated fan beams delivered from angles throughout the 0°–360° range – tomotherapy.

Axial Tomotherapy

Tomotherapy both pre- and post-dates fixed-field IMRT. Axial, or serial, tomotherapy was clinically implemented as early as 1994 [16] and it has been estimated that as late as the turn of the millennium, more patients had been treated using this technique than using fixed-field IMRT deliveries [17].

The equipment and associated quality assurance processes used to implement axial tomotherapy have been described thoroughly in the literature [16, 39–43]. Briefly, a MIMiC binary multileaf collimator (North American Scientific, NOMOS Radiation Oncology Division, Cranberry Township, PA) is attached to a conventional linac, either into or in place of the block tray. The collimator comprises two opposed banks of 20 pneumatically driven tungsten leaves, which modulate a fan beam of radiation produced by the linac. The leaf in–out drive direction is aligned perpendicular to the gantry rotational plane of the linac, with the fan beam lying parallel to the rotational plane. The fan-beam width in the direction perpendicular to the rotational plane can be set to a nominal 2 or 4 cm projected to isocentre, with the width of each leaf being nominally 1 cm at isocentre in the direction parallel to the rotational plane.

Patients are treated with rotational modulated deliveries, individual beam-modulation patterns being defined over each 5° interval of the treatment arc. Treatments are optimised using the Corvus planning system, also produced by NOMOS. Patients with planned target lengths (in the direction perpendicular to the gantry rotational plane) which exceed the fan-beam width are irradiated using multiple abutting arcs, reducing the delivery efficiency. Typically, each arc takes 2 min to deliver, with a further minute required between arcs to increment the treatment couch through a slice thickness, making the treatment time for a seven-arc delivery around 20 min. To limit slice-to-slice dosimetric junctioning errors to 5%, couch incrementation has to be accurate to about 0.2 mm [44], a level that can be achieved using the NOMOS CRANE couch indexer.

Helical Tomotherapy

Helical tomotherapy emerged after the development of fixed-field IMRT, the first patient being treated at the University of Wisconsin in 2002 [19]. Like the axial form of tomotherapy, radiation is delivered using a rotating intensity-modulated fan beam, the modulation varying with gantry angle. But whereas axial tomotherapy is delivered slice-by-slice, with patients being sequentially and discretely translated through the linac gantry rotational plane between slices, helical tomotherapy is delivered without interruption as patients are translated smoothly through the bore of the machine while its gantry continuously and synchronously rotates, the therapy equivalent of spiral computed tomography [18]. And while axial tomotherapy can be accomplished by adding a binary multileaf to the front of a conventional linac, the helical approach requires a completely re-engineered machine – because to achieve continuous beam rotation many major system components have to be placed on a ring gantry, coupled to the remaining non-rotating components using slip-ring technology. Hi-Art machines designed specifically to deliver helical tomotherapy have recently been built and commercialised by Tomotherapy, Inc. (Madison, WI).

Figure 4 shows the layout around the Hi-Art ring gantry of the major rotating system components, which are normally concealed under machine covers. The treatment head is schematically illustrated in Fig. 5. Much has been written elsewhere about Hi-Art design, dosimetry and quality assurance [45–53]. Notably, the Hi-Art system does not include a physical flattening filter; consequently its maximum dose rate is increased to around 8 Gy min^{-1} at isocentre, and the fluence of the 6 MV treatment fan beam is forward peaked until modulated by a single row of 64 binary tungsten multileaves, each of width 0.625 cm projected to isocentre. Individual modulation patterns are defined over rotational intervals ('projections') of just greater than 7°, corresponding to exactly 51 projections per gantry revolution, and are optimised by the Hi-Art planning system.

As for axial tomotherapy, the fan beam is aligned parallel to the gantry rotational plane and its width is held constant during treatment, generally at 1, 2.5 or 5 cm projected to isocentre. The gantry and the treatment couch on which patients are transported through the radiation beam both move at constant rates during treatment. The gantry rotates with a period of between 10 and 60 s, and during each rotation the couch translates patients through the beam by a constant fraction of the fan-beam width, known as the pitch of the delivery. Its value typically lies somewhere between 0.2 and 0.5, to some extent determines the resolution of the modulation in the couch-drive direction, and can be selected to minimise the thread effect [53] – a small dose perturbation resulting from the interplay between the helical delivery and the divergence of the fan beam.

Treatment times depend on the prescribed dose-per-fraction, the length of the target in the couch-drive direction, the depth of the target within the patient and the maximum degree of beam modulation used, but are essentially independent of pitch [52]. A 2 Gy-per-fraction prostate plan typically takes around 5 min to deliver.

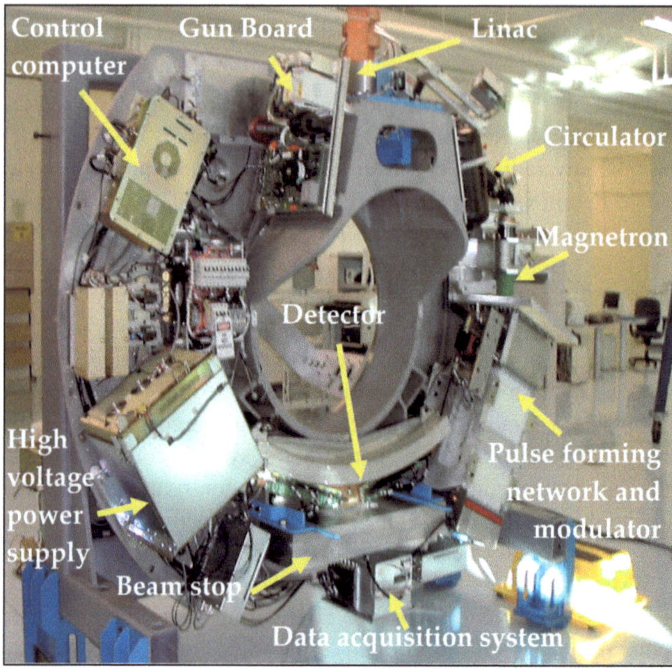

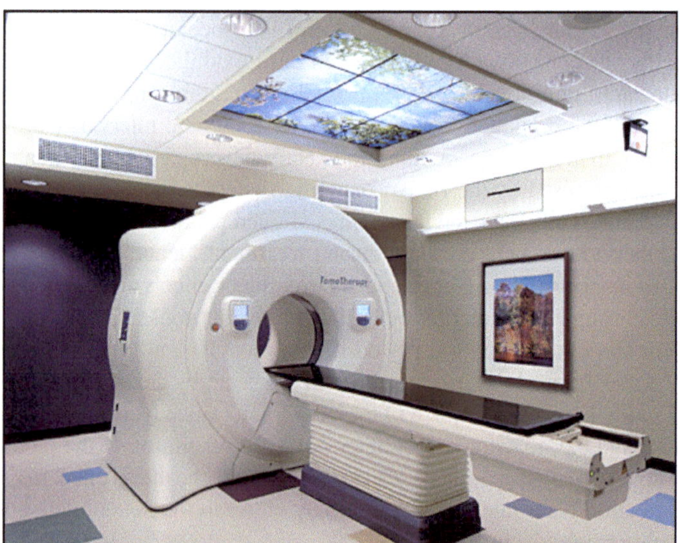

Fig. 4 (**a**) Distribution of machine subsystems around the ring gantry of a Hi-Art helical tomotherapy machine. (**b**) The fully assembled Hi-Art system

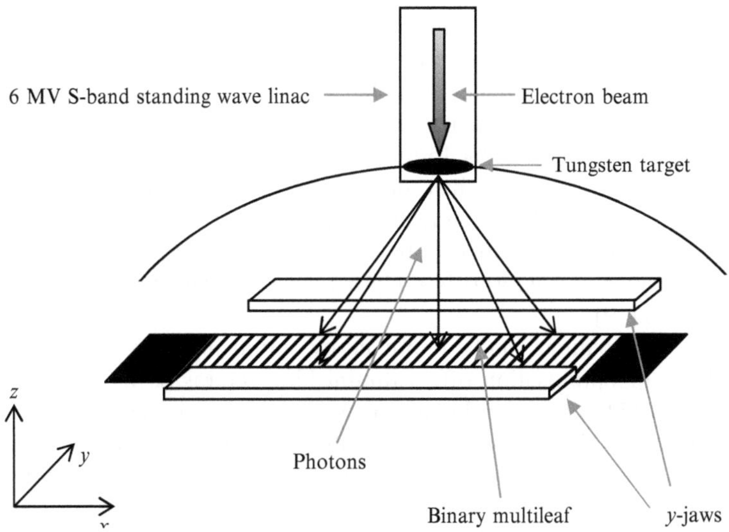

Fig. 5 A simplified schematic of the Hi-Art treatment head, pictured at a gantry angle of 0°. X-rays produced by a 6 MV linac are collimated down to a fan beam by a pair of jaws, and modulated laterally by a binary multileaf which is blocked off at both ends. The treatment head rotates around the *y*-axis, with an SAD of 85 cm

Tomotherapy Rationale

The development of tomotherapy was motivated both by the early pioneering IMRT papers which explored rotational treatment deliveries [1–3] and by the intuitive argument that plans comprising modulated beams delivered from many angles should be at least as good as, and perhaps rather better than, plans made up of fewer beams. Consequently, a first question arising, when assessing the advantages tomotherapy may offer over conventional IMRT, is whether rotational many-field IMRT dose distributions are in fact likely to substantially improve on plans generated using just a few coplanar modulated fields. As current tomotherapy treatment systems can only deliver coplanar radiation beams, a second question also arises: Are the gains achievable by delivering many fields ever outweighed by the loss of non-coplanarity?

Over the last decade, many papers have been written describing the effects of varying both the numbers of radiation beams used in fixed-field IMRT plans and the angles from which those beams are directed. The main findings of these studies are outlined briefly here. Intensity modulation allows the shape of at least one isodose line to be optimised even for three or four field plans [5], but the conformality of the overall dose distribution inevitably improves as more fields are added. The impact on prostate IMRT plans of progressively increasing the number of equispaced coplanar fields from 3 up to 15 has been studied [54]. At prescription dose levels of 70 and 76 Gy, target and critical structure dose distributions are improved by using nine fields rather than three, but no further gains are made by raising the number of fields to 15. However, at the 81 Gy prescription level, dose distributions are slightly improved by using 15 fields. The effect of increasing the number of coplanar fields further to the tomotherapy range, which can practically be considered to be of the order of 50, was not studied. Although the gains made by using 15 rather than nine fields are much less than those obtained using nine rather than three fields, further worthwhile improvements might still be achievable using really large numbers of fields [55]. A simple analysis suggests that large numbers of fields are needed if target dose uniformity is to be preserved whilst conformally sculpting dose distributions to avoid small critical structures [19].

IMRT dose distributions can be improved by optimising beam angles; however, this form of optimisation offers diminishing returns as the number of beams increases [54–59]. Tomotherapy planning can be viewed as a process which optimises the fluence of a large number of equispaced coplanar fixed fields, and thus essentially intrinsically optimises coplanar beam angles. Simply put, the technique raises the numbers of fields from the conventional 3–7 up to 51. Non-coplanar fields can sometimes be used to improve treatments of tumours in the brain, skull base and head-and-neck [58]. But in the body very little is gained using non-coplanar approaches, both because significant non-coplanarity is difficult to achieve below the head due to anatomic limitations, and because intensity-modulated coplanar treatment optimisation offers so many degrees of freedom that little is accomplished by adding non-coplanar beams, which by necessity have to traverse greater volumes of normal tissues before reaching the target [57].

In summary, the fixed-field IMRT optimisation literature suggests that tomotherapy is likely to offer enhanced control of dose distributions compared to IMRT treatments using a few (3–7) fields; that this enhanced control will take the form of preserving target dose uniformity whilst better avoiding critical normal structures; that dose distribution control may also be enhanced compared to IMRT planning using nine or more fields; and that although fixed-field non-coplanar IMRT plans will sometimes offer advantages over coplanar tomotherapy for treatment of targets above the clavicles, this is unlikely to be the case in the body.

Direct Comparisons with Fixed-Field IMRT

A number of papers have recently been published which directly compare treatment plans calculated for conventional and tomotherapy IMRT systems [60–71]. Results are summarised in Table 2 and agree well with the dose distribution differences suggested by the fixed-field IMRT literature. Broadly, these studies report that tomotherapy target volume dose distributions are more homogeneous than those of fixed-field IMRT plans, and that tomotherapy delivers lower doses to critical structures than does coplanar fixed-field IMRT. A comparison of tomotherapy and 7-field coplanar IMRT plans for a patient with oropharyngeal cancer treated at the University of Wisconsin is shown in Fig. 6.

Table 2 A comparison of tomotherapy and fixed-field IMRT plans

Study (number of patients planned)	Tumour site (stage when documented)	Tomo enhances target dose uniformity?	Comparison with fixed-field IMRT: Tomo delivers lower doses to –	Comparison with non-coplanar radiotherapy: Tomo delivers –
Rodriguez [60] (10)	Prostate (T1c-T3a)	Yes	Rectum, bladder, femurs	–
Wieland [61] (15)	Stomach (T3-4/N+)	Yes	–	Lower doses to spinal cord than fixed-field IMRT
Kron [62] (15)	Lung – NSCLC (Stage III)	–	Tomo improves dose quality index	–
Fiorino [63] (5)	Larynx, hypopharynx, oropharynx (T2–3/N0–2)	Yes	Parotids, mandible, spinal cord	–
van Vulpen [64] (5)	Oropharynx (T1–2/N1–2)	Yes	Parotids	–
Harari [65] (20)	Oropharynx	Yes	Contralateral parotid, spinal cord, oral cavity	–
Sheng [66] (10)	Oropharynx	Yes	Parotids, brainstem, larynx, spinal cord, oral cavity	–
Sheng [67] (10)	Nasal cavity, paranasal sinuses – (early and advanced)	Yes	–	Lower maximum doses to ipsilateral eye and both lenses than fixed-field IMRT
Soisson [68] (10)	Skull base – meningioma, pituitary adenoma, craniopharyngioma, osteosarcoma	Yes	Pituitary, chiasm, optic nerves	Lower doses to pituitary, chiasm, but higher doses to optic nerves, eyes than fixed-field IMRT/arc RT
Yartslev [69] (12)	Skull base – meningioma, pituitary adenoma, acoustic neuroma	Yes	Brainstem, chiasm	Higher doses to brainstem, chiasm, optic nerves and eyes than arc RT
Khoo [70] (5)	Brain – optic pathway glioma, astrocytoma, meningioma	–	–	Higher doses to lenses, and optic nerves than conformal RT
Han [71] (16)	Brain – irregularly shaped lesions	No	Fixed-field IMRT delivers lower doses to lenses, optic nerves than Tomo	Higher doses to brainstem, lenses and optic nerves than fixed-field IMRT

Non-coplanar fixed-field IMRT and tomotherapy plans have been compared for T3-4/N + gastric cancer, finding an advantage for tomotherapy [61]. This is currently the only comparative study of non-coplanar IMRT and tomotherapy techniques for tumour sites in the body or neck, presumably because non-coplanar approaches typically offer little advantage in this region. Higher up in the head, where non-coplanar techniques can be expected to be more advantageous, several studies have compared tomotherapy with unmodulated stereotactic arc radiotherapy and non-coplanar fixed-field 3D conformal and IMRT treatments. Tomotherapy of nasal cavity and paranasal sinus tumours improves on non-coplanar fixed-field IMRT [67], the advantage of the many tomotherapy fields outweighing the benefits of non-coplanarity at this site. And while tomotherapy treatments of skull-base tumours are better than coplanar fixed-field IMRT [68, 69], non-coplanar techniques have sometimes been found to offer advantages over tomotherapy: Soisson and colleagues [68] found that doses to some critical structures can be reduced using non-coplanar radiotherapy but that doses to other structures are raised, while Yartslev and coworkers [69] found for this site that non-coplanar stereotactic arcs on the whole produce lower critical structure doses than those calculated for tomotherapy. Similarly, it has been reported that non-coplanar treatments of intra-cranial tumours deliver lower doses to critical structures than does tomotherapy [70, 71].

Generally, then, these planning studies show that tomotherapy offers advantages over coplanar fixed-field IMRT, improving target dose homogeneity and reducing doses to critical structures, but for tumours located at the skull base or higher, the improvements which can be achieved by using non-coplanar techniques sometimes outweigh those made using tomotherapy.

Future Developments

The Hi-Art machine is the first commercially available helical tomotherapy system and further advances in machine design may remain to be made. For instance, by modifying the machine head to enable asymmetric setting of the jaws used to collimate the radiation fan beam, it should be possible to create dose distributions based on conic sections rather than slices, allowing non-coplanar tomotherapy treatments to be delivered.

Intensity-modulated arc therapy (IMAT) is a coplanar rotational delivery approach developed for conventional linac-plus-multileaf systems [72]. Modulation is achieved by delivering successive unmodulated conformal arcs, for each of which the multileaf-defined beam aperture changes with gantry angle in a different way. For instance, an IMAT delivery might begin with the multileaf tracking the silhouette of the target volume as the linac traverses its first arc, continue with a succession of arcs in which particular critical structures are blocked, and finish off with arcs designed specifically to make dose levels within the target volume as uniform as possible [73]. The technique has been implemented in several clinics [74–76] and development of IMAT optimisation algorithms is ongoing [77, 78].

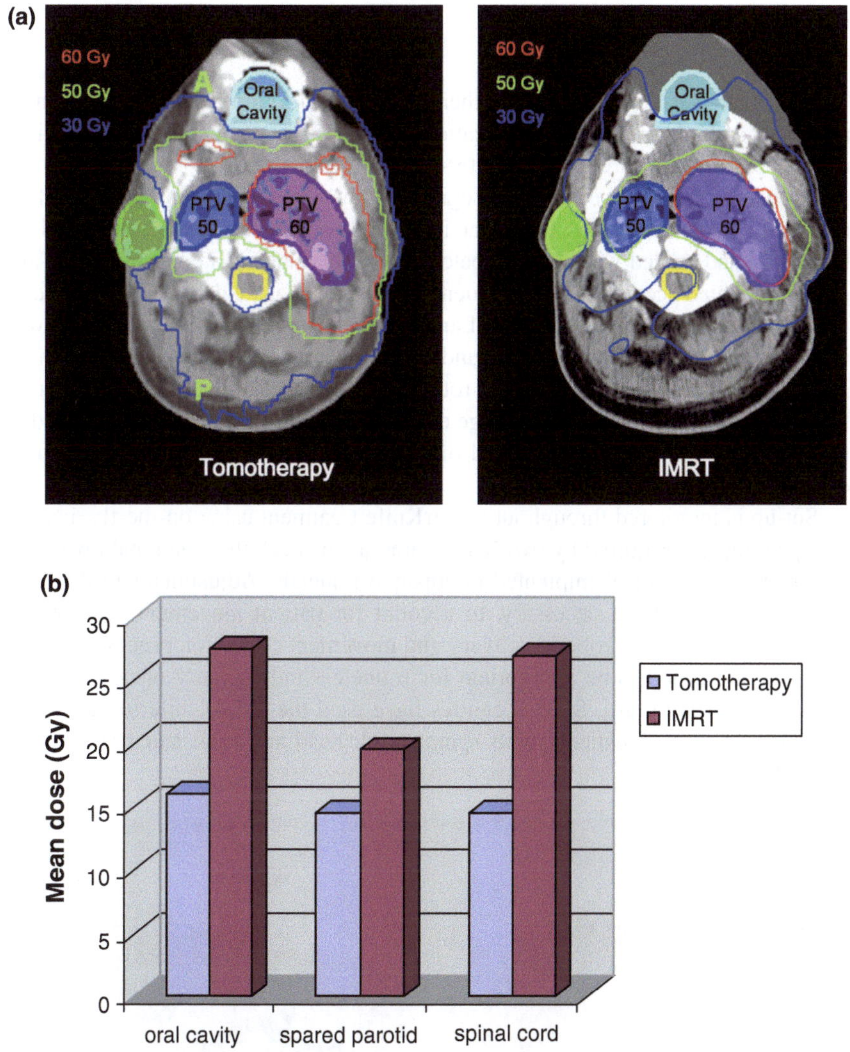

Fig. 6 **(a)** Axial CT slices showing planned Hi-Art and 7-field IMRT treatments of an oropharyngeal cancer. (**b**) A comparison of mean doses delivered to the oral cavity, spared parotid and spinal cord using the two techniques

Tomotherapy offers many more degrees of freedom for optimisation than IMAT, since the beam modulation of tomotherapy systems can be varied almost arbitrarily with gantry angle whereas IMAT modulation is constrained to change more gradually. How great an impact these additional tomotherapy degrees of freedom have on plan optimisation will determine how close IMAT can come to matching tomotherapy dose distributions. No comparison between IMAT and tomotherapy plans has yet been published and so this is an open question, analysable from both theoretical and practical standpoints.

CyberKnife

The CyberKnife is a modern radiotherapy system developed primarily for intra- and extra-cranial radiosurgery applications, comprising a light compact 6 MV linac carried on a highly precise computer-driven robotic arm [20–23] (Fig. 7). The position and orientation of the final segment of the arm is determined by six different mechanical subsystems. The linac is located on this final arm segment and can be moved and angled with much greater generality than can a conventional C-arm gantry-mounted accelerator. Consequently, non-coplanar fields can be delivered by the CyberKnife from a wide range of angles while patients lie still on a couch with the robot manoeuvring the linac around them – whereas using conventional linacs, non-coplanar field delivery requires rotation of the couch, which has the potential to disturb patient set-up, and the range of possible beam angles is circumscribed by the need to avoid colliding the head of the conventional linac with the patient or couch.

Set-up is monitored throughout CyberKnife treatment using on-the-fly analysis of repeat images acquired by two X-ray cameras to check the positional invariance either of the skull or of implanted radiopaque fiducials. Adjustments to the robot trajectory are made, if necessary, to account for patient movement. The overall spatial accuracy of the robotic delivery and movement correction process has been assessed and found to be appropriate for frameless radiosurgery of targets in the head and body [79, 80]. Several centres have used the CyberKnife to radiosurgically treat series of patients with spinal cord, head-and-neck and brain lesions [81–92].

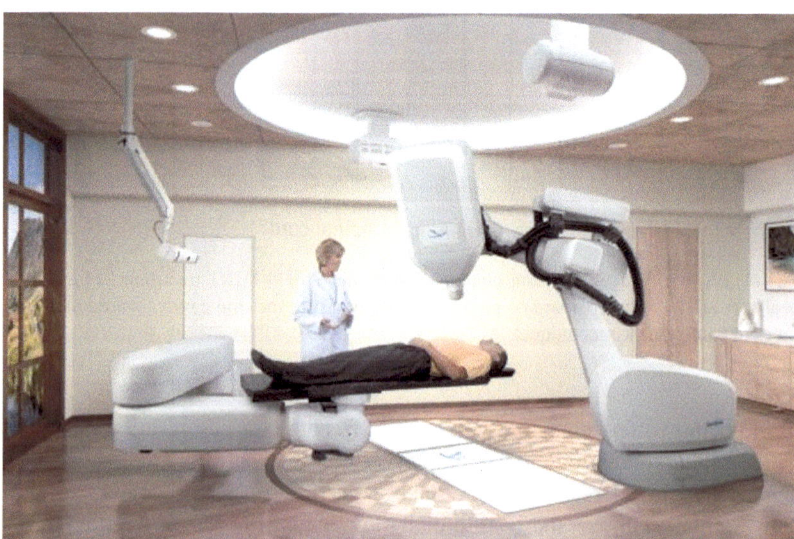

Fig. 7 The CyberKnife robotic linear accelerator (image used with permission from Accuray Incorporated)

Reflecting its radiosurgery origins, the CyberKnife radiation beam is shaped by one of twelve fixed cylindrical collimators with diameters between 5 and 60 mm [93, 94]. Interestingly, design differences between the CyberKnife and conventional linac-plus-multileaf systems are almost the mirror image of those between tomotherapy machines and conventional systems: Whereas a tomotherapy machine has an enhanced capability to deliver large number of modulated fields but limits the orientation of those fields to angles lying within the gantry rotation plane, the CyberKnife can be aimed from a vast range of angles but delivers unmodulated radiation.

Viewed narrowly, then, the CyberKnife is not an IMRT delivery system, since its radiation beam photon fluence is collimated but unmodulated. However, it can generate dose distributions similar to IMRT by delivering many unmodulated circular fields from a wide range of linac positions and angles, with robotic arm trajectories and beam weighting optimised using dedicated software [95] – an elegant 3D, non-coplanar, physical realisation of Birchoff's abstract line-drawing work [6]. Indeed, in principle, CyberKnife can do rather better than fixed-field IMRT since it is axiomatic that absolutely optimal photon beam dose distributions can be created by superposing very large numbers of suitably angled and weighted small fields [96].

How well CyberKnife dose distributions compare in practice will likely be determined by a range of technical considerations, such as the number of radiation beams that can be delivered by the system in reasonable treatment times. No comparisons between CyberKnife and conventional IMRT have yet been published for plans calculated for irregular target shapes and specific avoidance structures. And just as with tomotherapy, further CyberKnife design enhancements may remain to be made – for example, delivery options would be increased by replacing the fixed cylindrical collimators with adjustable jaws [97].

Summary

Fixed-field intensity-modulated treatments, delivered by conventional linac-plus-multileaf systems, have rapidly become the most common form of IMRT. Several innovative alternative IMRT options are also now available, including tomotherapy, CyberKnife and jaws-only linacs. These innovative approaches have divergent rationales. Jaws-only IMRT is being developed because it allows treatments to be delivered using conventional linacs without expensive multileaf collimators and not because it improves dose distributions. On the other hand, tomotherapy and CyberKnife systems have different geometric degrees of freedom, beam sizes and modulation techniques than those of conventional linacs, which may enable these innovative systems to deliver superior dose distributions to some treatment sites.

Because conventional linacs are themselves finely honed machines, enhancement of one aspect of machine performance is sometimes accompanied by diminution of another. For example, tomotherapy systems possess an enhanced rotational IMRT capability but currently can only deliver coplanar radiation beams. Thus the various delivery systems may prove optimal for different types of treatments, specific machine designs excelling for specific disease sites.

In practice, of course, IMRT delivery systems will be distinguished not just by the quality of the dose distributions they deliver but also by factors not discussed in this chapter, such as the efficiency of their treatment process, the integration of on-board imaging into that process, and their ability to measure, minimise and compensate for the effects of respiratory motion, a major detriment to accurate IMRT delivery.

References

1. Brahme A, Roos JE, Lax I: Solution of an integral equation in rotation therapy. Phys Med Biol 27:1221–1229, 1982
2. Cormack A: A problem in rotation therapy with X-rays. Int J Radiat Oncol Biol Phys 13:623–630, 1987
3. Cormack AM, Cormack RA: A problem in rotation therapy with X-rays: Dose distributions with an axis of symmetry. Int J Radiat Oncol Biol Phys 13:1921–1925, 1987
4. Bortfeld T, Bürkelbach J, Boesecke R, et al: Methods of image reconstruction from projections applied to conformation radiotherapy. Phys Med Biol 35:1423–1434, 1990
5. Bortfeld T: Optimized planning using physical objectives and constraints. Semin Radiat Oncol 9:20–34, 1999
6. Birkhoff GD: On drawings composed of uniform straight lines. J Math Pures Appl. 19:221–236, 1940
7. Brahme A: Optimization of stationary and moving beam radiation therapy techniques. Radiother Oncol 12:129–140, 1988
8. Webb S: Optimization of conformal radiotherapy dose distributions by simulated annealing. Phys Med Biol 34:1349–1370, 1989
9. Webb S: Optimization by simulated annealing of three-dimensional conformal treatment planning for radiation fields defined by multi-leaf collimator II. Inclusion of two-dimensional modulation of X-ray intensity. Phys Med Biol 37:1689–1704, 1992
10. Bortfeld T, Bürkelbach J, Schlegel W: Three-dimensional solution of the inverse problem in conformation radiotherapy, in Breit A: Advanced Radiation Therapy: Tumour Response Modelling and Treatment Planning. Berlin, Springer, 1992, pp 503–508
11. Wang X-H, Mohan R, Jackson A, et al: Optimization of intensity modulated 3D conformal treatment plans based on biological indices. Radiother Oncol 37:140–152, 1996
12. Ling CC, Burman C, Chui CS, et al: Conformal radiation treatment of prostate cancer using inversely-planned intensity-modulated photon beams produced with dynamic multileaf collimation. Int J Radiat Oncol Biol Phys 35:721–730, 1996
13. Memorial Sloan-Kettering Cancer Center Staff: A Practical Guide to Intensity-Modulated Radiation Therapy. Madison WI, Medical Physics Publishing, 2003
14. Convery DJ and Rosenbloom ME: The generation of intensity-modulated fields by dynamic collimation. Phys Med Biol 37:1359–1374, 1992

15. Galvin JM, Smith AR and Lally B: Combining multileaf fields to modulate fluence distributions. Int J Rad Oncol Biol Phys 25:181–192, 1993
16. Webb S: The physics of conformal radiotherapy – advances in technology. Bristol, UK, IOP Publishing, 1997
17. Webb S: Intensity-modulated radiation therapy. Bristol, UK, IOP Publishing, 2001
18. Kalender WA, Polacin A: Physical performance characteristics of spiral CT scanning. Med Phys 18:910–915, 1991
19. Mackie TR, Olivera GH, Kapatoes JM et al: Helical Tomotherapy, in Palta JR and Mackie TR: Intensity-Modulated Radiation Therapy – The State of the Art. Madison WI, Medical Phyics Publishing, 2003, pp 247–284
20. Adler JR, Chang SD, Murphy MJ, et al: The Cyberknife: A Frameless Robotic System for Radiosurgery. Stereotact Funct Neurosurg 69:124–128, 1997
21. Adler JR, Murphy MJ, Chang SD, et al: Image-guided Robotic Radiosurgery. Neurosurgery 44:1299–1306, 1999
22. Chang SD, Adler Jr: Robotics and Radiosurgery – The Cyberknife. Stereotact Funct Neurosurg 76:204–208, 2001
23. Kuo JS, Yu C, Petrovich Z, et al: The CyberKnife Stereotactic Radiosurgery System: Description, Installation, and an Initial Evaluation of Use and Functionality. Neurosurgery 53:1235–1239, 2003
24. Shepard DM, Earl MA, Li XA, et al: Direct aperture optimization: A turnkey solution for step-and-shoot IMRT. Med Phys 29:1007–1018, 2002
25. Battista JJ, Bauman GS: The Future of IMRT, in Palta JR and Mackie TR: Intensity-Modulated Radiation Therapy – The State of the Art. Madison WI, Medical Phyics Publishing, 2003, pp 843–873
26. Boyer AL: Static MLC IMRT (Step and Shoot), in Palta JR and Mackie TR: Intensity-Modulated Radiation Therapy – The State of the Art. Madison WI, Medical Physics Publishing, 2003, pp 285–317
27. Webb S: Contemporary IMRT. Bristol, UK, IOP Publishing, 1997
28. Keall P, Wu Q, Wu Y, et al: Dynamic MLC IMRT, in Palta JR and Mackie TR: Intensity-Modulated Radiation Therapy – The State of the Art. Madison WI, Medical Physics Publishing, 2003, pp 319–371
29. Patel R, Orton NP, Tomé WA, et al: Rectal dose sparing with a balloon catheter and ultrasound localization in conformal radiation therapy for prostate cancer. Radiother Oncol 67:285–294, 2003
30. Fenwick JD, Khoo VS, Nahum AE, et al: Correlations between dose-surface-histograms and the incidence of long-term rectal bleeding following conformal or conventional radiotherapy treatment of prostate cancer. Int J Radiat Oncol Biol Phys 49:473–480, 2001
31. Jackson A, Skwarchuk MW, Zelefsky MJ, et al: Late rectal bleeding after conformal radiotherapy of prostate cancer (II): Volume effects and dose–volume histograms. Int J Radiat Oncol Biol Phys 49:685–698, 2001
32. Scrimger RA, Tomé WA, Olivera G, et al: Reduction in radiation dose to lung and other normal tissues using helical tomotherapy to treat lung cancer, in comparison to conventional field arrangements. Am J Clin Oncol 26:70–78, 2003
33. Dai J-R, Hu Y-M: Intensity-modulation radiotherapy using independent collimators: an algorithm study. Med Phys 26:2562–2570, 1999
34. Earl M, Yu C, Jiang Z, et al: Clinical Feasibility of "jaws-only" IMRT using Direct Aperture Optimization. Med Phys 32:1973, 2005 (abstr)
35. Carol MP: Where we go from here: one person's vision, in Sternick ES: The Theory and Practice of Intensity-Modulated Radiation Therapy. Madison, WI, Advanced Medical Publishing, 1997, pp 243–252
36. Dawson D, Spies R and Carol MP: A volume delivery system for intensity modulation radiation therapy, in Leavitt DD and Starkshall G: Proc. 12th Int. Conf. on the Use of Computers in Radiation Therapy. Madison, WI, Medical Physics Publishing, 1997, p 481 (abstr)

37. Webb S: A new concept of multileaf collimator (the shuttling MLC) – an interpreter for high-efficiency IMRT. Phys Med Biol 45:3343–3358, 2000
38. Xu T, Shikhaliev PM, Al-Ghazi M, et al: Re-shapeable physical modulator for intensity modulated radiation therapy. Med Phys 30:2222–2228, 2003
39. Curran B: IMRT delivery using serial tomotherapy, in Palta JR and Mackie TR: Intensity-Modulated Radiation Therapy – The State of the Art. Madison WI, Medical Physics Publishing, 2003, pp 285–317
40. Low DA, Chao KSC, Mutic S, et al: Quality assurance of serial tomotherapy for head and neck patient treatments. Int J Radiat Oncol Biol Phys 42:681–692, 1998
41. Low DA, Mutic S, Dempsey JF, et al: Quantitative dosimetric verification of an IMRT planning and delivery system. Int J Radiat Oncol Biol Phys 49:305–316, 1998
42. Tsai JS, Rivard MJ and Engler MJ: Dependence of linac output on the switch rate of an intensity-modulated tomotherapy collimator. Med Phys 27:2215–2225, 2000
43. Woo SY, Grant III W, McGary JE, et al: The evolution of quality assurance for intensity-modulated radiation therapy (IMRT): sequential tomotherapy. Int J Radiat Oncol Biol Phys 56:274–286, 2003
44. Low DA, Mutic S, Dempsey JF, et al: Abutment region dosimetry for serial tomotherapy. Int J Radiat Oncol Biol Phys 45:193–203, 1999
45. Mackie TR, Holmes T, Swerdloff S, et al: Tomotherapy: A new concept for the delivery of dynamic conformal radiotherapy. Med Phys 20:1709–1719, 1993
46. Mackie TR, Balog J, Ruchala K, et al: Tomotherapy. Semin Radiat Oncol 9:108–117, 1999
47. Balog JP, Mackie TR, Reckwerdt P, et al: Characterization of the output for helical delivery of intensity modulated slit beams. Med Phys 26:55–64, 1999
48. Balog JP, Mackie TR, Wenman DL, et al: Multileaf collimator interleaf transmission. Med Phys 26:176–186, 1999
49. Balog JP, Mackie TR, Pearson D, et al: Benchmarking beam alignment for a clinical helical tomotherapy device. Med Phys 30:1118–1127, 2003
50. Balog J, Olivera G, Kapatoes J: Clinical helical tomotherapy commissioning dosimetry. Med Phys 30:3097–3106, 2003
51. Fenwick JD, Tomé WA, Jaradat HA, et al: Quality assurance of a helical tomotherapy machine. Phys Med Biol 49:2933–2953, 2004
52. Fenwick JD, Tomé WA, Kissick MW, et al: Modelling simple helically delivered dose distributions. Phys Med Biol 50:1505–1517, 2005
53. Kissick MW, Fenwick J, James JA, et al: The helical tomotherapy thread effect. Med Phys 32:1414–1423, 2005
54. Stein J, Mohan R, Wang X-H, et al: Number and orientations of beams in intensity-modulated radiation treatments. Med Phys 24:149–160, 1997
55. Webb S: Optimizing the planning of intensity-modulated radiotherapy. Phys Med Biol 39:2229–2246, 1994
56. Rowbottom CG, Nutting CM, Webb S: Beam-orientation optimization of intensity-modulated radiotherapy: clinical application to parotid gland tumours. Radiother Oncol 59:169–177, 2001
57. Ferreira BC, Svensson R, Löff J, et al: The Clinical Values of Non-Coplanar Photon Beams in Biologically Optimized Intensity Modulated Dose Delivery on Deep-Seated Tumours. Acta Oncol 42:852–864, 2003
58. Meedt G, Alber M, Nüsslin F: Non-coplanar beam direction optimization for intensity-modulated radiotherapy. Phys Med Biol 48:2999–3019, 2003
59. Gaede S, Wong E, Rasmussen H: An algorithm for systematic selection of beam directions for IMRT. Med Phys 31:376–388, 2004
60. Rodriguez G, Yartslev S, Chen J, et al: A comparison of prostate IMRT and helical tomotherapy class solutions. Radiother Oncol 80:374–377, 2006
61. Wieland P, Dobler B, Mai S, et al: IMRT for postoperative treatment of gastric cancer covering large target volumes in the upper abdomen: a comparison of a step-and-shoot and an arc therapy approach. Int J Radiat Oncol Biol Phys 59:1236–1244, 2004

62. Kron T, Grigorov G, Yu E, et al: Planning evaluation of radiotherapy for complex lung cancer cases using helical tomotherapy. Phys Med Biol 49:3675–3690, 2004
63. Fiorino C, Dell'Oca I, Pierelli A, et al: Significant improvement in normal tissue sparing and target coverage for head and neck cancer by means of helical tomotherapy. Radiother. Oncol. 78:276–282, 2006
64. van Vulpen M, Field C, Raaijmakers CPJ, et al: Comparing step-and-shoot IMRT with dynamic helical tomotherapy plans for head-and-neck cancer. Int J Radiat Oncol Biol Phys 62:1535–1539, 2005
65. Harari PM, Jaradat HA, Connor NP, et al: Refining target coverage and normal tissue avoidance with helical tomotherapy vs linac-based IMRT for oropharyngeal cancer. Int J Radiat Oncol Biol Phys 60:S160, 2004 (suppl 1) (abstr)
66. Sheng K, Molloy JA and Read PW: Intensity-modulated radiation therapy (IMRT) dosimetry of the head and neck: a comparison of treatment plans using linear accelerator-based IMRT and helical tomotherapy. Int J Radiat Oncol, Biol, Phys 65:917–923, 2006
67. Sheng K, Molloy JA, Larner JM, et al: A dosimetric comparison of non-coplanar IMRT versus Helical Tomotherapy for nasal cavity and paranasal sinus cancer. Radiother Oncol 82:174–178, 2007
68. Soisson ET, Tomé WA, Richards GM, et al: Comparison of linac based fractionated stereotactic radiotherapy and tomotherapy for treatment of skull-base tumors. Radiother Oncol 78:313–321, 2006
69. Yartslev S, Cozzi L, Fogliata A, et al: Tomotherapy planning of small brain tumours. Radiother Oncol 74:49–52, 2005
70. Khoo VS, Oldham M, Adams EJ, et al: Comparison of intensity-modulated tomotherapy with stereotactically guided conformal radiotherapy for brain tumors. Int J Radiat Oncol Biol Phys 45:415–425, 1999
71. Han C, Liu A, Schultheiss TE, et al: Dosimetric comparisons of helical tomotherapy treatment plans and step-and-shoot intensity-modulated radiosurgery treatment plans in intracranial stereotactic radiosurgery. Int J Radiat Oncol, Biol, Phys 65:608–616, 2006
72. Yu CX: Intensity modulated arc therapy with dynamic multileaf collimation: an alternative to tomotherapy. Phys Med Biol 40:1435–1449, 1995
73. Wong E, Chen JZ, Greenland J: Intensity-modulated arc therapy simplified. Int J Radiat Oncol Biol Phys 53:225–235, 2002
74. Yu CX, Li XA, Ma L, et al: Clinical implementation of intensity-modulated arc therapy. Int J Radiat Oncol Biol Phys 53:453–463, 2002
75. Duthoy W, de Gersem W, Vergote K, et al: Clinical implementation of intensity-modulated arc therapy (IMAT) for rectal cancer. Int J Radiat Oncol Biol Phys 60:794–806, 2004
76. Wong E, D'Souza DP, Chen JZ, et al: Intensity-modulated arc therapy for treatment of high-risk endometrial malignancies. Int J Radiat Oncol Biol Phys 61:830–841, 2005
77. Earl MA, Shepard DM, Naqvi S, et al: Inverse planning for intensity-modulated arc therapy using direct aperture optimization. Phys Med Biol 48:1075–1089, 2003
78. Bratengeier K: 2-Step IMAT and 2-Step IMRT: A geometrical approach. Med Phys 32:777–785, 2005
79. Chang SD, Main W, Martin DP, et al: An Analysis of the Accuracy of the CyberKnife: A Robotic Frameless Stereotactic Radiosurgical System. Neurosurgery 52:140–147, 2003
80. Yu C, Main W, Taylor D, et al: An Anthropomorphic Phantom Study of the Accuracy of CyberKnife Spinal Radiosurgery. Neurosurgery 55:1138–1149, 2004
81. Ryu SI, Chang SD, Kim DH, et al: Image-guided Hypo-fractionated Setereotactic Radiosurgery to Spinal Lesions. Neurosurgery 49:838–846
82. Pham CJ, Chang SD, Gibbs IC, et al: Preliminary Visual Field Preservation after Staged CyberKnife Radiosurgery for Perioptic Lesions. Neurosurgery 54:799–812, 2004
83. Gertzen PC, Ozhasoglu C, Burton SA, et al: CyberKnife Frameless Stereotactic Radiosurgery for Spinal Lesions: Clinical Experience in 125 Cases. Neurosurgery 55:89–99, 2004
84. Kajiwara S, Saito K, Yoshikawa K, et al: Image-guided stereotactic radiosurgery with the Cyberknife for pituitary adenomas. Minim Invasive Neurosurg 48: 91–96, 2005

85. Chang SD, Gibbs IC, Sakamoto GT, et al: Staged stereotactic irradiation for acoustic neuroma. Neurosurgery 56: 1254–1261, 2005
86. Gwak HS, Yoo HJ, Youn SM, et al: Hypofractionated stereotactic radiation for skull base and upper cervical chordoma and chondrosarcoma – preliminary results. Stereotact Funct Neurosurg 83: 233–243, 2005
87. Lim M, Cotrutz C, Romanelli P, et al: Stereotactic radiosurgery using CT cisternography and non-isocentric planning for the treatment of trigeminal neuralgia. Comput Aided Surg 11: 11–20, 2006
88. Dodd RL, Ryu MR, Kamnerdsupaphon P, et al: Cyberknife radiosurgery for benign intradural extramedullary spinal tumors. Neurosurgery 58: 674–685, 2006
89. Sinclair J, Chang SD, Gibbs IC, et al: Multisession Cyberknife radiosurgery for intramedullary spinal cord areteriovenous malformations. Neurosurgery 58: 1081–1089, 2006
90. Adler JR, Gibbs IC, Puataweepong P, et al: Visual field preservation after multisession cyberknife radiosurgery for perioptic lesions. Neurosurgery 59: 244–254, 2006
91. Voynov G, Heron DE, Burton S, et al: Frameless stereotactic radiosurgery for recurrent head and neck carcinoma. Technol Cancer Res Treat 5: 529–535, 2006
92. Nishizaki T, Saito K, Jimi Y, et al: The role of cyberknife radiosurgery/radiotherapy for brain metastases of multiple or large-size tumors. Minim Invasive Neurosurg 49: 203–209, 2006
93. Yu C, Jozsef G, Apuzzo MLJ, et al: Measurements of the Relative Output Factors for CyberKnife Collimators. Neurosurgery 54:157–162, 2004
94. Hamamoto Y, Manabe T, Nishizaki O, et al: Influence of Collimator Size on Three-dimensional Conformal Radiotherapy of the CyberKnife. Radiat Med 22:442–448, 2004
95. Tombropoulos RZ, Adler JR, Latombe J-C: CARABEAMER: a treatment planner for a robotic radiosurgical system with general kinematics. Med Image Analysis 3:237–264, 1999
96. Webb S: Conformal intensity-modulated radiotherapy (IMRT) delivered by robotic linac – testing IMRT to the limit? Phys Med Biol 44:1639–1654, 1999
97. Schweikard A, Adler JR: Robotic Radiosurgery With Non-cylindrical Collimators. Computer Aided Surgery 2:124–134, 1997

11
Image-Based Modeling of Normal Tissue Complication Probability for Radiation Therapy

Joseph O. Deasy and Issam El Naqa

Introduction

Radiation therapy dose distributions to eradicate tumor cells are typically constrained in extent or intensity to minimize the risk of injury to nearby critical normal tissues. With the widespread use of 3D image-based treatment planning systems, the question naturally arises how patient-specific anatomy and treatment differences affect outcome. It has long been known, that for many organs, variations in the fractional volume irradiated to high doses greatly alters the dose to achieve a given complication level (the "isoeffective dose") [1]. Smaller irradiated fractional volumes often lead to a much lower risk of complication; this is often referred to as the "volume-effect" in the literature, but would be more correctly referred to as the "dose–volume" effect. Normal tissue complication probability (NTCP) modeling is simply the ongoing effort to understand the risk of normal tissue injury as a function of the 3D dose distribution. Recently, there has been a steady accumulation of NTCP studies [2], and this is expected to continue or even accelerate in the future. NTCP models are particularly needed when the "volume-effect" becomes important (i.e., injury depends on the detailed dose distribution), such as for skin, lung, or liver. In this chapter we will review the basic principles of NTCP modeling, as well as publications related to selected endpoints (xerostomia, radiation pneumonitis, late rectal toxicity), and several issues related to the use of NTCP models, especially relating to their safe use. Other recent reviews which further discuss data on endpoints of interest in treatment planning include Deasy and Fowler [3], Moiseenko et al. [4], and the slightly older but still invaluable Seminars in Radiation Oncology issue, edited by Randy Ten Haken, devoted to dose–volume effects in normal tissues [2]. A useful review of models and model principles are the chapters by Jackson and Yorke [5], and Yorke [6]. Many technical issues in modeling dose–volume outcomes were also discussed by Deasy et al. [7].

This chapter describes standard NTCP models as well as our own approach, which is more data-driven and image-based [8]. This contrasts with the more common approach of assuming the validity of a specific model and then attempting to fit the model parameters to a given data set. The term "image-based" indicates

M.P. Mehta et al. (eds.), *Radiation Oncology Advances*.

that we require more than dose summary statistics, or even dose–volume histograms (which ignore spatial dose information).

NTCP Models: Tools or Toys?

Dose–volume-outcomes models have been criticized for their lack of biological realism, and radiobiologists have called some model assumptions "fanciful" [15, 16]. This criticism seems justified with respect to early models which on the one hand were detached from useful data sets and on the other were based on idealistic concepts regarding how treatment complications could arise, concepts that subsequently have not been validated by clinical or experimental observations. We write without exaggeration that there is not a single case in dose–volume-outcomes prediction in which a model has been proposed on purely a priori grounds that has been later validated in human studies. Moreover, models which tend to have any significant mechanistic basis tend to be too complicated to allow robust parameter estimation.

So far, the most widely used NTCP models have been phenomenological models such as the Lyman–Kutcher–Burman (LKB) model. This model has three parameters: one parameter relates to the local vs. global effect of the radiation damage and the other two parameters fix the steepness and location of the dose–response curve for uniform dose distributions [11]. The LKB model was developed as an empirical framework to summarize physician's dose–volume experience as captured as part of a collaborative effort on a large NCI funded project to develop 3D treatment planning in the late 1980s and early 1990s. Another common type of NTCP models relies on a "damage-injury" paradigm, in which the local damage to the tissue or organ is estimated as a function of the local absorbed dose, and this is subsequently translated into the probability of observing a specific complication [12–14]. Those models describe the overall function of the organ as a sum over local function and further estimate how this converts into a risk of clinically manifest injury. Other phenomenological models include the "relative seriality" model proposed by Brahme and co-workers, which models tissue response in a way that combines serial and parallel organization characteristics [15], and the probabilistic model for the so-called serial tissues, wherein the overall probability of a complication is simply the complement of the probability of no complication which is computed by multiplying the probability of no complication for each small subsection of the tissue (a model which has been challenged by recent data, as discussed below) [1, 16].

Currently, the most successful applications of NTCP models are those which have been data-driven, which increases the need to develop valid statistical model building tools. This chapter is a brief report on our efforts to do just that. Nevertheless, to answer the question of whether at least NTCP models can be tools rather than just toys, one needs to only look at recently achieved results that clearly separate patients who are at high risk for complications from those who are at low risk for complications for several endpoints, such as xerostomia due to head and neck cancer [17–19], radiation-induced liver damage [20, 21], acute esophagitis [22], or the risk of brain necrosis as a function of dose and volume [23]. Even for the difficult-to-model case of radiation pneumonitis, in which the Spearman's rank correlation coefficient of the model vs. the outcome is rather low (about 0.30), patients can typically be grouped or separated into high-risk vs. low-risk bins (see Fig. 1).

When applying radiobiological principles to radiotherapy treatment planning, one faces the conundrum of theory vs. data: When should expectations derived from outside the available data sets be allowed to guide selection and interpretation of treatment planning evaluation equations and parameters? Our approach is to rely on direct analysis of the most appropriate evidence for the endpoints in question and only when required, to resort to strongly supported principles (either radiobiological or physiological). These "strongly supported" principles include the applicability of the linear-quadratic fractionation model, along with some general trends which can be observed across multiple data sets and endpoints. The general trends include the importance of even rather low doses on function of the so-called parallel organs (e.g., parotid salivary glands, lung, liver); the probable importance of higher (>40–50 Gy) localized doses in creating ulcerative lesions or sites of

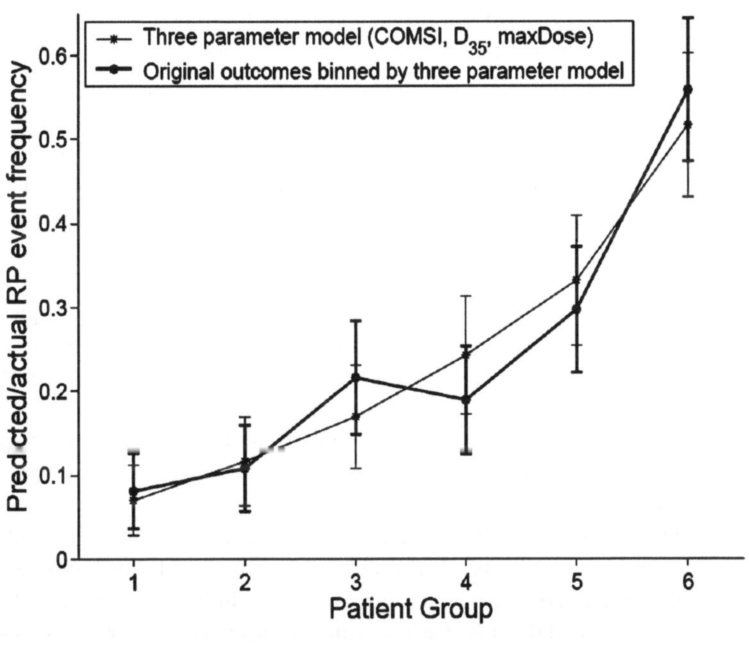

Fig. 1 Modeling of expected and observed rates of radiation pneumonitis (steroids or more intensive intervention) in the WUSTL data set (as published by Hope et al. [25]). Patients are grouped according to increasing modeled risk. The best performing three-parameter model selected included the tumor center-of-mass within the lung (more inferior is worse), D35 (lowest dose to the hottest 35% of the normal lung), and maximum dose (to a volume of at least 1 cm^3). It is clear that the model describes greatly increased risk for some patients (groups 5 and 6) compared to the low-risk patients (groups 1 and 2) (reproduced by permission from Hope et al. [25])

inflammation for endpoints such as acute esophagitis or late rectal bleeding; and the increase in tolerance for very small regions irradiated to high doses (less than about 1 cm^3). Some endpoints seem to be clearly related to lack of organ function (e.g., salivary gland function), whereas other endpoints, even for the so-called "parallel" organs, may be related to presence of a nonhealing/nonrepaired injury (probably including sporadic radiation pneumonitis [25]).

Why Image-Based NTCP Analysis?

Apart from these trends (we do not claim they are "principles"), our preference is to "let the data speak" while also realizing that "Although we often hear that data speak for themselves, their voices can be soft and sly." [26] To further motivate an open-ended data-mining and image-based approach to NTCP modeling, consider three recent, perhaps surprising, results.

De Crevoisier et al. [27] from M.D. Anderson Cancer Center (MDACC) recently reported that rectal distension due to stool, or bowel gas on the treatment planning CT scan, was strongly positively correlated with decreased probabilities of biochemical control, local control, and rectal toxicity in 127 prostate cancer radiotherapy patients. This was thought to be due to probable geographic target shifts during therapy when the rectum is usually not distended. Discovering this relationship would not have been possible if the authors had not explored the associated image data (CT scans and structure contours); nor would it have been discovered had the authors simply assumed they knew the functional form of the tumor control probability and normal tissue complication probability models to be related to the data.

As a second example, the WUSTL group recently reported on the relationship between tumor control probability for isolated lung tumors vs. dosimetric, spatial, and clinical factors (57 patients) [28]. They reported that the single most highly correlated factor for local failure was minimum distance from the tumor edge to the spinal cord, apart from all other planned dose distribution factors. The Spearman's rank correlation coefficient (R_s) for minimum distance to the spinal cord was 0.46. Similarly to the report by de Crevesior et al. [27], this raises the issue of whether treatment plan is an accurate representation of what was delivered for these patients.

As another example specific to NTCP analyses, a trend toward increasing radiation pneumonitis complication probability with an increasingly inferior tumor position has been detected and reported upon by several groups. In particular, the Amsterdam group accounted for a shift in NTCP risk with increasingly inferior tumor position that had not been expected in earlier investigations of radiation pneumonitis [29]. This relationship was also observed and reported on by the WUSTL group [24], who modeled it as a linearly increasing risk of radiation penumonitis from superior point to inferior point in the lung (further discussed below).

In these cases, the outcome has a somewhat or surprisingly different relation to the pretreatment image data sets than what might have been hypothesized a priori. Although we are only discussing NTCP modeling in detail here, these examples, nevertheless, illustrate the lesson that we will likely discover unexpected results as more data-driven, image-based, analyses of outcomes are performed.

Another important weakness of avoiding a unified data-mining (or even multivariate approach which considers all the potential predictors including models) is the importance of biological covariates. For example, one recent report by Cheng et al. [30] found that the risk of radiation-induced liver disease depends significantly, apart from dose–volume factors, on whether the patient is a carrier of the Hepatitis B virus.

Tissue Dose–Response Classification

Dose–volume analyses based on true 3D dose data sets have now become available for most dose-constraining organs. The earliest mechanistic ideas for likely dose–volume effects in the liver, lungs, and salivary parotid glands, for example, typically assumed that overall gland function would be the sum of remaining local function, and that local function would be a sigmoidally shaped function of local dose [10–12, 31]. A complication was not expected to occur unless and until organ function had decreased to below a critical threshold. On the whole, these models and their assumptions have not been validated above alternative approaches, with an important qualification: The delivery of small, focal, high dose–volumes of radiation, while inactivating organ function locally, may often be well tolerated. In particular, the experience of high-dose stereotactic lung radiosurgery for small T1 and T2 tumors has been impressive with respect to a lack of radiation pneumonitis events [32]. For external beam radiotherapy given in typical 1.8–2.0 Gy fractions, complication analyses for lung or liver based on the LKB model have been as or more successful than competing modeling based on parallel function ideas. Of course, this does not necessarily mean that the parallel function ideas are wrong.

Currently, most dose–volume analyses of the so-called parallel function organs have shown that the mean dose, or something close to it, is well correlated with treatment outcome (lung [33], liver [21], parotid salivary glands [19], brain [23]). The mean dose, unlike a dose–volume constraint, is sensitive to changes all along the DVH curve and is therefore more robust than a dose–volume constraint for treatment planning purposes.

The Concepts of "Serial" and "Parallel" Tissue Dose–Response

Organ architecture, with respect to dose–volume tolerance characteristics, has often been characterized as either "serial," or "parallel," or some combination. The metaphor is electrical: serial architecture means a complication can arise by breaking the tissue "circuit" anywhere; "parallel" architecture implies that function is related to number of "unbroken" elements. The distinction was further made by Marks between organizational structure (series vs. parallel) and functional distribution (homogeneous vs. heterogeneous) [34].

The basis of the classical serial organ concept is that (a) damage to any single small component results in a complication, and (b) the damage is only a function of the local dose and tissue characteristics (i.e., the response has no "parallel" component) [31]. These rather simplistic assumptions also formed the basis for the earliest dose–volume-outcomes models (Wolbarst, Schultheiss). Both of these assumptions are questionable based on more recent experimental results. The assumption of local response independence (b) results in complication predictions which have two general features: the threshold for a nonzero risk of a complication is independent of volume (length) irradiated (being just the threshold at which a so-called "functional subunit" [31] or "tissue rescuing unit" [35] might fail), and the slope of the response curve should become more shallow as the volume irradiated decreases, in a mathematically predictable way.

Powers et al. observed that, in 4 cm irradiated sections of Beagle dog spinal cords, pathological lesions often did not result in observable symptoms [36]. In comparison, lesions resulting from longer field irradiation (20 cm), at the same dose level, were typically larger and symptomatic. If the spinal cord were truly a classically serial tissue, then, as the early modeling papers hypothesize [1, 16], the probability of complication, at a given dose, for an irradiated length of 4 cm should be something like one-fifth the complication rate in a 20 cm length (for small rates of complication). This implies that the steepness of response with dose should be significantly reduced with smaller volumes. Not only is this not observed in the data of Powers et al., but also the steepness of the response at 4 cm is nearly equivalent to the steepness at 20 cm (for three separate types of lesions). The Powers et al. data imply that there is some component of spinal cord response which is "nonlocal" and "cooperative," such that tissue breakdown/injury tends to occur in a coordinated way (although this conclusion has recently been challenged by Alber et al. [37]).

Precise rat spinal cord irradiations performed by Bijl et al. also challenge the idea of a simple serial spinal cord dose–response [38, 39]: they reported that dose tolerance varies only slowly as field size is increased above 0.8 cm. Below that, tolerance climbs rapidly. They attribute this increase to the ability of cells from outside the field to migrate and rescue heavily damaged tissues. Moreover, the latent period significantly increases with smaller volume irradiated. This effect does not fit the classic "series" tissue idea as well. Further, elegant experiments by the same group show that the tolerance due to irradiation of 4-mm lengths of rat spinal cord can be reduced by irradiating the nearby region [39]. This effect is especially pronounced at 4 mm probably because the mean distance of migration is about 2 mm (cf. Fig. 4 in [38]).

Withers, however, interprets the Bijl et al. data as being entirely consistent with classical serial behavior if the migration of rescuing oligodendrocytes or ologidendrocyte precursors is presumed to occur over distances of the order of 2–3 mm [40]. Further, quantitative modeling will be required to understand the effect of cell migration in detail.

Clinical practice, however, is primarily concerned with the threshold of a very low probability of spinal cord complications. Thus it is the complication probability of large volumes of spinal cord irradiated in humans which is of greatest concern. It is well established, both from clinical experience and research reports, that the risk of radiation spinal cord injury is extremely small at doses of 45–50 Gy and fraction sizes of 1.8–2.0 Gy. The risk must clearly escalate if larger fractions are used, though accurate threshold dose data (especially near 1% risk) are absent. Rare complications may have been often due to nonideal radiation delivery, for example, field junction errors.

At very small volumes irradiated (less than 1 cm high-dose width), the brain stem also appears to have an increased tolerance. Debus et al. [41] present data that small brain stem volumes (<1 cm^3) have a higher dose tolerance (>60 CGE (Cobalt Gray Equivalents)) than larger volumes. They note: "Tolerance of brainstem to fractionated radiotherapy appears to be a steep function of tissue volume included in high dose regions rather than the maximum dose of brainstem alone." The relevance of tissue rescue and migration is supported in this data set as well, both by the steep impact of volume irradiated and by the statistically significant increase in complication risk due to surgical procedures.

Hence, the classical concept of a serial organ, originally thought to apply to structures such as the spinal cord, brain stem, small bowel, esophagus, and rectum, appears to be much too simple and does not apply except in very restrictive situations. Dose–response for tubular organs such as esophagus [22], rectum [42, 43], and small bowel is even less serial than for central nervous system tissue [44]. Tolerance in esophagus, rectum, and small bowel appears to depend significantly on volume irradiated to high doses as well as dose level, rather than just correlating with "maximum dose," or maximum dose to a small volume.

Local vs. Global Organ Injuries

Organ/tissue injuries can be approximately categorized as either (1) inflammatory or ulcerative in nature or (2) a reduction of physiological function. Figure 2 illustrates this suggested categorization endpoints by dose–volume effect. The classification of endpoints is not completely clear-cut, and some tissue endpoints may have both inflammatory and function-loss components (e.g., small bowel [46]). Complications further divide into early and late reactions, based on their latent period and their clinical course. Although the pathogenesis of early reaction seems well established, namely the loss of rapidly proliferating "target-cells," the pathogenesis of late reaction is much more complicated, involving cell loss (though delayed due to slower proliferation) as well as cascades of interrelating chemical signals and coordinated multicell-type responses to the radiation-induced "wound" [47]. Thus, our categorization is an oversimplification, but hopefully useful nevertheless.

Endpoints which are inflammatory/ulcerative appear more likely to relate to the absolute volume or absolute area irradiated (although this has not always been borne out in the literature, see the discussion on rectal complications below). Inflammatory endpoints may be more naturally modeled as a function of the area

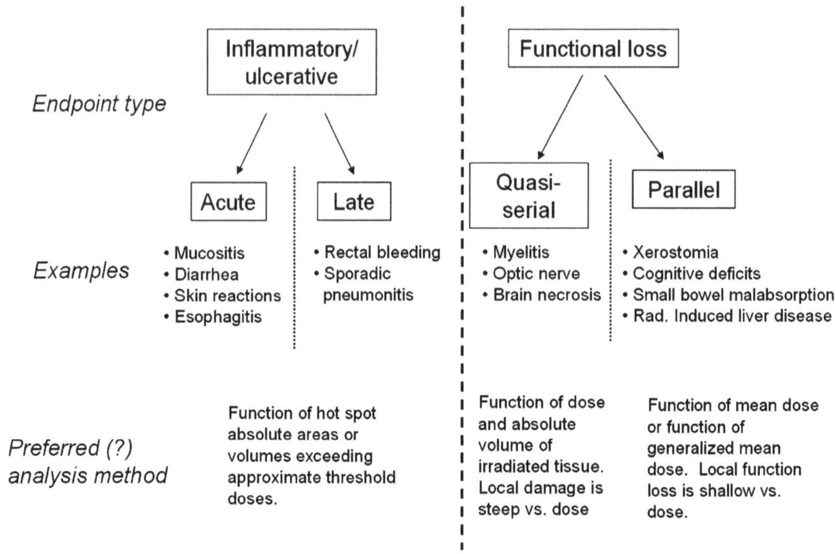

Fig. 2 A classification of tissue injury endpoints and the relation to (likely) preferred analysis methods. The main point is that volume effects associated with inflammation or ulcerative damage may need different analysis methods compared to volume effects associated with organ functional loss. Inflammatory or ulcerative endpoints may benefit from analyzing absolute areas or volumes exceeding some approximate critical dose threshold (cf. Bradley et al. [22]; or Thames et al. regarding cluster models [46]). Injury due to functional loss in the so-called parallel systems has often successfully been analyzed as a function of mean doses, or something close to it [2]. When functional loss is primarily due to structural damage, the endpoint is often discussed in terms of "serially" (or more accurately, "quasiserially") aligned functional subunits

or volume receiving dose above a threshold (or a graded model, as discussed below). The Lyman phenomenological model may therefore not be the best approach to these to the inflammatory endpoints (especially late rectal bleeding, acute esophagitis), as the volume of application must naturally coincide with the entire organ, whereas a complication may be produced only when, say, the region receiving more than 50 Gy reaches a given size.

NTCP Models

Early papers proposing models which could estimate complication probability based on dose distributions characteristics include those by Wolbarst et al. [16, 48, 49], Schultheiss and Orton [1], Lyman [50, 51], Kutcher et al. [52, 53], and Goitein and Niemierko [54]. However, these efforts were "data-poor" at best.

A seminal event in NTCP modeling was the publication by a multiinstitutional collaboration of estimates of partial volume tolerances to radiation in 1991 [55]. That group, including physicians and physicists, reviewed the (then sparse) literature and relied on extensive clinical experience as well to tabulate estimates of the tolerance of a wide-range of organs and tissues for partial volume irradiation. In the intervening years, it is perhaps surprising how usefully accurate their estimates have been even as more accurate evaluations have become available.

Necessarily, the early efforts were data-poor and rested on somewhat conjectural mechanistic or phenomenological hypotheses, as discussed for the serial models. Unfortunately, the underlying radiobiological mechanistic nature of the volume effect is still not well understood.

The first phenomenological model with just enough degrees of freedom to account for the volume effect was that proposed by Lyman [56], Kutcher [52], and Burman [11]. It is highly parsimonious, containing only three parameters, once the sometimes ambiguous choice of reference volume has been made. The wide-spread application of a power-law at even higher complication rates and for nonserial organs, first proposed by Lyman, was rooted in clinical experience, not mechanistic assumptions. Thus,

$$\mathrm{TD}(v) = \mathrm{TD}(1)/v^n, \tag{1}$$

where TD is the tolerance dose which results in a given rate of complications and v is the fraction of organ irradiated.

Withers and later followers, in particular, attempted to place partial volume effects on a more rational foundation by introducing the notion of a "functional subunit" (FSU) [31]. However, FSU-based models have typically overestimated the steepness of partial volume effects for organs which have a parallel functionality.

Understanding the use of NTCP functions requires consideration of several aspects, including: clinical endpoints, empirical basis, mathematical characteristics, and use in treatment planning.

The Generalized Equivalent Uniform Dose Equation

Although in varying mathematical formats, it was realized by several groups that the power-law given above could be generalized to apply to nonuniform dose distributions (or, to use the older phrase, "DVH reduction") [52, 57, 58]. The generalized equivalent uniform dose equation is given by:

$$\mathrm{gEUD}(d;a) = \left(\frac{1}{N}\sum_{i=1}^{N} d_i^a\right)^{1/a} = \left(\frac{1}{N}\sum_{i=1}^{N} d_i(d_i^{a-1})\right)^{1/a}, \tag{2}$$

This is just an exponential average of dose values over the N voxels of that structure (the gEUD goes by the name of generalized mean [59], or p-norm in other areas of application). The second line is written to emphasize that it is indeed just an exponential weighting. The key parameter is *a*. When *a* is large in magnitude but negative, the gEUD correlates with the low-dose part of the DVH; when *a* is large in magnitude but positive, the gEUD correlates with the high-dose part of the DVH; and when *a* is near one, the gEUD correlates with the mean dose (being equal to the mean dose when *a* equals exactly one). Thus, large positive values of *a* are appropriate for tissues which are thought to be damaged by even small volumes of high dose; large negative values of *a* are appropriate for tumors whose response is thought to be related primarily to the lower part of the DVH, and *a* is expected to be near one when the mean dose is important. We therefore refer to the exponential *a* parameter as the "localizing" parameter: When it is large in magnitude, damage (or treatment failure) is modeled as failing where the low/high doses are located. When *a* is small in magnitude, the damage is unlocalized, that is, it tends to extend across the tissue, in varying degree, in both high and low dose regions. Figure 3 demonstrates the relative change in tolerance expected vs. fractional organ volume irradiated, for differing localizing parameters.

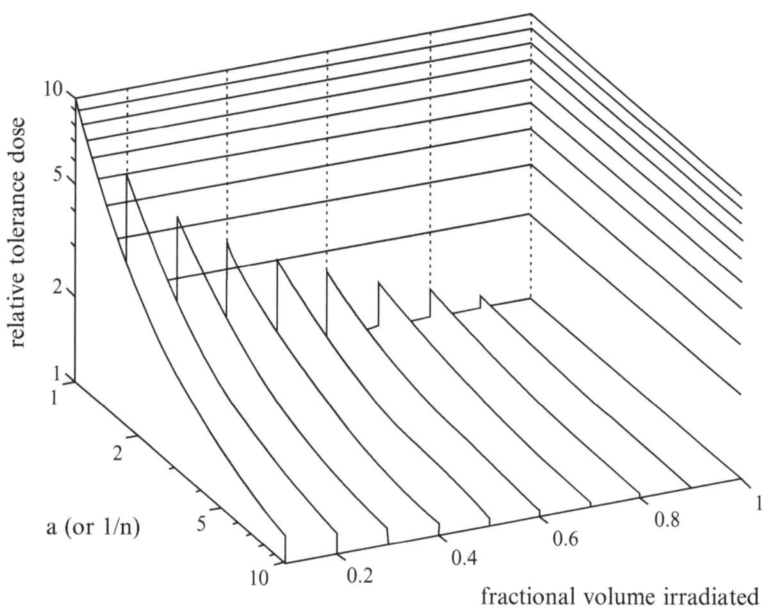

Fig. 3 Relative change in tolerance vs. fractional organ volume irradiated. This figure shows how the modeled expected tolerance varies in the idealized case when a fraction of the organ/tissue in question receives a uniform dose, the rest receiving zero dose. The important point is to observe that, when the localizing parameter (*a*) is small, the relative tolerance increases dramatically as irradiated volume is reduced from 100% to 10%. In contrast, when the localizing parameter is as large as 10, there is little change in tolerance as the volume irradiated is reduced by the same factor of 10 (reproduced with permission from Moiseenko et al. [4])

When a is less than or equal to 0, then gEUD equals zero if any dose equals zero [59]. In principle, there is nothing inherently wrong with a values less than one; they may indicate that it is the lower dose part of the DVH which is more important (e.g., due to functional sparing) [60]. Unfortunately, there are two notations for the gEUD equation which are sometimes used. The other notation often seen is the replacement of a with $1/n$.

Basic Mathematical Features of Common NTCP Functions

In this section we compare basic features of some common NTCP models (See also Moiseenko et al. for more detail on common NTCP models).

The Parallel-Function Model

Although our basic approach is to keep the models as simple as possible, the discussion would not be complete without considering the "parallel-function" model put forth by several groups [13, 14, 61]. This model is based on the previously mentioned paradigm of damage-injury: underlying radiation damage, if great enough, causes injury (complications). Although the model has some attractive properties, it has yet to be shown to be definitively superior to the LKB in clinical applications.

The parallel model proceeds in two steps: (1) it estimates local functional damage by assuming that local functional damage follows a sigmoidally shaped function and (2) the total volume-averaged functional damaged (f_{damage}) is then summed:

$$f_{\text{damage}} = \sum_{i=1}^{\text{voxels}} v_i p(D_i), \tag{3}$$

where $p(D_i)$ represents local functional reduction vs. local dose, and v_i is the volume of the ith voxel. The probability of local functional subunit incapacitation is given by a simple sigmoidal logistic equation:

$$p(D) = \frac{1}{[1+(D_{50}/D)^k]}, \tag{4}$$

where D_{50} is the dose to reach a 50% probability of inactivation, D again is the voxel or functional subunit dose (or the biologically transformed equivalent), and k is a constant determining the slope of the response (higher k values imply steeper slopes). Again following Jackson et al. [62], we have:

$$\text{NTCP}(f_{\text{damage}}) = \frac{1}{\sqrt{2\pi\sigma_u^2}} \int_0^{f_{\text{damage}}} \exp(-(f - f_{50})^2 / 2\sigma_f^2) \mathrm{d}f$$

where f_{50} is the mean level of functional damage required for 50% of the population to have a complication and σ_f is the standard deviation of this, which determines the slope of the response curve.

A key problem with this model is that, during the data-fitting stage, the steepness and position of the local function curve can trade off with the steepness and position of the population distribution (through D_{50} and m) [19].

For this reason, a related model is very helpful: the dose-threshold model (also called the "dose-cutoff" model) [63]. This is a simplification of the parallel-function model, where the local functional damage is binary: complete above the dose threshold, nonexistent below. The parameters to be estimated then are the f_{50} and σ_f, and the critical dose. Alternatively, Tucker has used the dose cutoff model for late rectal bleeding with the alternative formulation (relation between σ, s, and m).

The Lyman–Kutcher–Burman Model

In a slightly more convenient form than what is usually found in the literature, the three-parameter Lyman–Kutcher–Burman (LKB) model may be recast using the gEUD notation [64, 65]. One of the parameters, the reference volume is often not explicitly present because it is set to the volume of the organ or tissue to be evaluated in the gEUD formula. This model can be expressed as:

$$\mathrm{NTCP(gEUD)} = \frac{1}{\sqrt{2\pi}} \int_{-\infty}^{t} \exp(-u^2/2)\mathrm{d}u,$$

where $t = (\mathrm{gEUD}-D_{50})/(D_{50}m)$, D_{50} is the 50%-response dose, and the maximum slope of the response curve is inversely proportional to m.

The LKB model may be viewed as a model in which average functional damage (represented by gEUD) must accumulate above a given level (D_{50}) before a complication is likely.

Note how closely this model mathematically resembles the parallel-function model. In both cases, complications follow a sigmoidally shaped function defined by integrating over a Gaussian distribution of values which may be, but are not necessarily, interpreted as individual tolerance values.

Note that the volume effect parameter often quoted in analyses of the LKB model is n, which equals $1/a$. Our preference for a is due to increased intelligibility of the behavior as a changes, and, during data fitting, an increased likelihood that normal distributions of the parameter values are reasonable. When using n for fitting data, for example, the difference between an n of 2 vs. 1 is the difference between weighting doses quadratically or evenly, whereas the difference between n equal to a small number, say 0.01 vs. 1 is the difference between responding to the maximum dose only vs. responding to the mean dose. It is unlikely, therefore, that the usual Gaussian assumptions about the likelihood function really hold. In contrast, when using the a parameterization, similar numerical values yield similar dose-ranking behavior.

The Difference Between the LKB and the Parallel-Function Models

The LBK essentially responds according to the corresponding gEUD, which, as discussed above, depends critically on the exponential parameter, *a*.

Cluster Models

Recently, Thames and Tucker have argued that for some complication endpoints, it is not only the total volume or cross-sectional area receiving high doses which matters but also the shape of the high-dose region. To account for this effect, they proposed an innovative model based on the local shapes of the high-dose regions [45]. This "cluster" model is based on the radiobiologically reasonable concept that a high dose–volume which forms a concentrated region of damage is more likely to give rise to a complication compared to, say, multiple disconnected subvolumes of high dose of the same total volume. Potentially, this may be superior to purely gEUD approaches. More research on this important issue will be needed to understand the potential value of such models.

A Data-Mining/Data-Driven Approach to NTCP Modeling

A data-driven and exploratory approach to NTCP analyses allows for consideration of a wider range of dosimetric, spatial, and clinical factors within the same model-building exercise than is typically done. Potentially this can lead to the problem of model overfitting where too many variables are included within the model fit, because addition of new variables and the fine tuning of the constants for those variables could continually increase the agreement between the model and the data which are used for the model fitting. Our approach to this problem is to use cross-validation techniques (supplemented by information theoretic measures discussed below). In a recent publication, El Naqa et al. [8] examined several cross-validation techniques: bootstrap base methods, 90/10 cross-validation methods, and leave-one-out (jackknife) cross-validation methods. For all these, modeling is performed on a subset (or bootstrap pseudodata set) of data. Prediction power is tested by applying the model to the out-of-sample data points. In most cases, all of these methods when used correctly gave similar answers (for the test data sets) as to the proper size of the model (number of parameters). This model-based approach facilitates inclusion of a very wide range of dosimetric, spatial, and clinical factors. Figure 4 shows a self-correlation matrix amongst many of the factors which were considered for the analysis of acute esophagitis at WUSTL [22]. This figure illustrates well the problem of intercorrelation amongst the potentially predictive factors included in the analyses. The fact that so many of these factors, such as V20 vs. V30 for example, are so highly correlated means that it is nearly impossible to

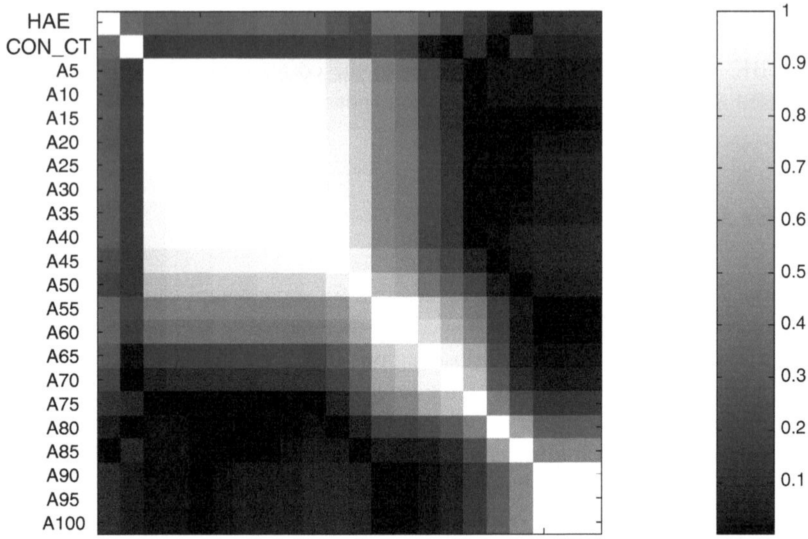

Fig. 4 This is a gray-scale figure of Spearman's rank correlations between different dosimetric statistics, within a data set for acute esophagitis [22]. HAE = highest acute esophagitis score; CON_CT = concurrent chemotherapy; V5, V10,...,V100 are absolute volumes receiving, respectively, at least 5, 10,..., 100 Gy dose. Each row is assigned a given variable, as listed. To find the correlation with another variable, starting on the row of the first variable, find the column on that row which numerically equals the row number of the second variable. The figure clearly shows that many Vx values are very highly correlated with neighboring Vx values, thus making it impossible to distinguish their effects in an outcomes model (reprinted with permission from El Naqa et al. [8])

isolate crucial dose levels with high precision (if indeed they exist). To understand these sensitive interrelationships and also the effect of having a finite size data set, we have developed and introduced a method of performing regression analyses on bootstrap resamples of the original data set [8]. Thus, the stepwise process of selecting statistically significant variables and fitting their coefficients to the present training data set is repeated using pseudodata sets created according to the bootstrap principle, as further discussed below.

Data Collection

The identification of the potential explanatory variables, whether they are dose–volume variables (e.g., Vx, Dx, mean dose) or clinical factors such as age, gender, treatment type, etc., is usually done as part of the experimental design of the study. Generally speaking, the process of experimental design of any clinical study is very involved and is beyond the scope of this chapter. Nevertheless, it should be done in consultation with a biostatistician.[1] Historically, NTCP modeling has been considered as a dose–volume effect; however, recent studies have focused on incorporating other clinical and biological potential contributing factors. In this context of data-driven modeling of outcomes, the observed treatment outcome (e.g., NTCP) is considered as the result of functional mapping of several dosimetric and clinical input variables, which could mathematically be expressed as: $f(\mathbf{x};\mathbf{w}^*)$: $X \rightarrow Y$, where $x_i \in \mathbb{R}^N$ are the input explanatory variables (dose–volume metrics, patient disease-specific prognostic factors) and $y_i \in Y$ are the corresponding observed treatment outcome (TCP or NTCP), and $\mathbf{w}^*$ includes the optimal parameters of model $f(\cdot)$ obtained by optimizing a certain objective functional. Hence, there are three basic building blocks for any modeling exercise, which are: (1) the observed treatment endpoints, (2) the input variables, and (3) the functional form of the model itself.

Extraction of Data from Clinical Sources: CERR

Although the advent of 3D treatment planning has made dose–volume outcomes NTCP studies possible, the process of extracting data from clinical sources is still technically complex. We have developed and continue to maintain a set of software tools which are designed to make this sort of data extraction feasible, efficient, and reliable. CERR (a computational framework for radiotherapy research, pronounced "sir"), is a system based on the widely used and flexible Matlab data analysis, visualization, and programming environment [66]. The process of using CERR for NTCP analyses is schematically represented in Fig. 5. The primary motivation for creating CERR was the practical impossibility of verifying the correctness of any newly computed dose or image-based variables extracted from treatment planning systems (such as DVHs) without extensive graphical visualization tools. Furthermore, the ability to actually recontour certain structures is sometimes crucial, either to maintain consistency, correct small flaws, or to work around treatment planning limitations such as the inability to have overlapping targets and normal structures (a painful limitation of one commercial system). The current release of CERR (3.0) extends the capabilities of the system to include the use of multiple image data sets. CERR is free to use or modify for research use, and the current version is always maintained by WUSTL (currently at http://radium.wustl.edu/cerr). Several outcome analyses have been published to data which used CERR [67–71]. CERR has also been used for other types of radiotherapy research projects [72–75]. Furthermore, some of the modeling tools discussed in the chapter are available in an open-source package available from the authors.

[1]Sir Ronald Fisher mentioned in an address to Indian Statistical Congress (1938): "To consult the statistician after an experiment is finished is often merely to ask him to conduct a post mortem examination. He can perhaps say what the experiment died of."

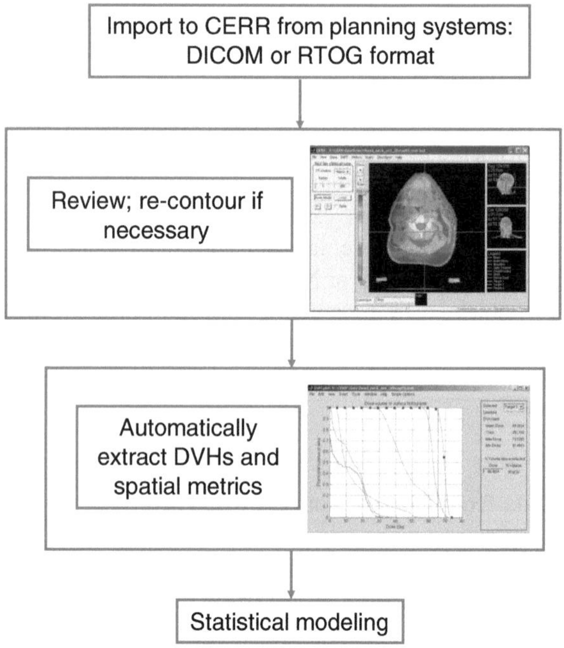

Fig. 5 Flow chart for building statistical outcomes models with CERR. The correctness of treatment plan extraction can be verified graphically. Image data sets (CT, PET, MRI) as well as dose distributions, beam definitions, and any precomputed DVHs can be imported [70]. If necessary, anatomical contours can be modified or created. CERR and the underlying Matlab environment thus provide powerful tools for conveniently extracting a wide range of treatment plan characteristics which can then be used as candidate variables in statistical modeling. The current version of CERR is always available at a Web page supported by WUSTL (currently http://radium.wustl.edu/cerr). Some of the modeling tools discussed in the chapter are available in an open-source package available from the authors

Selection of End Points

Complications are chronologically divided into early (acute) and late (chronic) effects. Acute effects usually occur within days or few weeks after treatment and are usually episodic but in some cases contribute to the risk of chronic complications [76]. On the other hand, late effects may cause irreversible damage to slowly proliferating tissues and result in chronic complications which are more difficult to manage. The relation is typically monotonic, meaning higher the dose (given the same number of fractions), the more intense the damage will be.

Complications are defined according to a categorical grading system. The National Cancer Institute has usefully encouraged standardized outcomes terminology (Common Terminology Criteria for Adverse Events version 3.0) [77].

It is always important to consider uncertainties in the grading measurements, especially whether they are likely to vary significantly between physicians, institutions, or even patient populations, which certainly contribute to potential model/data variations. Typically, patients are divided into dichotomous endpoints (with a grade threshold), although analyses that preserve grade order are certainly possible. There is typically a tradeoff between the severity/importance of the threshold complications considered as "events" (say, Grade 2 and greater) and statistical needs; including lower grades nearly always improves the modeling. A related issue is that low-grade complications may even have a different cause than typical higher-grade complications. Moreover, the complications in any given grade may form a heterogeneous continuum with a variety of related biological etiologies.

Selection of Relevant Input Variables

Traditional NTCP modeling such as the popular LKB is based on a priori assumptions about the functional form of dose–volume effects [4, 53, 56]. However, the pool of candidate variables would span other dose–volume metrics that are extracted from the dose–volume histogram such as Vx (the percentage volume that got x Gy), Dx (the minimum dose to the hottest $x\%$ volume), mean dose, maximum and minimum dose, generalized equivalent uniform dose [57], clinical and patient specific data such as age, gender, ethnicity, date of treatment start, treatment technique, treatment aim, chemotherapy, disease stage, treatment duration, histological features, and even genetic markers [8, 68, 78–81]. The previously mentioned set of variables are generic to most complication types. Moreover, for each type of normal tissue complication there are more specific variables that could be identified, such as measurements of forced expiratory volume in 1 s (FEV1) or forced vital capacity (FVC) in lung cancer, or prostate specific antigen (PSA) readings in prostate cancer.

However, selection of relevant variables from a large pool of variables is a challenging problem. This is particularly true in radiation oncology, where the data are multidimensional, the "true" model (or very good approximation to response) is unknown, and the number of observations is limited. Therefore, dimensionality reduction or subset selection techniques aim to find the "significant" set of features. An ideal modeling method should marginalize redundant variables which usually complicate data exploration without adding significance. This problem is especially acute with respect to the presence of highly correlated variables (such as V20 and V30, as discussed above). One method which we have used is to recursively eliminate one partner from each variable duo which shows a correlation greater than a given threshold (0.75 in our case).

In any given pattern recognition/machine-learning problem (or which outcomes modeling is one example), there are a large number of features that could be extracted from patients' data; therefore it is necessary to select a finite subset of features that has the most discriminating power for the problem. Univariate analysis could be used as a starting screening step; however, it is hard to determine the role of the variable based solely on univariate analysis due to the interplay between variables. An optimal subset could be determined by exhaustive search, but this yields an exponential explosion of possible variable sets. Other alternatives [82] include making an educated guess based on experience and domain knowledge, and then applying a feature transformation (e.g., principle component analysis (PCA) [83]), or using a conventional organized search such as sequential forward selection, or sequential backward selection, or a combination of both [82]. We typically use sequential forward selection after determining model order (discussed below). In any case, the pool of variables should be constrained to those which may potentially have causal relevance. Note, however, that often it is hard to know where to draw this line.

The role of exploratory data analysis should not be neglected: if a simple transformation of the data leads to a highly interpretable response surface in low dimensions (as for example observed by Chao et al. [18] for mean dose to left and right parotid glands, discussed below), such a reduction may greatly reduce the noise in the data, in addition to adding to human interpretability.

Selection of Model Functional Form

The selection of the functional form of the model is closely related to the prior knowledge of the problem. In mechanistic models, the shape of the functional form is selected based on the clinical or biological process at hand. In phenomenological modeling, the objective is usually to find a functional form that fits the data. Guidelines for model selection would depend on the problem itself. In NTCP modeling, the response will usually follow an S-shaped curve. This suggests that models with sigmoidal shape are more appropriate to use. A commonly used sigmoidal form is the logistic model, which also has nice numerical stability properties. The logistic model is [84, 85]

$$P(\mathbf{x}_i) = \frac{e^{g(\mathbf{x}_i)}}{1+e^{g(\mathbf{x}_i)}}, \quad i = 1,\ldots,n, \tag{5}$$

where n is the number of cases (patients), $\mathbf{x}_i$ is a vector of the input variable values used to predict $P(\mathbf{x}_i)$ for outcome y_i of the i_{th} patient. $P(\cdot)$ is referred to as the logistic transformation. The "x-axis" summation $g(\mathbf{x}_i)$ is given by:

$$g(\mathbf{x}_i) = \beta_0 + \sum_{j=1}^{s} \beta_j x_{ij}, \quad i = 1,\ldots,n,\ j = 1,\ldots,s, \tag{6}$$

where s is the number of model variables and the βs are the set of model coefficients that are determined by maximizing the probability that the data gave rise to the observations (i.e., the likelihood function). Many commercially available software packages, such as SAS, SPSS, and Stata, provide estimates of the logistic regression model coefficients and their statistical significance. However, it is the analyst's responsibility to test for interaction effects on the estimated response, which can potentially be corrected by adding cross terms to (6). Note that the variable x_{ij} could be replaced by a more general polynomial fractional form x_{ij}^{r}, where r is any real number giving rise to many possible options that should adhere again to the underlying clinical or biological knowledge.

Other more complicated forms have been used in the literature, such as using an architecture of neural networks, which are a class of machine-learning methods that are massively parallel distributed nonlinear elements arranged in patterns reminiscent of a simplistic biological neuron [86]. Neural networks have been used to model postradiation treatment outcomes for cases of lung injury (pneumonitis) [87–89], in prostate cancer (prostatic adenocarcinoma) [90, 91]. They offer potentially superior performance at the expense of increased computational complexity in comparison with the logistic regression approach. We have reported elsewhere on our use of neural networks [89]. Generally, we find there is some improvement in outcome prediction (typically, Spearman's increases by roughly 0.1) at the cost of reduced model transparency and interpretability.

Selection of Model Order

The specific definition of model order changes depending on the functional form of the model order. It could be identified by the number of parameters in logistic regression as in (6), or by the number of neurons and layers in the case of neural networks, etc. However, in any of these forms, the model order creates a balance between complexity (increased model order) and the model ability to generalize to unseen data. Finding this balance is referred to in statistical theory as the bias-variance dilemma (see Fig. 6), in which an oversimple model is expected to underfit the data (large bias and small variance), whereas a too complex model is expected to overfit data (small bias and large variance) [92]. Hence, the objective is to achieve an optimal parsimonious model, i.e., a model with the correct degree of complexity to fit the data and thus a maximum ability to generalize to new, unseen, data sets.

Model Order Based on Information Theory

Information theory provides two easy-to-use measures of model order optimality: Akaike information criteria (AIC) and the Bayesian information criteria (BIC) [93]. AIC is an estimate of predictive power of a model, which includes both the maximum likelihood principle and a model complexity term that reasonably penalizes models with an increasing number of parameters (to avoid overfitting the data). BIC is derived from Bayesian theory which results in a penalty term that increases linearly with the number of parameters. Sample results for BIC and AIC metrics to define esophagitis NTCP model selection are shown in Fig. 7. Our experience has been that BIC tends to agree better with resampling methods (discussed below).

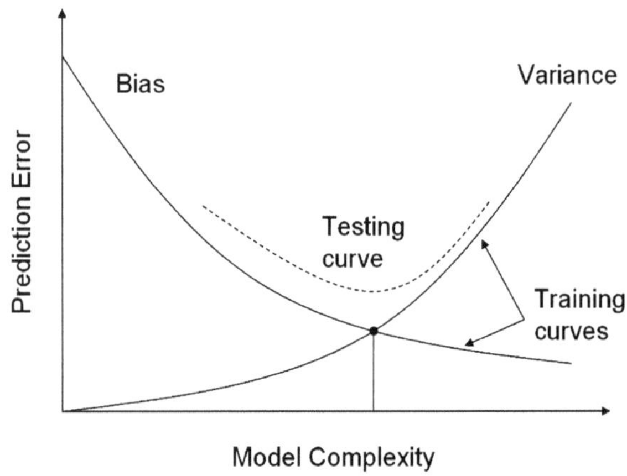

Fig. 6 This figure illustrates a common tradeoff in model predictive power (assuming the model is capable of describing the data) between prediction bias (average error) and prediction variance (square error). As model complexity increases, the average prediction error (bias) tends to decrease while the average square error tends to decrease. The point of optimal complexity tends to be near the point when average and square error are of similar magnitude (reprinted with permission from El Naqa et al. [8])

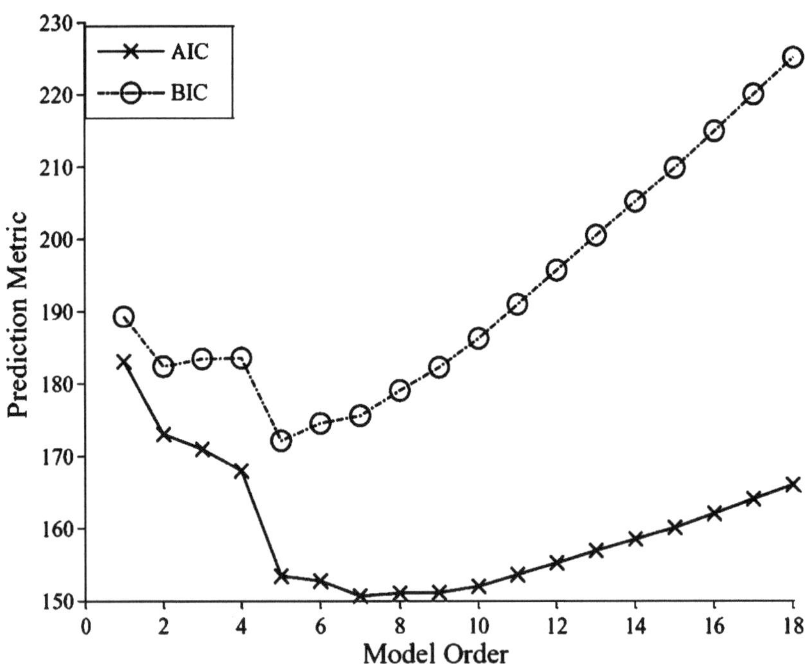

Fig. 7 A plot of Akaike and Bayesian information criteria for esophagitis logistic models. While the AIC metric shows a very strong preference for a complex model with seven or more variables, BIC shows a preference for a smaller model of five variables (reprinted with permission from El Naqa et al. [8])

Model Order Based on Cross-validation Methods

Resampling techniques are used for model selection and performance comparison purposes to provide statistically sound results when the available data set is limited (which is always the case). We use two types of fit-then-validate methods: cross-validation methods and bootstrap resampling techniques. *Cross-validation* [82] uses some of the data to train the model and some of the data to test the model validity. The type we most often use is the "leave-one-out" procedure (also known as the "jackknife"). In each leave-one-out iteration, all the data are used for training/fitting except for one data point left out for testing, and this is repeated so that each data point is left out exactly once. The overall success of predicting the left-out data is a quantitative estimate of model performance on new data sets. *Bootstrapping* [94] is an inherently computationally intensive procedure but generates statistically sound results. Typically, a bootstrap pseudodata set is generated by making copies of original data points, selected randomly, until the number of data points in the pseudodata set equals the number of original data points. This means that an original data point may be included in the pseudodata set zero or multiple times, with a probability of inclusion of 63%. The bootstrap often works acceptably well even when data sets are small or unevenly distributed. Using the bootstrap, data are fitted to the bootstrap pseudodata set, but then tested on the data points where they are not contained in the pseudodata set to predict performance on new data. To achieve valid results, this process must be repeated many times, typically several hundred times. Figure 8 shows results of resampling to determine model order for the same esophagitis data set used in Fig. 7.

Model Variable Stability

Model variable selection for the final model is unfortunately not straightforward. The standard method of conducting a single multivariate analysis gives little guidance as to the stability of the results. One is always left asking whether the variables selected were perhaps selected accidentally, i.e., due to data size limitations. We commonly use forward-variable-selection on bootstrap data replications to evaluate the stability and robustness of the "best" set of variables. Visual display of the results is a powerful way to examine potential variable interactions.

Model Parameter Fitting

After optimal model order and variable selection is determined, the fitting of the model parameters is the next to last step of model building.[2] Following the selection of the variables, determination of the functional form, and estimation of the model

[2]The last step would be model feasibility and interpretation.

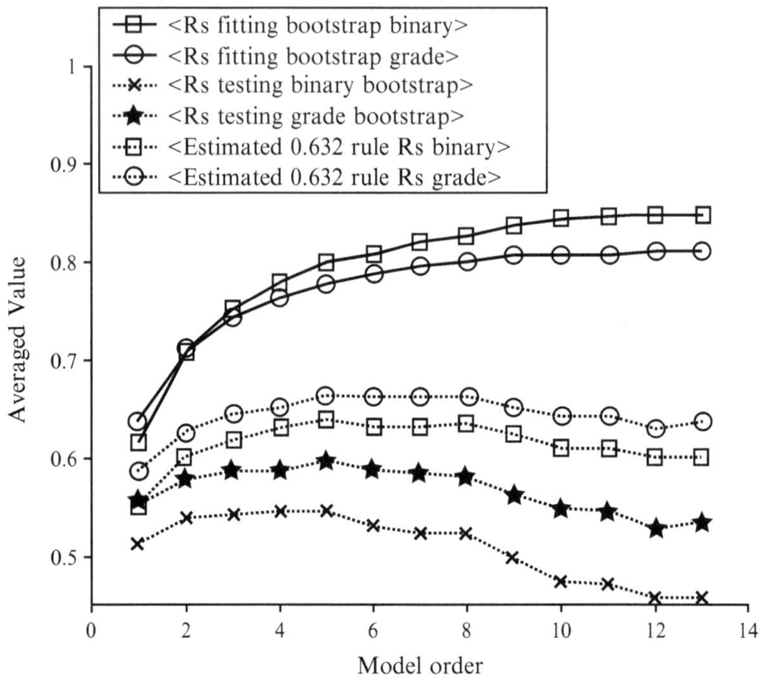

Fig. 8 A comparison of bootstrap-based methods to investigate the predictive power of xerostomia models, including: (**a**) refitting bootstrap replicates, (**b**) testing the refit models on data left out of that bootstrap replicate, and (**c**) the "0.632" method which combines results from each cohort*. In each case, the average Spearman's coefficient is tabulated for all replicates. As expected, the refitting results simply increase with increasing terms, whereas the testing and 0.632 methods show no improvement above five or six terms (reprinted with permission from El Naqa et al. [8])

order, the optimal set of parameters $\mathbf{w}^*$ is estimated. The fitting process itself is usually posed as an optimization problem, with a cost function related to the likelihood. For example, in logistic regression, the objective is to maximize the likelihood function that arises from a binomial distribution; whereas, in neural networks, more complicated objective functions are usually proposed.

Image-Based Factors and Radiosensitivity Predictors

This approach allows one to mix all the potential prognostic factors, image-based or clinical, into the same outcome analysis. It should be emphasized that when outcome analysis does not include the potentially important variations in dose distributions between patients, then potentially the known large affects of any variations in dose distribution may swamp potentially useful prognostic marker outcome correlations. The previous lack of inclusion of dose–volume-outcome factors may be one reason why the clinical application of biological prognostic markers has not been more successful.

Some Critical NTCP Endpoints

A broader review of data relating to plan ranking and dose–volume effects has recently been published by Moiseenko et al. [4]. Here, in addition to the previous discussion of spinal cord and brain stem dose–volume effects, we focus on three critical endpoints to illustrate NTCP modeling and application issues: radiation pneumonitis due to lung irradiation, late rectal toxicity due to prostate irradiation, and xerostomia resulting from head and neck irradiation.

Late Rectal Toxicity Due to External Beam Prostate Cancer Treatment

With the advent of 3D conformal RT and IMRT, the type of rectal complications has changed from strictures and stenoses (often requiring surgical intervention), to, less severe complications, such as chronic rectal bleeding [3]. Typically, late rectal bleeding has been reported to be correlated with the dose values above 50 Gy, with modest evidence that even increasing volume in the 30–40 Gy region may also increase risk. More recently, Rancati et al. reported that the best-fit localizing parameter (a) of the gEUD equation was higher for higher grades of bleeding, "...suggesting that for severe bleeding the rectum is more serial [i.e., a is higher]" [95]. We take this to be consistent with the ulcerative nature of this radiation injury. However, Tucker et al. observed that, for their data set ($n = 127$), no model was better than using gEUD (inside the LKB model) with a fixed a of 1 (i.e., a "mean dose" model) [63]. Dale et al. ($n = 66$) found a preference for a higher value of a for rectal-related endpoints reported via a questionnaire, but the overall correlation between NTCP calculations and late rectal endpoints was low [96]. Hartford et al. observed that DVH curves ($n = 41$) could be statistically successfully grouped into low, medium, and high risk categories, and that a parallel-function model could be fit which tracked increasing risk (although the model parameters were not given) [97].

As shown by Fiorino et al. [98], fraction-to-fraction relative motion of rectal tissue with respect to the high dose–volume causes significant uncertainty in the actual delivered rectal DVH. It seems clear that there is a strong need for image-guided techniques (in addition to effective immobilization, if possible) to better define true rectal DVHs.

Radiation Pneumonitis Due to Thoracic Irradiation for Lung Cancer

There have been many reports on dose–volume and clinical factors associated with radiation pneumonitis [33, 56, 61, 62, 64, 65, 99–104]. The most common dose–volume factors associated with RP have been mean dose to the normal lung tissue or Vx values, such as V20 or V30. Other prognostic factors include anatomical dose location (inferior tumor location is usually riskier) [29, 101–107], fractionation [108], age [109–111], smoking [102, 113], weight loss [102], pulmonary function [112–118], gender [116], chemotherapy [105, 106, 118–122], performance status [112, 116], and circulating cytokines during and after therapy [103].

Miller et al. have recently elaborated on “A Practical Approach to Pulmonary Risk Assessment in the Radiotherapy of Lung Cancer” [123]. Treatment doses are potentially restricted based on recommended limited mean dose and V25 to non-gross tumor volume lung tissue. Furthermore, the proposed limits depend on the pulmonary status (based on pulmonary function tests) and tumor location (central lesions considered riskier). In their review, they consider the many confounding factors (smoking, highly nonuniform lung function, tumor effect on lung perfusion, etc.) which contribute to the poor predictive power of current radiation pneumonitis predictors.

RP risk has also been correlated with the spatial distribution of functional capacity (as evaluated by SPECT) [29]. Travis et al. demonstrated in a mouse model that lower lobe irradiation, for the same volume irradiated, was associated with increased risk of pneumonitis [124, 125]. Khan et al demonstrated regional differences in DNA-damage in a rat radiotherapy model [126].

The WUSTL group recently analyzed both their own institutional data with respect to multiple risk factors including dose, volume, and tumor location ($n = 57$) [81]. Tumor location was the strongest single factor on univariate analysis (inferior location was worse), and survived as part of the strongest multivariate models (see Figs. 9 and 10. Using multivariable data-mining methods [8], they found that D35 (the minimum dose to the hottest 35% of the lung) was also consistently selected, but only weakly, over other dose–volume factors such as mean dose and V20 (see also the model vs. observations, in Fig. 1). Those results demonstrated both the strengths and the weaknesses of the data-mining approach which looks at many factors: small, nearly insignificant factors were identified, yet such factors may be the result of the model “tuning” to the data set under consideration.

A test of the robustness of the WUSTL single-institution model was afforded by an analysis by the same group of radiation pneumonitis data from RTOG trial 93–011, a Phase I/II dose escalation trial based on volume of tissue receiving greater than 20 Gy [127]. Perhaps surprisingly, the strongest multivariate model based on the WUSTL data set did not predict for pneumonitis in the RTOG 93–11 data set, even though some factors, such as superior–inferior tumor position and D15, were similar to the WUSTL analysis results (as mentioned, a combined analysis is ongoing).

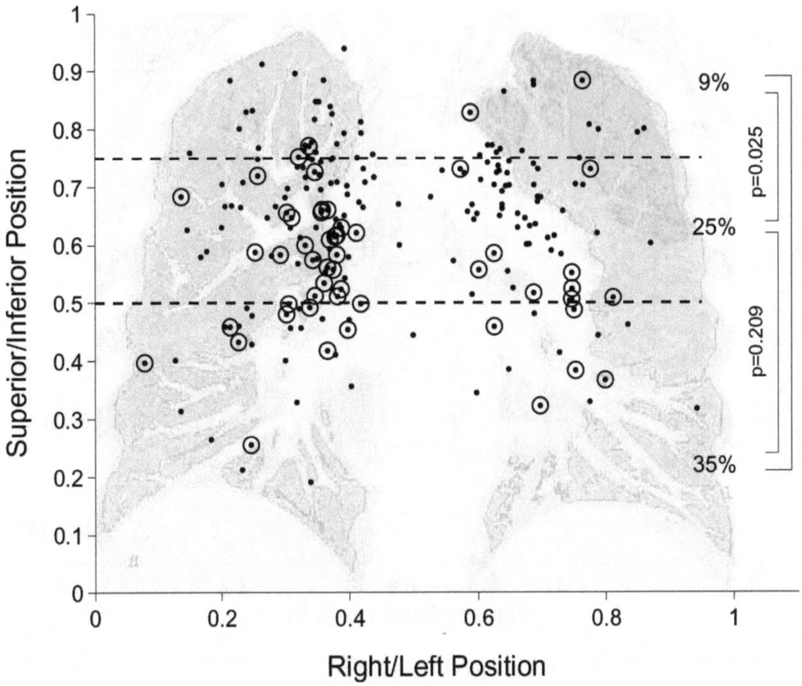

Fig. 9 The distribution of lung tumor centers of mass within a normalized lung coordinate space (WUSTL data set, 219 patients). Patients who experienced radiation pneumonitis (steroids or more intensive intervention required) are circled. An increased risk of RP is visually apparent and statistically validated for increasingly inferior tumor locations. A potential correlation between medial vs. lateral position was also explored, but was not found to be an independent predictor within a multivariate framework (reproduced with permission from Hope et al. [85])

Seppenwoolde et al. recently reviewed data sets from two institutions ($n = 382$) to assess DVH-based NTCP models [104]. They found that a mean-dose model (i.e., with a localizing parameter of 1) performed as well as other models with a tuned localizing parameter fitted to the data (best fit, $a = 1.01$).

Yorke et al. recently reported statistical correlations for a cohort of lung cancer patients enrolled in a single-institution clinical trial ($n = 78$). They confirmed correlations between mean lung dose and pneumonitis, but also that "the most significant correlations were for (V05–V13) in ipsilateral lung."

Viewed in light of the trend toward fits which confirm the importance of the mean dose, the results of Kwa et al. are notable: they pooled 540 patient data points from five institutions including breast, lymphoma, and lung cancer patients and correlated mean lung dose (transformed using the linear-quadratic model to a 2 Gy per fraction equivalent) [33]. To achieve the best agreement, institution-specific "baseline" rates (i.e., rate of "pneumonitis" at low mean dose) were modeled explicitly (typically near 11%).

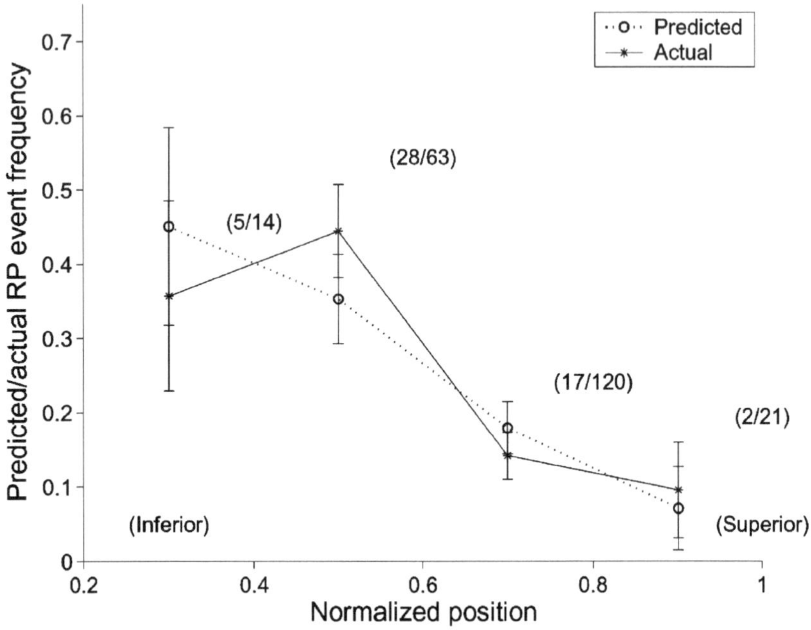

Fig. 10 Radiation pneumonitis risk vs. position of the GTV center (inferior to superior, 0 to 1): the solid line is observed, the dotted line is our model prediction, based on a three-term model (GTV normalized position, D35, and a smaller effect from maximum dose). The figure demonstrates consistency between the model and data with respect to the effect of tumor position (reproduced with permission from Hope et al. [85])

Open questions with respect to radiation pneumonitis risk factors include: (1) the potential effect of breathing on DVHs; (2) the effect of dose calculation accuracy; (3) does anatomic position affect risk in a more complicated way than modeled to date; and (4) how much does interpatient biological susceptibility impact RP risk.

Xerostomia Due to Head and Neck Cancer Treatment

Dry mouth (xerostomia) is a critical late side effect of radiation to the head and neck area and is cited by patients as the primary cause of decreased quality of life after radiotherapy. Decreased saliva output causes alterations in speech and taste and increases the potential for secondary nutritional deficiencies. Oral mucosal dryness creates a predisposition to fissures and ulcers, and changes in the composition of the oral flora increase the risk of dental caries and infections. As Amosson et al. report: "Xerostomia affects every aspect of life including speech, nutrition, taste, and sleep. Patients live with a constant reminder of their diminished quality of life" [128].

Xerostomia has often been defined as salivary flow capability for either stimulated (via lemon juice or some other stimulant) or unstimulated conditions of less than 25% of the pre-RT salivary flow capability [129]. However, this is somewhat arbitrary, and a more comprehensive picture is obtained by measuring and modeling salivary flow itself and relating it to endpoints such as quality of life.

Salivary production is mostly due to major glands (parotid, submandibular, and sublingual) but also contributions from minor glands (mostly located in the oral cavity) [130]. The treatment of xerostomia has previously been unsatisfactory or expensive [131, 132].

IMRT has recently been shown to enable partial parotid gland sparing [133]. IMRT allows the treatment planner to "sculpt" the high-dose region to largely avoid the parotid glands yet still cover target volumes which may include gross disease or a surgical bed, along with lymphatic drainage pathways. However, some irradiation of the parotid glands is typically unavoidable. A quantitative model of the reduction of parotid function for varying possible dose distributions is therefore highly desirable as a guide to whether a dose distribution will be well tolerated.

Amosson et al. [128] analyzed the response of 30 patients to xerostomia-related questions. They found that patients typically believed they had "adequate" saliva when the contralateral (less irradiated) gland mean dose was 16.2 Gy or less in 25 fractions. Patients felt they had "too little" saliva at a mean dose of 22.5 Gy or greater.

Eisbruch et al. [134] reported the Michigan experience of contralateral sparing of parotid glands during 3D conformal head and neck irradiation. The mean dose thresholds for both unstimulated and stimulated parotid saliva flow rates to reduce to $<25\%$ of pretreatment levels were 24 and 26 Gy (in approximately 35 fractions), respectively. Using the same data set, Roesnik et al. [135] modeled the reduction in individual parotid flow rates using the LKB model. They originally derived an exponential parameter $a<1$, but fixed it at one. They derived a TD50 mean dose of 35–39 Gy in 25–35 fractions.

The WUSTL xerostomia data set, reported by Chao et al. [18] and Blanco et al. [67], consists of 55 patients, with pretreatment and posttreatment measurements of relative whole-mouth salivary function (at 6 months post-RT and a smaller data set at 12 months). The radiation delivery method was primarily IMRT [18]. Quality-of-life questionnaire data were collected. Figure 11 summarizes measured stimulated salivary flow 6 months after the end of radiotherapy relative to pretreatment values. The figure clearly shows the main trend as a function of gland mean doses. Based on the clear trends shown in Fig. 11, modeling showed that the data could be described with a simple "mean-dose-exponential" equation [18, 136]:

$$\text{Relative total flow} = \frac{\left[\exp[-A\bar{d}_{\mathrm{L}}] + \exp[-A\bar{d}_{\mathrm{R}}]\right]}{2}. \tag{7}$$

This model simply says that salivary flow is reduced exponentially, for each gland individually, according to the value of that gland's mean dose ($\bar{d}_{\mathrm{L}}$ or $\bar{d}_{\mathrm{R}}$). The coefficient A was found to be 0.054/Gy (95% CIs: 4.6, 6.7; $n = 55$). Thus, parotid glands lose function at a rate of approximately 5% per Gy. This coefficient yields a

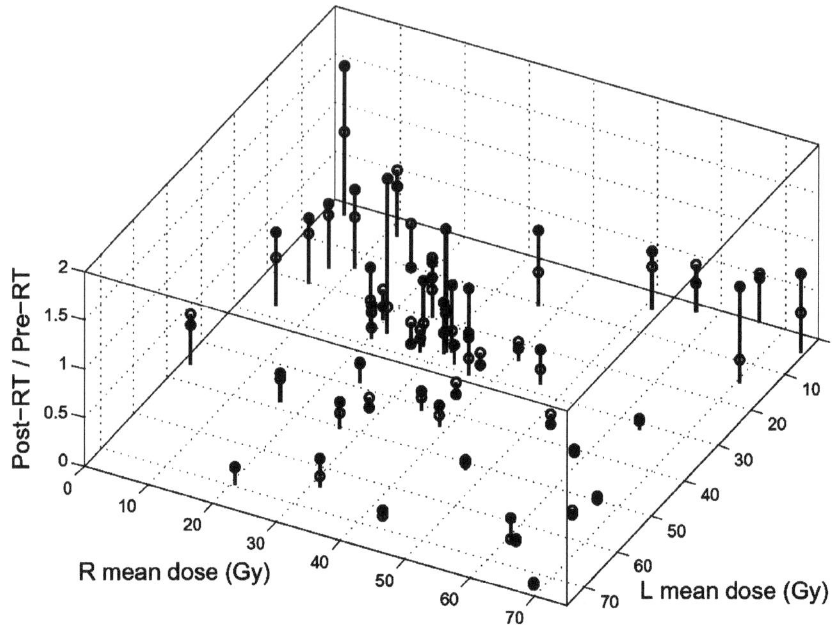

Fig. 11 Stimulated whole-mouth salivary function over 5 min, 6 months. after the end of RT divided by the pre-RT result, as a function of the mean dose to the left and right parotid glands. Closed circles are measurements; open circles are the result of the exponential mean dose equation [18]. The model prediction appears to classify the results fairly well. However, in the region where both parotid glands receive between 20 and 30 Gy, the model tends to underpredict salivary function; a more complicated parallel-function model reported by Blanco et al. [19] works better in that region. This figure supports the simple observation that if one or the other parotid gland receives <20 Gy, xerostomia (drop below 25% pretreatment level) is unlikely (current Washington University data)

"threshold dose" (for 25% function, on average) of 25.8 Gy (in 35 fractions), which is consistent with Michigan's data (28 Gy, determined at 1-year follow-up), but lower than Roesnik et al.'s value (35–39 Gy). Figure 11 is clearly consistent with the 26 Gy threshold value: if both glands receive more than about 25–30 Gy, salivary flow is poor, whereas if both glands receive less (or even one gland receives significantly less), salivary flow is significantly higher. The mean-dose-exponential model also statistically significantly correlated with QOL answers 6 months after the end of radiotherapy.

Although this model captures the main trends described in the WUSTL data set, more complicated models can improve the fit, especially when both glands receive 15–25 Gy mean dose (see Fig. 11). In particular, in the analyses reported by Blanco et al. [19], a slight preference was shown for a model which incorporated a parallel function model with a sigmoidally shaped summed local function vs. salivary function response curve. Other groups have also recently reported on the incorporation of a sigmoidal response curve [137, 138]. Furthermore, linear-quadratic dose effects cannot be incorporated into the mean-dose-exponential model, but can be incorporated into more parallel models [19].

The data and model, both imply that attempting to minimize parotid mean doses, when consistent with adequate target coverage, may help protect salivary function. Ideally, this objective would be included in the IMRT objective function, consistent with desired target doses. It is important to note that salivary function is likely to improve for mean dose reductions down to 10–15 Gy. The 26 Gy threshold should not be taken as the "magic number"! At that dose, 50% of irradiated glands are expected to fall below 25% function, not a particularly desirable outcome (of itself) from the patient's point of view.

Drawbacks to Treatment Planning Based on Dose–Volume Limits

Typical criteria in judging IMRT treatment plans include dose–volume limits on normal structures [139] (e.g., rectum V40 and V65, and target D95). Unfortunately, basing treatment planning on dose–volume constraints can be inherently risky, for several related reasons. Consider an arbitrary dose–volume cut point, such as V20, which has often been cited in the radiation pneumonitis literature. Firstly, V20, as noted above and seen in Fig. 4, is likely to be highly correlated to other Vx values, such as V10, V30, mean dose, etc. Thus, it is unlikely that V20 can be clearly distinguished as the key variable, *even if it truly is*. Secondly, treatment-specific characteristics of the dose distribution may favor some particular Vx or Dx value as highly useful to split patients into two groups, almost apart from underlying radiobiological effects. Thirdly, it is unlikely that, a priori, in any tissue with a significant volume effect, there is a magic dose level, below which damage is negligible and above which it is severe. That is, single dose–volume constraints could be radiobiologically realistic only if local damage to the organ in question is very high above the cut point and very low below the cut point. Lastly, if this metric is used to drive treatment planning, the computer (or human planner) may be tempted to "pile-up" dose in increasing volumes just below 20 Gy, trusting what is certainly an unrealistic feature of the metric. Alternative metrics, such as the generalized equivalent uniform dose (gEUD) or the mean dose, are not as susceptible to this as they do not have the built-in "on–off" feature of dose–volume constraints.

Some other points to keep in mind when comparing gEUD to dose–volume constraint point, include:

- A dose–volume point may remain constant while the volume irradiated to higher doses increases; the gEUD would be sensitive to such an increase.
- A dose–volume point may remain constant while volumes at lower doses are increased in dose (but still below the dose–volume point itself), whereas the gEUD would continue increasing.
- Using dose–volume points as constraints may create a potentially complex search space (a "nonconvex feasibility space") such that the computer-determined

solution may not be the best available [140]. The gEUD function leads to convex (simpler) search spaces [141].

New functions may emerge which are both useful for outcomes analyses, treatment plan evaluations, and driving treatment planning. In particular, Romeijn et al. [142] have introduced "conditional value-at-risk" constraints, or more clearly, "mean-upper-tail" constraints in IMRT treatment planning, which have their origin in financial optimization. We will refer to these as upper-mean-dose (denoted MDU, mean dose of the hottest v fractional volume of a defined structure) or the lower-mean-dose (MDL, the mean dose to the coldest v fractional volume). MDU and MDL may be particularly useful for NTCP modeling given the proposed categories of dose–volume effects shown in Fig. 2, which emphasizes that some complications are likely related to both the volume and mean dose of the tissue "hot spot." MDU should be more sensitive than dose–volume constraints to increases in the dose above the dose–volume constraint dose cutoff point, being discrete in only one variable (volume), not two. We expect MDL to be particularly useful as a simpler substitute for the often-used D95 (lowest dose to the hottest 95%) target evaluation criteria. In that case, the fractional volume parameter could be set to 5% or so. MDU and MDL furthermore have the advantage of being implementable using purely linear variables and constraints, thus being very computationally tractable. We expect significant work to continue which examines potential candidate functions in addition to gEUD which may be particularly useful in driving treatment planning in an outcomes-relevant fashion.

Uncertainties in NTCP Models

It can be argued that the uncertainty in NTCP models should explicitly include the uncertainty in the parameter values. After all, NTCP is only our best estimate as to the probability of the endpoint. Typically, NTCP models are determined such that the model parameters best fit the data set at hand. The term "best fit" typically means some kind of peak has been found in either the likelihood function or something similar, such as a variance function. These "best fit" parameters are then often plugged into the model, along with the dose distribution at hand and any clinical factors that have been included in the modeling, to yield the prediction of the risk of complication. However, the actual risk of a complication should take into account the probability that the true parameters that go into the model are uncertain, even if the model is perfectly representative of the functional form of the outcome. That is, the true parameters are always determined by a finite data set. *The true risk of a complication, especially if even a small risk might be considered unacceptable, should take into account the probability that the true parameters may have a lower tolerance threshold than the "maximum likelihood" parameters.* Thus, the true probability of a complication is essentially an average of the NTCP model values over the uncertainty distribution of the parameters.

This theme was developed by Schilstra et al. [143] in the likelihood framework and also separately by Deasy et al. [144] using bootstrap resamples. In both cases, the authors make the argument that the true probability of the complication cannot be said to be accurately represented by using only the maximum likelihood parameters determined in a model. This observation is simply related to the larger observation that for any analysis the true model and the true parameters have not been determined. The actual implementation of this philosophy requires larger associated data sets to be propagated from the fitting process to the treatment plan evaluation process (which can be done conveniently with bootstrap parameter fits). This addresses the often-heard remark that one would like to know "NTCP plus or minus something." This plus or minus something should be built into the actual NTCP estimate whenever possible, from any source of uncertainty, to produce a more accurate NTCP.

Incorporating Fractionation Sensitivity

The in situ fractionation sensitivity appropriate to a given endpoint depends on the fraction of cells cycling and their relative distribution within the cycle. This is the likely source of the difference in fractionation sensitivity for late- and early-responding tissues, though other causes have been hypothesized [145]. Nonetheless, it seems likely (though not inevitable) that the principle of linear quadratic fractionation sensitivity is carried through at a mechanistic level even when dose delivery is nonuniform. The issue is complicated by the fact that fractionation sensitivity for normal tissues has previously been derived *in the presence of dose nonuniformity*. The effect of dose heterogeneity (both intraorgan and interpatient) on the observable fractionation sensitivity is an open question. The data from well-characterized animal experiments, however, are quite clear: late-responding endpoints tend to higher dose-per-fraction sensitivity [146].

For example, consider a two-bin dose distribution (0/1) to a given organ. For the same organ mean dose, consider the possible effect of a constant mean dose to the whole organ vs. concentrating the effect in a fraction of the volume. The important point is that, as the entire integral dose is concentrated into a smaller and smaller volume, the linear-quadratic transformation to biologically equivalent dose has a correspondingly greater effect, and thus *the fractionation sensitivity of the organ would be expected to increase*. Hence, fractionation sensitivity cannot be completely isolated from volume effects. The situation is greatly complicated by the fact that human normal tissue data are normally obtained under conditions of nonuniform irradiation.

Despite all this, based on animal experiments, it is reasonable to expect that an NTCP model will have a natural role for linear-quadratic fractionation sensitivity. Generally, the most obvious procedure is to replace the voxel-by-voxel dose variable by a transformation, either to biologically equivalent dose (BED, dose of an equivalent effect if given in man small fractions) or nominal tissue dose (NTD, dose of an equivalent effect if given in standard, usually 2 Gy, fractions). Alternatively, Lyman has suggested transforming the parameter defining the 50% level of the dose–response curve, for any shape dose-distribution, but with little justification [147].

In some cases, the inability to incorporate linear-quadratic behavior, and reasonably estimate an alpha/beta ratio, is evidence that the model is flawed, and perhaps should be discarded. A good example is given by Blanco et al. [19] who showed that a parallel-function model allowed for a reasonable estimate of alpha/beta (about 6), whereas simpler nonmechanistic models did not.

Model Robustness vs. Model Sensitivity: Generalizability

It is important to distinguish the issue of generalizability of a statistical model from goodness-of-fit for the data set that was used. As Schultheiss has previously noted, applying models derived on the basis of one data set to another data set is inherently risky [148]. Nevertheless, the long-term goal of outcomes model building is to produce models which have the widest possible range of applicability. This goal can only be reached by considering the widest possible range of possible delivered dose distributions and their associated outcomes, from multiple institutions. It may often be the case that producing models of wide applicability conflicts with the goal of producing models which are sensitively tuned to a feature in a particular institution's underlying data set. This could be due to factors which may be of some importance clinically for that particular institution (or just that data set), but which cannot be generalized to multiple institutions due to, for example, details of the types of dose distributions delivered. Thus, there is an inherent competition between model tuning and complexity and model applicability. The key to escaping this trap is to eventually gather data sets which are extremely inclusive with respect to treatment types, patient characteristics, and treatment characteristics (including dose distribution characteristics).

As a specific example of the value of interinstitutional data, we return to our experience with radiation penumonitis modeling. In the recently published paper by Hope et al. [81], it was found that the best pneumonitis model for the WUSTL data set typically contains up to five terms and, if based on nonheterogeneity corrected dose distributions, contains a maximum dose term (to at least 1 cm^3), as well as D35, and the target center of mass position between most superior possible and most inferior possible (increasing risk with a more inferior position). We note however, that retrospective Monte Carlo-based dose corrections by our group reduced the importance of the maximum dose factor. Moreover, we recently obtained permission to analyze dose–volume factors related to pneumonitis for RTOG Trial 93-11. There a somewhat different model was produced compared to the best-performing model for the WUSTL data, as reported at the 2005 ASTRO meeting [149]. For the 93-11 data, the best performing statistical model included D15, as well as positional terms (superior–inferior, inferior being riskier, as well as anterior–posterior, posterior being riskier). Both models gave similar Spearman coefficients on the fitted data. Again, RTOG 93-11 was a dose escalation trial based on the size of the target.

In particular, as the size of the target was reduced, dose escalation was pursued. We see from our analysis that 93-11 cases tended to have smaller tumors which received higher doses compared to typical WUSTL tumors.

In further work, which we only briefly discuss here (in press), we combined the WUSTL data set and the RTOG data sets and used our full data-mining techniques. Briefly, the optimal two-term model contains a mean, normal lung dose term and a positional term relative of the center of mass of the lung tumor (again inferior position being riskier). Radiation pneumonitis is defined here as requiring the use of steroids or anything more intensive. The Spearman's rank correlation coefficient for this two-term model applied to both data sets was similar to the rank correlation coefficient obtained by the best-performing models for each data set ($R_s = 0.30$). We believe this type of combined analysis across a broader range of treatment and disease characteristics is very helpful in creating models that are more generalizable to larger populations. As mentioned, we believe NTCP and even TCP analyses must be based on, or tested against, large, combined interinstitutional data sets.

Extrapolation vs. Interpolation: Models and Regions of Validity

It is a seldom-recognized yet universal problem that NTCP models may be applied to dose distributions which are unlike the characteristics of the data which gave rise to the NTCP model [7]. That is, there is currently no barrier to applying NTCP models in regions for which the NTCP model has not been validated. Thus, one might think of an NTCP model as always having a "valid zone" within the space of possible dose distributions, fractionation schedules, and patient characteristics (and even variable goodness of fit within that region). Currently there is little research that has been done on methods which could be used to automatically warn the user when NTCP models are being applied to dose distributions which are "foreign" or "uncharacteristic" of the basis data set. However, it is clear that such methods need to go hand-in-hand with any potential widespread use of NTCP models either for simply reviewing treatment plans or for driving treatment planning within the so-called radio-biologically guided optimization. This will undoubtedly be an area of active research for some time to come. The problem is especially acute when outcomes models are used as objective functions to drive automated intensity modulated radiation therapy treatment planning. In that case, the planning system may easily drive the system outside the valid zone, creating plans with characteristics unlike those the model was validated against.

The Need to Create Long-Lived Interinstitutional Databases

Many of the hurdles toward creating and testing meaningful outcomes models in radiation oncology can at least partly be surmounted with the creation and evolution of long-lived, publicly available databases of treatment plans, imaging data, patient data, and resulting outcomes. Whereas clinical trials are often designed to give the most unambiguous answer possible to a given single question, the need to model treatment response over a wide range of possible treatment and anatomy types means that it is desirable to collect a maximum range of dose distributions and relate those to treatment outcomes. This can only be done by combining data sets from various sources because institutions or even interinstitutional databases related to a single clinical trial all have systematic trends which hamper any type of extrapolation. Our experience combining the WUSTL and RTOG data sets supports this view. It is our belief that long-lived, publicly available archives of treatment plans and associated clinical and outcomes data represent the best tool for validating image-based outcomes models which can be used across a wide range of treatment delivery techniques and patient types.

Summary

We therefore conclude that NTCP models, at least in some cases, are definitely tools not toys. However, like any good tool, they can be abused and in fact could lead to injury with misuse. In particular, we have pointed out that it is risky indeed to apply NTCP models to dose distributions which are very dissimilar to the dose distributions for which the NTCP model has been validated. While this warning is somewhat fuzzy, it is clear that more research needs to be done in this area. We believe that ultimately for NTCP models to be used routinely in treatment planning in a safe and effective way, the actual application will need to be closely related to the characteristics of the data sets and the uncertainties of the treatment parameters in the models under consideration. Another sign that NTCP models are becoming tools rather than toys is that there is often good agreement as to what constitutes a correct direction of improving the reduced risk for that particular complication endpoint. Thus, for example, mean dose to normal lung almost always comes out as being the most predictive or nearly most predictive factor in the analysis of radiation pneumonitis.

Acknowledgments Many colleagues contributed directly or indirectly to data or analyses shown in this chapter, including: Jeff Bradley, MD, Cliff Chao, MD, Milos Vicic, PhD, James Alaly, BS, Dan Mullen, DDS, Patricia Lindsay, PhD, Andrew Hope, MD, Dan Mullen, DVM, MS, and Gita Suneja, BS. This research was largely supported by NIH R01 grant CA85181. The authors also thank Soeren Bentzen for a critical review and useful suggestions.

References

1. Schultheiss TE, Orton CG, Peck RA. Models in radiotherapy: volume effects. Med Phys 1983; 10:410–415.
2. Ten Haken RK. Partial organ irradiation. Semin Radiat Oncol 2001; 11.

3. Deasy JO, Fowler JF. Radiobiology of IMRT Intensity Modulated Radiation Therapy: A Clinical Perspective, edited by A.J. Mundt, Roeske, J. (BC Decker, Hamilton, Ontario, 2005), pp. 53–74.
4. Moiseenko V, Deasy JO, Van Dyk J. Radiobiological modeling for treatment planning The Modern Technology of Radiation Oncology: A Compendium for Medical Physicists and Radiation Oncologists, edited by Jacob Van Dyk (Medical Physics Publishing, Madison, WI, 2005), Vol. 2, pp. 185–220.
5. Jackson A, Yorke E. NTCP and TCP for treatment planning, in A Practical Guide to Intensity Modulated Radiation Therapy. Madison: Medical Physics Publishing, 2003.
6. Yorke ED. Biological indices for evaluation and optimization of IMRT in Intensity-Modulated Radiation Therapy: The State of The Art, edited by J.R. Palta, Mackie, T.R. Madison: Medical Physics Publishing, 2003.
7. Deasy JO, Niemierko A, Herbert D, Yan D, Jackson A, Ten Haken RK, Langer M, Sapareto S. Methodological issues in radiation dose-volume outcome analyses: summary of a joint AAPM/NIH workshop. Med Phys 2002; 29:2109–2127.
8. El Naqa I, Bradley J, Blanco AI, Lindsay PE, Vicic M, Hope A, Deasy JO. Multivariable modeling of radiotherapy outcomes, including dose-volume and clinical factors. Int J Radiat Oncol Biol Phys 2006; 64:1275–1286.
9. Hopewell JW. The volume effect in radiotherapy–its biological significance. Br J Radiol 1997; 70(Spec No.):S32–S40.
10. Hopewell JW, Trott KR. Volume effects in radiobiology as applied to radiotherapy. Radiother Oncol 2000; 56:283–288.
11. Burman C, Kutcher GJ, Emami B, Goitein M. Fitting of normal tissue tolerance data to an analytic function. Int J Radiat Oncol Biol Phys 1991; 21:123–135.
12. Jackson A., Ten Haken RK, Robertson JM, Kessler ML, Kutcher GJ, Lawrence TS. Analysis of clinical complication data for radiation hepatitis using a parallel architecture model. Int J Radiat Oncol Biol Phys 1995; 31:883–891.
13. Jackson A, Kutcher GJ, Yorke ED. Probability of radiation-induced complications for normal tissues with parallel architecture subject to non-uniform irradiation. Med Phys 1993; 20:613–625.
14. Niemierko A, Goitein M. Modeling of normal tissue response to radiation: the critical volume model. Int J Radiat Oncol Biol Phys 1992; 25:135–145.
15. Kallman P, Agren A, Brahme A. Tumour and normal tissue responses to fractionated non-uniform dose delivery. Int J Radiat Biol 1992; 62:249–262.
16. Wolbarst AB. Optimization of radiation therapy II: the critical-voxel model. Int J Radiat Oncol Biol Phys 1984; 10:741–745.
17. Chao KS, Bosch WR, Mutic S, Lewis JS, Dehdashti F, Mintun MA, Dempsey JF, Perez CA, Purdy JA, Welch MJ. A novel approach to overcome hypoxic tumor resistance: Cu-ATSM-guided intensity-modulated radiation therapy. Int J Radiat Oncol Biol Phys 2001; 49:1171–1182.
18. Chao KS, Deasy JO, Markman J, Haynie J, Perez CA, Purdy JA, Low DA. A prospective study of salivary function sparing in patients with head-and-neck cancers receiving intensity-modulated or three-dimensional radiation therapy: initial results. Int J Radiat Oncol Biol Phys 2001; 49:907–916.
19. Blanco AI, Chao K.S.C, El Naqa I, Franklin GE, Zakarian K, Vicic M, Deasy J O. Dose-volume modeling of salivary function in patients with head and neck cancer receiving radiation therapy. Int J Radiat Oncol Biol Phys 2005; 62:1055–1069.
20. Dawson LA, Normolle D, Balter JM, McGinn CJ, Lawrence TS, Ten Haken RK. Analysis of radiation-induced liver disease using the Lyman NTCP model. Int J Radiat Oncol Biol Phys 2002; 53:810–821.
21. Dawson LA, Ten Haken RK, Lawrence TS. Partial irradiation of the liver. Semin Radiat Oncol 2001; 11:240–246.
22. Bradley J, Deasy JO, Bentzen S, El Naqa I. Dosimetric correlates for acute esophagitis in patients treated with radiotherapy for lung carcinoma. Int J Radiat Oncol Biol Phys 2004; 58:1106–1113.

23. Levegrun S, Ton L, Debus J. Partial irradiation of the brain. Semin Radiat Oncol 2001; 11:259–267.
24. Hope AJ, Lindsay P, El Naqa I, Bradley JD, Vivic M, Deasy JO. Clinical, dosimetric, and location-related factors to predict local control in non-small cell lung cancer. Int J Rad Oncol Biol Phys 2006; 63:S231.
25. Abratt RP, Morgan GW. Lung toxicity following chest irradiation in patients with lung cancer. Lung Cancer 2002; 35:103–109.
26. Mosteller F, Fienberg SE, Rourke RER. Beginning Statistics with Data Analysis. Reading, MA:Addison-Wesley; 1983.
27. de Crevoisier R, Tucker SL, Dong L, Mohan R, Cheung R, Cox JD, Kuban DA. Increased risk of biochemical and local failure in patients with distended rectum on the planning CT for prostate cancer radiotherapy. Int J Radiat Oncol Biol Phys 2005; 62:965–973.
28. Hope AJ, Lindsay PE, El Naqa I, Bradley JD, Vivic M, Deasy JO. Clinical, dosimetric, and location-related factors to predict local control in non-small cell lung cancer. Int J Rad Onc Bio Phys 2005; S231.
29. Seppenwoolde Y, De Jaeger K, Boersma LJ, Belderbos JS, Lebesque JV. Regional differences in lung radiosensitivity after radiotherapy for non-small-cell lung cancer. Int J Radiat Oncol Biol Phys 2004; 60:91–98.
30. Cheng JC, Liu HS, Wu JK, Chung HW, Jan GJ. Inclusion of biological factors in parallel-architecture normal-tissue complication probability model for radiation-induced liver disease. Int J Radiat Oncol Biol Phys 2005; 62:1150–1156.
31. Withers HR, Taylor JM, Maciejewski B. Treatment volume and tissue tolerance. Int J Radiat Oncol Biol Phys 1988; 14:751–759.
32. Fowler JF, Tome WA, Fenwick JD, Mehta MP. A challenge to traditional radiation oncology. Int J Radiat Oncol Biol Phys 2004; 60:1241–1256.
33. Kwa SL, Lebesque JV, Theuws JC, Marks LB, Munley MT, Bentel G, Oetzel D, Spahn U, Graham MV, Drzymala RE, Purdy JA, Lichter AS, Martel MK, Ten Haken RK. Radiation pneumonitis as a function of mean lung dose: an analysis of pooled data of 540 patients. Int J Radiat Oncol Biol Phys 1998; 42:1–9.
34. Marks LB. The impact of organ structure on radiation response. Int J Radiat Oncol Biol Phys 1996; 34:1165–1171.
35. Hendry J, Thames HD. Correspondence: the tissue-rescuing unit. Br J Radiol 1986; 59: 628–630.
36. Powers BE, Thames HD, Gillette SM, Smith C, Beck ER, Gillette EL. Volume effects in the irradiated canine spinal cord: do they exist when the probability of injury is low? Radiother Oncol 1998; 46: 297–306.
37. Alber M, Belka C. A normal tissue dose response model of dynamic repair processes. Phys Med Biol 2006; 51: 153–172.
38. Bijl HP, van Luijk P, Coppes RP, Schippers JM, Konings AW, van der Kogel AJ. Dose-volume effects in the rat cervical spinal cord after proton irradiation. Int J Radiat Oncol Biol Phys 2002; 52: 205–211.
39. Bijl HP, van Luijk P, Coppes RP, Schippers JM, Konings AW, van der Kogel AJ. Unexpected changes of rat cervical spinal cord tolerance caused by inhomogeneous dose distributions. Int J Radiat Oncol Biol Phys 2003; 57:274–281.
40. Withers R. Migration and myelination. Int J Radiat Oncol Biol Phys 2003; 57: 9–10.
41. Debus J, Hug EB, Liebsch NJ, O'Farrel D, Finkelstein D, Efird J, Munzenrider JE. Brainstem tolerance to conformal radiotherapy of skull base tumors. Int J Radiat Oncol Biol Phys 1997; 39:967–975.
42. Jackson A, Skwarchuk MW, Zelefsky MJ, Cowen DM, Venkatraman ES, Levegrun S, Burman CM, Kutcher GJ, Fuks Z, Liebel SA, Ling CC. Late rectal bleeding after conformal radiotherapy of prostate cancer. II. Volume effects and dose-volume histograms. Int J Radiat Oncol Biol Phys 2001; 49: 685–698.
43. Jackson A. Partial irradiation of the rectum. Semin Radiat Oncol 2001; 11:215–223.
44. Roeske JC, Bonta D, Mell LK, Lujan AE, Mundt AJ. A dosimetric analysis of acute gastrointestinal toxicity in women receiving intensity-modulated whole-pelvic radiation therapy. Radiother Oncol 2003; 69: 201–207.

45. Thames HD, Zhang M, Tucker SL, Liu HH, Dong L, Mohan R. Cluster models of dose-volume effects. Int J Radiat Oncol Biol Phys 2004; 59:1491–1504.
46. Hauer-Jensen M, Wang J, Denham JW. Bowel injury: current and evolving management strategies. Semin Radiat Oncol 2003; 13: 357–371.
47. Bentzen SM. Preventing or reducing late side effects of radiation therapy: radiobiology meets molecular pathology. Nat Rev Cancer 2006; 6(9):702–713.
48. Wolbarst AB, Sternick ES, Curran BH, Dritschilo A. Optimized radiotherapy treatment planning using the complication probability factor (CPF). Int J Radiat Oncol Biol Phys 1980; 6: 723–728.
49. Wolbarst AB, Chin LM, Svensson GK. Optimization of radiation therapy: integral-response of a model biological system. Int J Radiat Oncol Biol Phys 1982; 8:1761–1769.
50. Lyman JT, Wolbarst AB. Optimization of radiation therapy, III: a method of assessing complication probabilities from dose-volume histograms. Int J Radiat Oncol Biol Phys 1987; 13: 103–109.
51. Lyman JT, Wolbarst AB. Optimization of radiation therapy, IV: a dose-volume histogram reduction algorithm. Int J Radiat Oncol Biol Phys 1989; 17: 433–436.
52. Kutcher GJ, Burman C, Brewster L, Goitein M, Mohan R. Histogram reduction method for calculating complication probabilities for three-dimensional treatment planning evaluations. Int J Radiat Oncol Biol Phys 1991; 21:137–146.
53. Kutcher GJ, Burman C. Calculation of complication probability factors for non-uniform normal tissue irradiation: the effective volume method. Int J Radiat Oncol Biol Phys 1989; 16:1623–1630.
54. Goitein M, Niemierko A. Biologically based models for scoring treatment plans; 1988.
55. Emami B, Purdy JA, Manolis J, Barest G, Cheng E, Coia L, Doppke K, Galvin J, LoSasso T, Matthews J, et al. Three-dimensional treatment planning for lung cancer. Int J Radiat Oncol Biol Phys 1991; 21:217–227.
56. Lyman JT. Complication probability as assessed from dose–volume histograms. Radiat Res Suppl 1985; 8:S13–S19.
57. Niemierko A. A generalized concept of Equivalent Uniform Dose (abstr.). 1999; 26: 1100.
58. Mohan R, Mageras GS, Baldwin B, Brewster LJ, Kutcher GJ, Leibel S, Burman CM, Ling CC, Fuks Z. Clinically relevant optimization of 3-D conformal treatments. Med Phys 1992; 19: 933–944.
59. Abramowitz M, Stegun I. Handbook of Mathematical Functions. New York: Dover Publications, Inc; 1970.
60. Deasy JO. Comments on the use of the Lyman-Kutcher-Burman model to describe tissue response to nonuniform irradiation. Int J Radiat Oncol Biol Phys 2000; 47: 1458–1460.
61. Yorke ED, Kutcher GJ, Jackson A, Ling CC. Probability of radiation-induced complications in normal tissues with parallel architecture under conditions of uniform whole or partial organ irradiation. Radiother Oncol 1993; 26: 226–237.
62. Yorke ED, Jackson A, Rosenzweig KE, Merrick SA, Gabrys D, Venkatraman ES, Burman CM, Leibel SA, Ling CC. Dose–volume factors contributing to the incidence of radiation pneumonitis in non-small-cell lung cancer patients treated with three-dimensional conformal radiation therapy. Int J Radiat Oncol Biol Phys 2002; 54:329–339.
63. Tucker SL, Cheung R, Dong L, Liu HH, Thames HD, Huang EH, Kuban D, Mohan R. Dose-volume response analyses of late rectal bleeding after radiotherapy for prostate cancer. Int J Radiat Oncol Biol Phys 2004; 59:353–365.
64. Willner J., Jost A, Baier K, Flentje M. A little to a lot or a lot to a little? An analysis of pneumonitis risk from dose-volume histogram parameters of the lung in patients with lung cancer treated with 3-D conformal radiotherapy. Strahlenther Onkol 2003; 179:548–556.
65. Yorke ED, Jackson A, Rosenzweig KE, Braban L, Leibel SA, Ling CC. Correlation of dosimetric factors and radiation pneumonitis for non-small-cell lung cancer patients in a recently completed dose escalation study. Int J Radiat Oncol Biol Phys 2005; 63:672–682.
66. Deasy JO, Blanco AI, Clark VH. CERR: a computational environment for radiotherapy research. Med Phys 2003; 30:979–985.

67. Blanco AI, El Naqa I, Franklin GE, Zakarian K, Vicic M, Deasy JO, Chao KSC. Dose-volume modeling of salivary function in patients with head-and-neck cancer receiving radiotherapy. Int J Radiat Oncol Biol Phys 2005; 62: 1055.
68. Bradley J, Deasy JO, El Naqa I, Bentzen S. Dosimetric correlates for acute esophagitis in patients treated with radiotherapy for lung carcinoma. Int J Radiat Oncol Biol Phys 2004; 58: 1106.
69. Chao KSC, Ozyigit G, Blanco AI, Thorstad WL, Deasy JO, Haughey BH, Spector GJ, Sessions DG. Intensity-modulated radiation therapy for oropharyngeal carcinoma: impact of tumor volume. Int J Radiat Oncol Biol Phys 2004; 59: 43.
70. El Naqa I, Bradley J, Blanco AI, Lindsay PE, Vicic M, Hope A, Deasy JO. Multivariable modeling of radiotherapy outcomes, including dose-volume and clinical factors. Int J Radiat Oncol Biol Phys 2006; 64: 1275.
71. El Naqa I, Lindsay PE, Wickerhauser MV, Vicic M, Zakarian K, Deasy JO, Kawrakow I, Fippel M, Siebers JV, Kauffmann N. A comparison of Monte Carlo dose calculation denoising techniques. Phys Med Biol 2005; 50: 909.
72. Gladwish A, Kron T, McNiven A, Bauman G, Van Dyk J. Asymmetric fan beams (AFB) for improvement of the craniocaudal dose distribution in helical tomotherapy delivery. Med Phys 2004; 31: 2443.
73. Hamilton CS, Ebert MA. Volumetric uncertainty in radiotherapy. Clin Oncol 2005; 17: 456.
74. Wieslander E Knöo?s T. A virtual-accelerator-based verification of a Monte Carlo dose calculation algorithm for electron beam treatment planning in homogeneous phantoms. Phys Med Biol 2006; 51: 1533.
75. Zhang M, Moiseenko V, Liu M, Craig T. Internal fiducial markers can assist dose escalation in treatment of prostate cancer: result of organ motion simulations. Phys Med Biol 2006; 51: 269.
76. Dorr W. Hendry JH. Consequential late effects in normal tissues. Radiother Oncol 2001; 61: 223–231.
77. Trotti A., Colevas AD, Setser A, Rusch V, Jaques D, Budach V, Langer C, Murphy B, Cumberlin R, Coleman CN, Rubin P. CTCAE v3.0: development of a comprehensive grading system for the adverse effects of cancer treatment. Semin Radiat Oncol 2003; 13:176–181.
78. Levegrun S. Jackson A, Zelefsky MJ, Skwarchuk MW, Venkatraman ES, Schlegel W, Fuks Z, Leibel SA, Ling CC. Fitting tumor control probability models to biopsy outcome after three-dimensional conformal radiation therapy of prostate cancer: pitfalls in deducing radiobiologic parameters for tumors from clinical data. Int J Radiat Oncol Biol Phys 2001; 51:1064–1080.
79. Marks LB. Dosimetric predictors of radiation-induced lung injury. Int J Radiat Oncol Biol Phys 2002; 54:313–316.
80. Blanco AI, Chao KS, El Naqa I, Franklin GE, Zakarian K, Vicic M, Deasy JO. Dose-volume modeling of salivary function in patients with head-and-neck cancer receiving radiotherapy. Int J Radiat Oncol Biol Phys 2005; 62:1055–1069.
81. Hope AJ, Lindsay PE, El Naqa I, Alaly JR, Vicic M, Bradley JD, Deasy JO. Modeling radiation pneumonitis risk with clinical, dosimetric, and spatial parameters. Int J Radiat Oncol Biol Phys 2006; 65: 112–124.
82. Kennedy R, Lee Y, Van Roy B, Reed CD, Lippman RP. Solving data mining problems through pattern recognition. Prentice Hall; 1998.
83. Dawson LA, Biersack M, Lockwood G, Eisbruch A, Lawrence TS, Ten Haken RK. Use of principal component analysis to evaluate the partial organ tolerance of normal tissues to radiation. Int J Radiat Oncol Biol Phys 2005; 62.
84. Hosmer DW, Lemeshow S. Applied Logistic Regression. 2nd ed. John Wiley; 2000.
85. Vittinghoff E. Regression methods in biostatistics: linear, logistic, survival, and repeated measures models. New York: Springer; 2005.
86. Haykin S. Neural Networks: A Comprehensive Foundation. 2nd ed. Prentice Hall; 1999.
87. Munley MT, Lo JY, Sibley GS, Bentel GC, Anscher MS, Marks LB. A neural network to predict symptomatic lung injury. Phys Med Biol 1999; 44:2241–2249.
88. Su M, Miftena M, Whiddon C, Sun X, Light K, Marks L. An artificial neural network for predicting the incidence of radiation pneumonitis. Med Phys 2005; 32:318–325.

89. El Naqa I Bradley J, Deasy J. Machine learning methods for radiobiological outcome modeling. in AAPM Symposium Proceedings, edited by M. Mehta, B. Paliwal, and S. Bentzen (Medical Physics Publishing, 2005), Vol. 14.
90. Gulliford SL, Webb S, Rowbottom CG, Corne DW, Dearnaley DP. Use of artificial neural networks to predict biological outcomes for patients receiving radical radiotherapy of the prostate. Radiother Oncol 2004; 71: 3–12.
91. Lennernas B, Sandberg D, Albertsson P, Silen A, Isacsson U. The effectiveness of artificial neural networks in evaluating treatment plans for patients requiring external beam radiotherapy. Oncol Rep 2004; 12:1065–1070.
92. Hastie T, Tibshirani R, Friedman JH. The Elements of Statistical Learning: Data Mining, Inference, and Prediction: with 200 Full-Color Illustrations. New York: Springer; 2001.
93. Burnham KP, Anderson DR. Model Selection and multimodal inference: a practical information-theoretic approach. 2nd ed. New York: Springer; 2002.
94. Efron B, Tibshirani R. An introduction to the bootstrap. New York: Chapman & Hall; 1993.
95. Rancati T, Fiorino C, Gagliardi G, Cattaneo GM, Sanguineti G, Borca VC, Cozzarini C, Fellin G, Foppiano F, Girelli G, Menegotti L, Piazzolla A, Vavassori V, Valdagni R. Fitting late rectal bleeding data using different NTCP models: results from an Italian multi-centric study (AIROPROS0101). Radiother Oncol 2004; 73:21–32.
96. Dale E, Olsen DR, Fossa SD. Normal tissue complication probabilities correlated with late effects in the rectum after prostate conformal radiotherapy. Int J Radiat Oncol Biol Phys 1999; 43:385–391.
97. Hartford AC, Niemierko A, Adams JA, Urie MM, Shipley WU. Conformal irradiation of the prostate: estimating long-term rectal bleeding risk using dose-volume histograms. Int J Radiat Oncol Biol Phys 1996; 36:721–730.
98. Fiorino C, Foppiano F, Franzone P, Broggi S, Castellone P, Marcenaro M, Calandrino R, Sanguineti G. Rectal and bladder motion during conformal radiotherapy after radical prostatectomy. Radiother Oncol 2005; 74:187–195.
99. Abraatt RP. Clinical dose-volume histogram and lung toxicity after irradiation for lung cancer. Int J Radiat Oncol Biol Phys 2000; 47:1461.
100. Armstrong JG. Three-dimensional conformal radiotherapy. Precision treatment of lung cancer. Chest Surg Clin N Am 1994; 4.
101. Kwa SL, Theuws JC, Wagenaar A, Damen EM, Boersma LJ, Baas P, Muller SH, Lebesque JV. Evaluation of two dose-volume histogram reduction models for the prediction of radiation pneumonitis. Radiother Oncol 1998; 48:61–69.
102. Hernando ML, Marks LB, Bentel GC, Zhou SM, Hollis D, Das SK, Fan M, Munley MT, Shafman TD, Anscher MS, Lind PA. Radiation-induced pulmonary toxicity: a dose-volume histogram analysis in 201 patients with lung cancer. Int J Radiat Oncol Biol Phys 2001; 51:650–659.
103. Fu XL, Huang H, Bentel G, Clough R, Jirtle RL, Kong FM, Marks LB, Anscher MS. Predicting the risk of symptomatic radiation-induced lung injury using both the physical and biologic parameters V(30) and transforming growth factor beta. Int J Radiat Oncol Biol Phys 2001; 50.
104. Seppenwoolde Y, Lebesque JV, de Jaeger K, Belderbos JS, Boersma LJ, Schilstra C, Henning GT, Hayman JA Martel MK, .Ten Haken RK. Comparing different NTCP models that predict the incidence of radiation pneumonitis. Normal tissue complication probability. Int J Radiat Oncol Biol Phys 2003; 55:724–735.
105. Yamada M, Kudoh S, Hirata K, Nakajima T, Yoshikawa J. Risk factors of pneumonitis following chemoradiotherapy for lung cancer. Eur J Cancer 1998; 34.
106. Tsujino K, Hirota S, Endo M, Obayashi K, Kotani Y, Satouchi M, Kado T, Takada Y. Predictive value of dose-volume histogram parameters for predicting radiation pneumonitis after concurrent chemoradiation for lung cancer. Int J Radiat Oncol Biol Phys 2003; 55:110–115.

107. Yu X, Zhou SM, Khan D, Ahn S, Shafman TD, Hollis D, Light K, Tisch A, Folz RJ, Jaszczak R, Coleman RE, Marks JE. Predicting RT-induced pulmonary symptoms based on the dose to the superior vs. inferior lung in patients irradiated for lung cancer. Int J Radiat Biol 2003; 57:S415.
108. Roach M 3rd, Gandara DR, Yuo HS, Swift PS, Kroll S, Shrieve DC, Wara WM, Margolis L, Phillips TL. Radiation pneumonitis following combined modality therapy for lung cancer: analysis of prognostic factors. J Clin Oncol 1995; 13.
109. Koga K, Kusumoto S, Watanabe K, Nishikawa K, Harada K, Ebihara H. Age factor relevant to the development of radiation pneumonitis in radiotherapy of lung cancer. Int J Radiat Oncol Biol Phys 1988; 14:367–371.
110. Schild SE, Stella PJ, Geyer SM, Bonner JA, McGinnis WL, Mailliard JA, Brindle J, Jatoi A, Jett JR. The outcome of combined-modality therapy for stage III non-small-cell lung cancer in the elderly. J Clin Oncol 2003; 21:99–109.
111. Claude L, Perol D, Ginestet C, Falchero L, Arpin D, Vincent M, Martel I, Hominal S, Cordier JR, Carrie C. A prospective study on radiation pneumonitis following conformal radiation therapy in non-small-cell lung cancer: clinical and dosimetric factors analysis. Radiother Oncol 2004; 71:175–181.
112. Monson JM, Stark P, Reilly JJ, Sugarbaker DJ, Strauss GM, Swanson SJ, Decamp MM, Mentzer SJ, Baldini EH. Clinical radiation pneumonitis and radiographic changes after thoracic radiation therapy for lung carcinoma. Cancer 1998; 82:842–850.
113. Abratt RP, Willcox PA. The effect of irradiation on lung function and perfusion in patients with lung cancer. Int J Radiat Oncol Biol Phys 1995; 31.
114. Boersma LJ, Damen EM, de Boer RW, Muller SH, Valdes Olmos RA, van Zandwijk N, Lebesque JV. Estimation of overall pulmonary function after irradiation using dose-effect relations for local functional injury. Radiother Oncol 1995; 36:15–23.
115. Marks LB, Munley MT, Spencer DP, Sherouse GW, Bentel GC, Hoppenworth J, Chew M, Jaszczak RJ, Coleman RE, Prosnitz LR. Quantification of radiation-induced regional lung injury with perfusion imaging. Int J Radiat Oncol Biol Phys 1997; 38:399–409.
116. Robnett TJ, Machtay M, Vines EF, McKenna MG, Algazy KM, McKenna WG. Factors predicting severe radiation pneumonitis in patients receiving definitive chemoradiation for lung cancer. Int J Radiat Oncol Biol Phys 2000; 48:89–94.
117. Brooks BJ Jr, Seifter EJ, Walsh TE, Lichter AS, Bunn PA, Zabell A, Johnston-Early A, Edison M, Makuch RW, Cohen MH, et al. Pulmonary toxicity with combined modality therapy for limited stage small-cell lung cancer. J Clin Oncol 1986; 4.
118. Rancati T, Ceresoli GL, Gagliardi G, Schipani S, Cattaneo GM. Factors predicting radiation pneumonitis in lung cancer patients: a retrospective study. Radiother Oncol 2003; 67:275–283.
119. Byhardt RW, Scott C, Sause WT, Emami B, Komaki R, Fisher B, Lee JS, Lawton C. Response, toxicity, failure patterns, and survival in five Radiation Therapy Oncology Group (RTOG) trials of sequential and/or concurrent chemotherapy and radiotherapy for locally advanced non-small-cell carcinoma of the lung. Int J Radiat Oncol Biol Phys 1998; 42:469–478.
120. Fernando IN, Powles TJ, Ashley S, Grafton D, Harmer CL, Ford HT. An acute toxicity study on the effects of synchronous chemotherapy and radiotherapy in early stage breast cancer after conservative surgery. Clin Oncol (R Coll Radiol) 1996; 8:234–238.
121. Segawa Y, Takigawa N, Kataoka M, Takata I, Fujimoto N, Ueoka H. Risk factors for development of radiation pneumonitis following radiation therapy with or without chemotherapy for lung cancer. Int J Radiat Oncol Biol Phys 1997; 39.
122. Taghian AG, Assaad SI, Niemierko A, Kuter I, Younger J, Schoenthaler R, Roche M, Powell SN. Risk of pneumonitis in breast cancer patients treated with radiation therapy and combination chemotherapy with paclitaxel. J Natl Cancer Inst 2001; 93.
123. Miller KL, Shafman TD, Marks LB. A practical approach to pulmonary risk assessment in the radiotherapy of lung cancer. Semin Radiat Oncol 2004; 14:298–307.

124. Liao ZX, Travis EL, Tucker SL. "Damage and morbidity from pneumonitis after irradiation of partial volumes of mouse lung." Int J Radiat Oncol Biol Phys 1995; 32.
125. Travis EL, Liao ZX, Tucker SL. Spatial heterogeneity of the volume effect for radiation pneumonitis in mouse lung. Int J Radiat Oncol Biol Phys 1997; 38.
126. Khan MA, Van Dyk J, Yeung IW, and Hill RP. Partial volume rat lung irradiation; assessment of early DNA damage in different lung regions and effect of radical scavengers. Radiother Oncol 2003; 66:95–102.
127. Bradley J, Deasy J, El Naqa I, Lindsay P, Hope A, Bosch W, Matthews J, Sause W, Graham M. Predictors of Lung Toxicity from the RTOG 9311 Radiation Dose Escalation Trial: GTV Position is Important (abstr.). Int J Rad Onc Bio Phys 63:S40.
128. Amosson CM, Teh BS, Van TJ, Uy N, Huang E, Mai WY, Frolov A, Woo SY, Chiu JK, Carpenter LS, Lu HH, Grant, 3rd HH, Butler EB. Dosimetric predictors of xerostomia for head-and-neck cancer patients treated with the smart (simultaneous modulated accelerated radiation therapy) boost technique. Int J Radiat Oncol Biol Phys 2003; 56:136–144.
129. Pavy JJ, Denekamp J, Letschert J, Littbrand B, Mornex F, Bernier J, Gonzales-Gonzales D, Horiot JC, Bolla M, Bartelink H. EORTC Late Effects Working Group. Late effects toxicity scoring: the SOMA scale. Radiother Oncol 1995; 35:17–60.
130. Dawes C. Circadian rhythms in human salivary flow rate and composition. J Physiol 1972; 220:529–545.
131. Brizel DM, Light K, Zhou SM, Marks LB. Conformal radiation therapy treatment planning reduces the dose to the optic structures for patients with tumors of the paranasal sinuses. Radiother Oncol 1999; 51:215–218.
132. Johnson JT, Ferretti GA, Nethery WJ, Valdez IH, Fox PC, Ng D, Muscoplat CC, Gallagher SC. Oral pilocarpine for post-irradiation xerostomia in patients with head and neck cancer. N Engl J Med 1993; 329:390–395.
133. Chao KS. Protection of salivary function by intensity-modulated radiation therapy in patients with head and neck cancer. Semin Radiat Oncol 2002; 12:20–25.
134. Eisbruch A, Ten Haken RK, Kim HM, Marsh LH, Ship JA. Dose, volume, and function relationships in parotid salivary glands following conformal and intensity-modulated irradiation of head and neck cancer. Int J Radiat Oncol Biol Phys 1999; 45:577–587.
135. Roesink JM, Moerland MA, Battermann JJ, Hordijk GJ, Terhaard CH. Quantitative dose-volume response analysis of changes in parotid gland function after radiotherapy in the head-and-neck region. Int J Radiat Oncol Biol Phys 2001; 51:938–946.
136. Blanco AI, Chao KSC, El Naqa I, Franklin GE, Zakarian, K., Vicic, M., Deasy, J.O. Dose-volume modeling of salivary function in patients with head and neck cancer receiving radiation therapy. Int J Radiat Oncol Biol Phys 2005; 62:1055-1069.
137. Johnson TD, Taylor JM, Ten Haken RK, Eisbruch A. A Bayesian mixture model relating dose to critical organs and functional complication in 3D conformal radiation therapy. Biostatistics 2005; 6:615–632.
138. Scrimger RA, Stavrev P, Parliament MB, Field C, Thompson H, Stavreva N, Fallone BG. Phenomenologic model describing flow reduction for parotid gland irradiation with intensity-modulated radiotherapy: evidence of significant recovery effect. Int J Radiat Oncol Biol Phys 2004; 60:178–185.
139. Huang EH, Pollack A, Levy L, Starkschall G, Dong L, Rosen I, Kuban DA. Late rectal toxicity: dose-volume effects of conformal radiotherapy for prostate cancer. Int J Radiat Oncol Biol Phys 2002; 54:1314–1321.
140. Deasy JO. Multiple local minima in radiotherapy optimization problems with dose-volume constraints. Med Phys 1997; 24:1157–1161.
141. Choi B, Deasy JO. The generalized equivalent uniform dose function as a basis for intensity-modulated treatment planning. Phys Med Biol 2002; 47:3579–3589.
142. Romeijn HE, Ahuja RK, Dempsey JF, Kumar A, Li JG. A novel linear programming approach to fluence map optimization for intensity modulated radiation therapy treatment planning. Phys Med Biol 2003; 48:3521–3542.

143. Schilstra C, Meertens H. Calculation of the uncertainty in complication probability for various dose-response models, applied to the parotid gland. Int J Radiat Oncol Biol Phys 2001; 50:147–158.
144. Deasy JO, Chao KS, Markman J. Uncertainties in model-based outcome predictions for treatment planning. Int J Radiat Oncol Biol Phys 2001; 51:1389–1399.
145. Deasy JO, Fowler JF. The radiobiology of intensity modulated radiation therapy. in Intensity Modulated Radiation Therapy: A Clinical Perspective, edited by A.J. Mundt, Roeske, J.C. BC Decker: Hamilton, 2005.
146. Thames HD, Hendry JH. Fractionation in Radiotherapy. New York: Taylor & Francis; 1987.
147. Lyman JT. Normal tissue complication probabilities: variable dose per fraction. Int J Radiat Oncol Biol Phys 1992; 22:247–250.
148. Schultheiss T. The controversies and pitfalls in modeling normal tissue radiation injury/damage. Semin Radiat Oncol 2001; 11:210–214.
149. Bradley J, Graham MV, Winter K, Purdy JA, Komaki R, Roa WH, Ryu JK, Bosch W, Emami B. Toxicity and outcome results of RTOG 9311: a phase I–II dose-escalation study using three-dimensional conformal radiotherapy in patients with inoperable non-small-cell lung carcinoma. Int J Radiat Oncol Biol Phys 2005; 61.

12 Optimization of Radiotherapy Using Biological Parameters

Yusung Kim and Wolfgang Tomé

Introduction

Most early stage cancers can be cured with either radiotherapy or surgery; however, tumor control for many locally advanced tumors has been unsatisfactory in spite of combined-modality treatments. It has been observed that local recurrence of tumors happens in high-risk tumor subvolumes such as hypoxic tumor subvolumes [1, 2] or regions that contain a large number of highly proliferation-capable clonogens [2, 3]. In an effort to overcome local recurrence, radiation dose boosting techniques have been widely studied. Clinical evidence exists that tumor control can be enhanced using boosting techniques for the following disease sites: head-and-neck (H & N) cancer [4–6], prostate cancer [7, 8], lung cancer [9–11], and liver cancer [12, 13]. Moreover, it has been shown that improved locoregional tumor control is associated with an increased survival rate [14, 15]. For example, Thames et al. [15] have conjectured that a boost dose from 10 to 20% to target volumes (TV) could result in a measurable increase in survival for a cohort of 50–200 patients having high-risk primary tumors. However, this clearly depends on the natural history of disease: In the EORCT trial for breast cancer it was estimated that only one in 34 patients would have benefited from an additional boost above baseline in terms of increased locoregional control. Applying the whole boosting technique to all patients carries the risk of incurring added side effects at no benefit to most patients [16].

Therefore, "selective" boosting based on patient-specific information obtained from functional tumor imaging in which only tumor subvolumes that are at risk for local recurrence will be boosted is clearly of interest. Using mathematical modeling, several investigators explored the benefit of selective boosting [17–20]. For instance, Tomé and Fowler found that selective boosting of tumor subvolumes could result in an increase in tumor control probability (TCP) by up to 20% if 60–80% of the tumor volume can be boosted to 20–30% above the minimal peripheral prescription dose [17]. Recent progress in functional and molecular imaging allows recording of information at the physiological and cellular level. Image-guided, intensity-modulated radiotherapy (IG-IMRT) allows one to minimize

M.P. Mehta et al. (eds.), *Radiation Oncology Advances.*

geometric uncertainties [21] and therefore allows one to improve physical conformality and target localization, even at the tumor subvolume level [22–24].

As a result of this progress, efforts are currently on the way to integrate biological information into radiotherapy treatment planning with the aim of boosting high-risk tumor subvolumes for H & N cancer [22, 24], cervical cancer (cf. [22] and reference there in), nonsmall cell lung cancer (NSCLC) (cf. [22] and reference there in), and prostate cancer [23, 25]. To achieve selective boosting based on biological information, three requirements have to be met: (1) a highly conformal radiotherapy delivery technique (e.g., IG-IMRT) needs to be available, (2) functional or molecular imaging of the target needs to possible, and (3) a method to decide on a boosting level needs to be available that is based on the information obtained from functional or molecular imaging. The majority of present approaches determine the boosting level for high-risk tumor subvolumes based on clinical experience (cf. [24, 25, 26]). Therefore, the selective boosting regions are patient-specific but the boosting level is still based on clinical data obtained from the patient population cohort.

The following question therefore arises: How can the boost dose be based on *patient-specific* information for high-risk tumor subvolumes while avoiding injury to normal tissues? One approach is to prescribe physical dose and add a nonuniform boosting component that corresponds to a companion functionally based risk image intensity. This nonuniform component can have discrete dose levels (cf. [27]) or a continuously varying dose to each voxel called "dose painting by numbers" as proposed by Bentzen [28]. These approaches essentially determine the patient-specific boosting level according to an image intensity map. Thus, accurate information of voxel intensity and robust geometric reproducibility at the voxel level are required. All these approaches assume that there exists a monotonic relation between functional image intensity and some high-risk tumor characteristic. In addition, it is noted that this image-intensity-based selective boosting approach also uses dose–volume-based objective functions.

An alternative and equivalent way to boost the dose level based on patient-specific information is to use radiobiological models – e.g., TCP, normal tissue complication probability (NTCP), and an objective function that is a combination of TCP and NTCP such as uncomplicated tumor control probability (UTCP). As remarked by Brahme and colleagues [29, 30], biologically optimized treatment planning has the potential to strike the right balance between cure and complications. Therefore, we present what follows a biological optimization strategy that is based on the possible risk characteristics for local recurrence in *tumor subvolumes* rather than in individual tumor voxels and treatment plans are optimized using *biological objective functions that are region-specific, rather than voxel specific*. This approach has been termed "Risk-Adaptive Optimization" by Kim and Tomé [31]. In addition, we suggest that the risk characteristics for local recurrence could be identified and quantified using functional imaging or functional imaging and biopsy data. In this chapter, we present the framework of this risk-adaptive, selective boosting strategy, referred to as "risk-adaptive radiotherapy" in the following.

The Need for Optimization Based on Biological Parameters

Presently, most IMRT optimization systems use dose–volume-based objective functions. The majority of boosting trials have also employed these dose–volume-based objective functions in which boosting doses are determined from retrospective population-based data. More recently, selective boosting strategies based on biological information have been considered and the issue of the most effective way of selective boosting is emerging as a topic of interest. Functional-image-guided selective boosting allows one to target high-risk tumor subvolumes according to their risk characteristics with the aim of reducing the risk of tumor recurrence. Essentially, this approach aims to incorporate personalized, radiobiological information into IMRT planning. Hence, the inherent limitations of dose–volume-based optimization become an issue when it is employed in selective boosting strategies based on biological information that require highly inhomogeneous dose patterns.

In contrast to a dose–volume-based optimization, radiobiological-model-based optimization can effectively produce dose patterns for the following reasons. First, biological objective functions can reflect a personalized inhomogeneity of tumor risk and normal tissue toxicity, while a dose–volume-based optimization pursues a homogeneous dose to the highly inhomogeneous tumor cell organization. This occurs because radiobiological objective functions include to some degree the volume dependence of organs to radiation injury as well as their internal structural organizations (albeit in a limited way) in terms of functional subunits (FSU). More importantly, a radiobiological objective function allows one to include directly the possible physiological characteristics of different tumor subvolumes. Secondly, using radiobiological objective functions, one can find the optimal biological trade-off between tumor cure and normal tissue complications by using radiobiological integration methods like UTCP rather than the mechanical summation of the objective values from target volumes (TV) and organs at risk (OAR), which are employed in dose–volume-based IMRT optimization. Using radiobiological objective functions in the optimization process therefore allows one to directly incorporate the concepts of tumor control probability and normal tissue tolerance into the optimization process rather than having to use surrogate physical dose objectives to find an optimal solution. As proposed by Munro and Gilbert, a tumor is controlled if and only if all subtumor regions of the tumor are controlled, since tumors can be viewed as the ultimate parallel structures [32]. With regard to the normal tissue, the most sensitive OAR governs the overall objective values for OAR. In section "Subvolume-Based Radiobiological Models", a method to strike an optimal biological balance between tumor control and normal tissue toxicity using UTCP is presented. Lastly, it is well known that both tumor and normal tissue dose–response curves have a sigmoid (i.e., "S") shape [33]. Therefore, since the dose–response curve is clearly nonlinear, it can only be locally replaced with a linear response over a narrow dose range. Hence, as remarked by Tanderup et al. [34], it is suboptimal simply to add boosting dose in a linearly proportional fashion to the image intensity since we do not have proven clinical evidence for this specific relation apart from the fact that a linear dependence is the simplest approximation to any correlation. In contrast, risk-adaptive radiotherapy reflects high-risk tumor subvolumes by using a sigmoid shape dose–response model.

Furthermore, Thorwarth et al. [35] have recently suggested a possible way of obtaining patient-specific TCP parameters from functional image information. Thorwarth et al. [35] clinically verified a high correlation of hypoxia-perfusion patterns (from ^{18}F-FMISO-PET) and RT treatment outcome ($p < 0.01$) for H & N cancer, and have presented "TCP – Risk Level" modeling based on functional image information.

Radiobiological Models

As mentioned above, risk-adaptive radiotherapy employs radiobiological models for its objective function, and therefore requires radiobiological models that reflect the dose–response of tumor and normal tissue to radiation insult. In 1936, Holthusen [33] in his seminal paper entitled "Erfahrungen über die Verträglichkeitsgrenze für Röntgenstrahlen und deren Nutzanwendung zur Verhütung von Schäden" showed that dose–response curves for local tumor control and normal tissue reactions have a sigmoid shape. He, furthermore, suggested that the aim of radiotherapy should be to maximize tumor control while at the same time minimizing normal tissue complications which has remained the core goal of radiotherapy to this day, and is also the exact aim of risk-adaptive optimization [33]. To this end he proposed the use of a function called "Heilung" to find the optimal trade-off between local tumor control and normal tissue tolerance, which he obtained as the difference between the dose–response curve for "Leistungsziffer der Tumorvernichtung" (TCP) and the dose–response curve for "Wahrscheinlichkeit für die Entwicklung einer Dauerschädigung" (NTCP) (cf. Bild 5 and 6 in [33]). Clearly, Holthusen [33], in his visionary paper, has proposed the concept of probability of complication-free tumor control (P_+).

To quantify dose–response relationships, several investigators have proposed a number of biomathematical models incorporating both the response of cells to radiation and the organization of cells into FSU. Among them, the Poisson model, the Logistic model, and the Probit model are widely used as standard formulations [cf. 36]. The Lyman model uses the Probit model as the underlying model to describe the sigmoid shape of dose–response relationships.

Although all three models can be employed for tumor control and normal tissue complications, there are different radiobiological characteristics that need to be considered prior to modeling. First, the organization of the FSU must be addressed. For a tumor, a FSU is a single clonogen and therefore tumors are the ultimate parallel structures [32]. A parallel structure (e.g., the kidney and the lung) is defined as having a FSU organization in which the inactivation of a small number of FSU does not lead to loss of organ function and so the functional damage will not occur until a critical number of FSU has been eliminated. In a serial structure (e.g., the intestine and spinal cord), the FSU are organized such that the inactivation of one FSU may cause loss of function in the whole organ. In general, however, normal tissues typically consist of a combination of serial and parallel structure components. Moreover, normal tissue complications are strongly governed by the volume irradiated to high doses. The presence of volume effects in normal tissue has led to several biomathematical formulations of dose–response curves for partial-volume irradiation that employ nonuniform dose–volume histograms (DVH) that characterize the highly inhomogeneous dose distributions in normal tissues.

When considering inhomogeneous dose patterns, one converts the DVH to an equivalent uniform DVH. For this purpose two methods have been proposed: the effective volume method proposed by Kutcher and Burman [37] and the generalized-EUD (*g*EUD) method [38, 39]. Using these DVH-reduction methods, all three standard radiobiological models can be employed for calculating NTCP, along with TCP. It is important to note that when Rancati and colleagues fitted late rectal bleeding data from 547 patients using different NTCP models (Poisson, Logistic, Lyman), they found that the resulting NTCP curves were quite similar. All the models provided similar likelihood values indicating that the simplest model (i.e., Logistic) would describe the data as accurately as more complex models. In the following sections, each model is briefly presented.

Poisson Model

In 1961, Munro and Gilbert [32] derived the Poisson model from the clonogen hypothesis and the random nature of cell killing, and it has widely influenced radiotherapy as well as radiobiology (i.e., Poisson distribution with $n = 0$ [40]). The tumor control probability is simply given by:

$$\mathrm{TCP} = \mathrm{e}^{-\lambda}, \tag{1}$$

where λ refers to the average number of surviving clonogens per tumor after irradiation. This formula has become the standard model of tumor control probability when combined with the linear quadratic model:

$$\mathrm{TCP} = \exp\left[-N_0 \exp\left(-\alpha D - \beta d D + \lambda(T - T_k)\right)\right], \tag{2}$$

where N_0, α, β, λ, T, T_k are the initial number of clonogens, the linear and quadratic coefficients of cell kill, the proliferation rate of clonogens, overall treatment time, and the kickoff time, respectively. The term $\exp(-\alpha D - \beta d D + \gamma(T - T_k))$ refers simply to the surviving fraction of clonogens after total dose (D) (i.e., $D = nd$; n = fraction number, and d = fraction size) has been delivered.

Logistic Model

The Logistic model was introduced into radiobiology by Suit and colleagues [41] and the probability of an event is expressed as:

$$P(u) = \frac{e^u}{1 + e^u}, \tag{3}$$

where $u = a_o + bD$ when treating with a fixed dose per fraction. The parameterized Logistic model is given in (4a). When using the logarithm of the dose as the covariate, the more widely used formulation of this model is given by (4b) (cf. [36]):

$$P(D) = \frac{1}{1 + \exp\left[4\gamma_{50}\left(1 - \frac{D}{D_{50}}\right)\right]} \tag{4a}$$

$$P(D) = \frac{1}{1 + \left(\frac{D_{50}}{D}\right)^{4\gamma_{50}}} \tag{4b}$$

where $P(D)$ is the responding probability as a function of dose, D.

In spite of being a phenomenological model without any biomechanical background, its simplicity and flexibility make the Logistic model very useful for the modeling of response to therapy, and a recent comparison study for NTCP models suggested that it yields results similar to that of the Lyman model [42].

Bentzen and Tucker [36] reparametrized all three standard dose–response models including (2) in terms of parameters (D_{50} and γ_{50}) which are directly related to the observed dose–response data (cf. Table 1 in [36]). The parameter, D_{50}, refers to the dose yielding a 50% dose–response for a specific end point to either tumor control or normal tissue complications. With regard to the steepness of the dose–response curve, the normalized dose–response gradient, γ_{50}, proposed by Brahme is widely used and represents the increase in response in percentage points with regard to a 1% increase in dose at the position of D_{50}.

Probit Model

The Probit model has been introduced into radiobiology by Holthusen [33]. In fact, Holthusen [33] suggested that the sigmoid shape of the dose–response curve could be interpreted as a cumulative distribution function (CDF). When assuming a normal distribution of the radiosensitivities and no threshold, the CDF can be expressed in terms of the error function:

$$\mathrm{CDF}(x) = \frac{1}{\sqrt{2\pi}}\int_{-\infty}^{x} e^{-u^2/2}\,du = \frac{1}{2}\left(1 + \mathrm{erf}\frac{x}{\sqrt{2}}\right), \tag{5}$$

where the mean μ and the variance σ have values of 0 and 1, respectively. Just as the Logistic model, the Probit model is a phenomenological dose–response model. The advantage of phenomenological models is that their mathematical simplicity makes them easy to use when analyzing clinical data.

The Lyman Model for Normal Tissue Complications

Lyman [43] fitted this Probit model to NTCP and derived the so-called Lyman model that requires three parameters.

$$\mathrm{NTCP}(D,v) = \frac{1}{\sqrt{2\pi}}\int_{-\infty}^{t} \mathrm{e}^{-x^2/2}\mathrm{d}x,$$
$$t(D,v) = \frac{D - D_{50}(v)}{mD_{50}(v)}, \tag{6}$$
$$D_{50}(v) = \frac{D_{50}(1)}{v^n},$$

where $D_{50}(1)$ is the dose to the whole organ that leads to a complication probability of 50%. The value of ν represents the fraction of the organ irradiated to the uniform dose (D). The parameter, n, denotes the volume-effect parameter. Here, volume effect refers to the volume of tissue that is irradiated and is an important determinant of clinical tolerance without having any influence on tissue sensitivity per unit volume. When n is near 1, the volume effect is large and when it is near 0, the volume effect is small. The third parameter, m, is related to the normalized slope of the dose–response curve through the relation $m = 1/(\sqrt{2\pi}\gamma_{50})$ [44]. One possible DVH-reduction technique that has been suggested by Kutcher and Burman [37] uses the effective volume (v_{eff}) concept to reduce the inhomogeneous normal tissue DVH to an equivalent uniform one in which the effective volume is irradiated to the maximum dose. The combination of this DVH-reduction method with the Lyman model is referred to as the Lyman–Kutcher–Burman (LKB) model. The effective volume (v_{eff}), irradiated to the maximum dose (D_{max}), is calculated by assuming that the bin-dose in each bin follows the dose–response relationship for the whole organ:

$$v_{\mathrm{eff}} = \sum_{i=1}^{N} v_i \left(D_i \big/ D_{\max} \right)^{1/n}, \tag{7}$$

where v_i denotes the fractional volume of the ith dose-bin whose dose value is denoted by D_i.

Niemierko [38, 39] has suggested the concept of the generalized-EUD (gEUD) as an alternative DVH-reduction method. Rancati et al. [42] have shown that the gEUD concept is equivalent to the LKB when coupled with Lyman model parameters.

$$\mathrm{gEUD} = \left(\sum_i v_i D_i^{1/n} \right)^n, \tag{8}$$

where v_i and D_i again denote the fractional volume and the bin-dose at the ith-bin of DVH, and n refers to the volume-effect parameter of the Lyman model.

Uncomplicated Tumor Control Modeling

The integrated probability concept (i.e., probability of complication-free tumor control (P_+)) for tumor control and normal tissue toxicity was proposed by Ågren et al. [45] in 1990 from general statistics and was followed by biophysical modeling studies by Källman et al. [29]. Ågren [45] presented the probability of complication-free tumor control (P_+) as:

$$P_+ = P(B) - P(IB), \tag{9}$$

where $P(B)$ denotes the probability of benefit (TCP), and $P(IB$ refers to the probability of having both tumor control and normal tissue complications. There are two limiting cases for which P_+ can be expressed in a simple equation in terms of TCP and NTCP. The first limiting case assumes that the tumor control is independent of normal tissue complications; in this case P_+ is known as the UTCP:

$$\mathrm{UTCP} = \mathrm{TCP}(1 - \mathrm{NTCP}). \tag{10}$$

In the second limiting case, normal tissue complications and tumor control are totally correlated, i.e., an occurring normal tissue complication will always be connected to tumor control; in this case P_+ is obtained as the difference of TCP and NTCP, as proposed by Holthusen [33]. Hence, P_+ = TCP − NTCP. A more general expression of P_+ can be obtained by forming a linear combination of these two limiting cases that we call generalized UTCP (UTCP_δ):

$$\mathrm{UTCP}_\delta = \mathrm{TCP} - \mathrm{NTCP} + \delta \mathrm{NTCP}[1 - \mathrm{TCP}], \tag{11}$$

where the correlation parameter, δ, is the estimated fraction of patients for which tumor and normal tissue response are statistically independent ($0.0 \le \delta \le 1.0$). This definition implies that for a correlation parameter, $\delta = 0$, the genetic radio-characteristics (susceptibility or resistance) to radiation are the same for both tumor and normal tissue, i.e., all patients may suffer normal tissue complications in the attempt to achieve local tumor control.

Biological Optimization

Subvolume-Based Radiobiological Models

Subvolume-Based TCP Model

In our implementation of risk-adaptive radiotherapy, we have chosen to work with a phenomenological Logistic TCP model that has been described above in (4b):

$$\mathrm{TCP}(D) = \frac{1}{1 + \left(\frac{D_{50}}{D}\right)^{4\gamma_{50}}}, \tag{12}$$

where the two parameters D_{50} and γ_{50} are determined from clinical data. D_{50} is the dose that yields a tumor control probability of 50%. This model strictly applies to tumors that receive a uniform dose, D. We assume that D_{50} and γ_{50} can be determined for different tumor types using either biopsies or functional imaging techniques. If we think of our tumor or target as being composed of R different risk regions each receiving a uniform dose D_j, then the overall expected TCP will be the product of the expected TCP for each individual risk region:

$$\mathrm{TCP} = \prod_{j=1}^{R} [\mathrm{TCP}(D_j)]^{v_j}, \tag{13}$$

where v_j is the fractional volume of the jth subvolume of the tumor (cf. [31] for the proof), and R denotes the total number of tumor subvolumes. Since tumors are the ultimate parallel structures, a tumor is controlled if and only if all tumor subvolumes are controlled [32]. In what follows, let us now assume that we have in subvolume j an inhomogeneous dose distribution, $\{D_i^j, v_i^j\}_{i=1}^k$, where v_i^j is the fractional volume of subvolume j receiving the constant total dose, D_i^j, then the expected TCP for subregion j is given by:

$$\mathrm{TCP}_j(\{D_i^j, v_i^j\}) = \prod_{i=1}^{k} \left[\frac{1}{1 + \left(\frac{D_{50}^j}{D_i^j} \right)^{4\gamma_{50}^j}} \right]^{v_i^j}, \text{ where } \sum_{i=1}^{k} v_i^j = 1, \tag{14}$$

where D_i^j is constant across the tumor voxels having a fractional volume of v_i^j. In (14), we have made the generalization that each of the R-subvolumes may have a different D_{50}^j and γ_{50}^j that are based on the physiological tumor risk make-up. This approach assumes of course that we have a method to estimate the different D_{50}^j and γ_{5C}^j either from population-based clinical data or from individual tumor-based assessments particular to each patient. Therefore, the overall tumor subvolume-based TCP is given by:

$$\mathrm{TCP}(\{D\}) = \prod_{j=1}^{R} [\mathrm{TCP}_j(\{D_i^j, v_i^j\})]^{v_j} = \prod_{j=1}^{R} \left(\prod_{i=1}^{k} \left[\frac{1}{1 + \left(\frac{D_{50}^j}{D_i^j} \right)^{4\gamma_{50}^j}} \right]^{v_i^j} \right)^{v_j} \tag{15}$$

where $\{D\}$ denotes the inhomogeneous dose distribution in the entire tumor. The detailed derivations of this subvolume-based TCP and the gradient of the TCP function needed for risk-adaptive optimization using inverse planning are given in [31]. To summarize, in our expression for the overall subvolume-based TCP of a tumor, we hypothesize that each of the R-tumor-subvolumes has different D_{50}^j and γ_{50}^j

values that are based on the make-up of the tumor subvolume and that these values can be obtained from clinical data. Therefore, the subvolume-based TCP model presented in (15) represents one possible way of formulating a phenomenological TCP function for personalized risk-adaptive radiation therapy.

Voxel-Based NTCP Model

Again, for simplicity, we have chosen to work with a phenomenological Logistic NTCP model that has been presented in (4b). To employ the clinical data fitted to the LKB model, γ_{50} was simply replaced by $1/(\sqrt{2\pi}m)$.. This can be derived straightforwardly from the LKB model by simply evaluating the dose gradient at $D = D_{50}$. We have assumed no volume effect across individual normal tissue voxels. Hence, our phenomenological NTCP is given by:

$$\mathrm{NTCP} = \frac{1}{1+\left(\frac{D_{50}}{D}\right)^{4/\sqrt{2\pi}m}}, \tag{16}$$

where D_{50} and m are again determined from clinical data fitted using the LKB model. Of course it is well known that with the substitution for γ_{50}, the Logistic model becomes equivalent to the LKB model with no volume effect (i.e., $n = 0$). Intuitively, this equivalence is clear since we have simply reparametrized one cumulative probability function to match another. Given Q different OARs, the overall NTCP can be expressed as the product of the expected NTCP for the individual OAR:

$$\mathrm{NTCP} = 1 - \prod_{j=1}^{Q}[1 - \mathrm{NTCP}(\{D_i^j, v_i^j\})], \tag{17}$$

where Q refers to the number of OARs. In our formulation of NTCP, all complications have an equal likelihood of occurrence if their probabilities to manifest are equal. As a result, the overall NTCP is governed by the most sensitive OAR rather than the lowest value of NTCP. Equation (17) also avoids the problem of zero overall NTCP if one of the OARs has a zero NTCP. Given a number of $\{\mathrm{OAR}_j\}_{j=1}^{Q}$, let us now assume that we have in OAR_j the inhomogeneous dose distribution, $\{D_i^j, v_i^j\}_{i=1}^{I}$, where v_i^j is the fractional volume of OAR_j receiving the constant total dose, D_i^j, then the expected NTCP for OAR_j is given by:

$$\mathrm{NTCP}(\{D_i^j, v_i^j\}) = 1 - \prod_{i=1}^{I}(1 - \mathrm{NTCP}(D_i^j))^{v_i^j}, \tag{18}$$

where,

$$\mathrm{NTCP}(D_i^j) = \frac{1}{1+\left(\frac{D_{50}^j}{D_i^j}\right)^{4/\sqrt{2\pi}m^j}},$$

$$\sum_{i=1}^{I} v_i^j = 1.$$

Thus, the overall voxel-based NTCP for Q organs at risk is given by:

$$\mathrm{NTCP}(\{D\}) = 1 - \prod_{j=1}^{Q}\left[1 - \left(1 - \prod_{i=1}^{I}(1 - \mathrm{NTCP}(D_i^j))^{v_i^j}\right)\right] \tag{19}$$

where $\{D\}$ denotes the inhomogeneous dose distribution in the entire irradiated volume. The derivation of the gradient calculation for NTCP that is required to carry out inverse treatment planning is given in [31].

Biological Objective Function UTCP$_\delta$

We have chosen the P_+ model that we have presented in (11) as our objective function for risk-adaptive optimization. As discussed above, there are two limiting cases for P_+. In the first one every cure leads to a complication, i.e., $\delta = 0$, and P_+ is called $UTCP_0$:

$$\mathrm{UTCP}_0(\{D\}) = \mathrm{TCP}(\{D\}) - \mathrm{NTCP}(\{D\}). \tag{20}$$

In the second limiting case, cure and the induction of a complication are uncorrelated, i.e., $\delta = 1.0$, and P_+ is called UTCP, denoted by $UTCP_1$, and which is given by:

$$\mathrm{UTCP}_1(\{D\}) = \mathrm{TCP}(\{D\})[1 - \mathrm{NTCP}(\{D\})]. \tag{21}$$

Using (15) and (19), the subvolume- and voxel-based $UTCP_1$ is given by:

$$\mathrm{UTCP}_1(\{E\}) = \prod_{j=1}^{R} \mathrm{TCP}(\{D_i^j, v_i^j\})^{v_j}\left[1 - \left\{1 - \prod_{j=1}^{Q}[1 - \mathrm{NTCP}(\{D_i^j, v_i^j\})]\right\}\right] \tag{22}$$

The gradient of UTCP$_1$ that has been employed in risk-adaptive optimization has been derived in [31]. We have shown in [31] that the value of δ influences risk-adaptive optimization only weakly and that it is, therefore, sufficient to work either with UTCP$_0$ or UTCP$_1$. As one can see from Fig. 1, the function UTCP$_0$ minorizes all objective functions with a value for $0 < \delta < 1$, while UTCP$_1$ majorizes them. Furthermore, working with UTCP$_1$ is advantageous since it can be transformed into a convex objective function, and hence a globally optimal solution can be found (cf. [46]).

Example: Risk-Adaptive Radiotherapy applied to Prostate Cancer

Prostate cancer is the second leading cause of cancer deaths in men [47]. With regard to local relapse after radiotherapy of prostate cancer, it has been reported that biopsy-proven local relapses after definitive radiotherapy occur in 19–65% of patients treated for stage T1–T3 disease [8]. Relapses mostly happen at the original

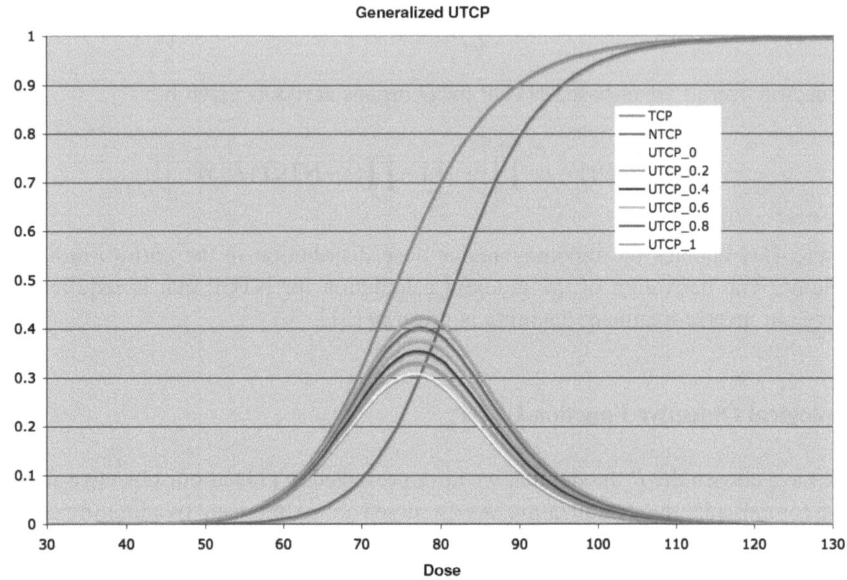

Fig. 1 Generalized UTCP$_\delta$ for values of δ ranging from 0 to 1.0 in 0.2. The curve of TCP was modeled for a high-risk tumor with moderate slope (i.e., D_{50} = 74.5 and γ_{50} = 2.0). We modeled the NTCP curve with the parameters for rectum (i.e., D_{50} = 81.9, m = 0.19, and n = 1.0)

tumor location within the PTV [23, 48]. Furthermore, several investigators have demonstrated that local relapse is associated with a significant increase in the risk of metastatic disease [49, 50], and have suggested a cause-and-effect relationship between these phenomena [50, 51].

Hence, the rationale of risk-adaptive optimization for prostate cancer in targeting local relapse regions is threefold. First, locoregional tumor control rates for prostate cancer can be increased with dose boosting [7, 8]. Therefore, it is of benefit to focus on intraprostatic lesions such as the original tumor nodules. Second, a low α/β -ratio, 1.5 Gy, as remarked by Fowler et al. [52], implies high fractionation sensitivity if higher doses per fractions are given (cf. also [53]). Lastly, the slope of tumor control curves is frequently less steep than those for normal tissue injury. This in effect limits the toxicity-free dose boosting and the ability to optimize local tumor control [8, 15, 54]. Several authors suggested that a shallow slope of tumor control curves could be thought of as a composite of steeper curves, corresponding to tumor subvolumes with different tumor risk [6, 15, 54]. Thus, risk-adaptive optimization using the "selective" boosting scheme has the potential to maximize local tumor control and therefore could minimize local relapse. Levegrün et al. [55] have identified D_{50} values for low-risk, intermediate-risk, and high-risk prostate cancer. Based on the values found by Levegrürn and colleagues [55], we have carried out a number of risk adaptive optimizations (for complete details the reader is referred to [31]). The result of one of these risk-adaptive optimizations assuming that the nodule exhibits high-risk characteristics, while the remainder of the PTV exhibits intermediate risk characteristics is shown in Fig. 2.

As one can see from Fig. 2, risk-adaptive optimization allows one to significantly increase the dose in high-risk tumor subvolumes above the minimal peripheral dose without violating normal tissue constraints.

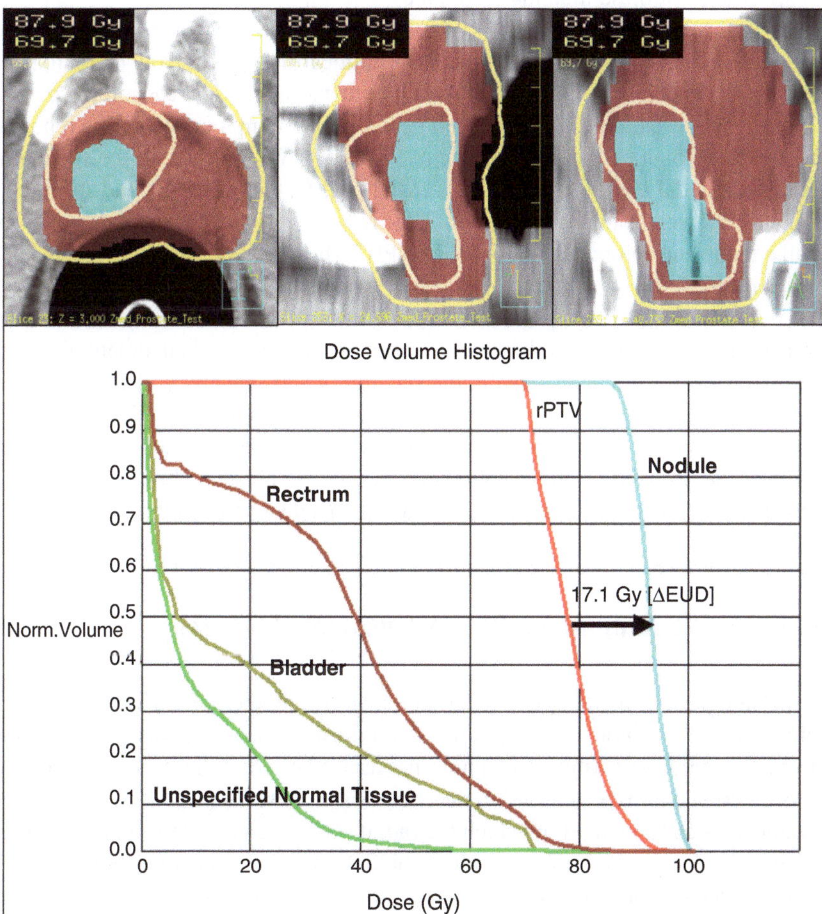

Fig. 2 Isodose maps and dose–volume histograms for a single nodule assumed to exhibit high-risk characteristics, while the remainder of the PTV is assumed to exhibit intermediate-risk characteristics

Impact of Diagnostic Accuracy on Biological Optimization

Functional Imaging in Oncology

The functional imaging modalities positron emission tomography (PET), single-photon-emission CT (SPECT), and functional MRI techniques play a central role in oncology. In particular, these functional imaging modalities have been employed in general oncology mainly for tumor diagnosis [56, 57], tumor staging [58, 59], and assessment of the therapeutic response [58, 59]. For these applications, the sensitivity and specificity of a functional imaging technique is clearly of importance, and therefore a lot of effort has been focused on the assessment of the sensitivity and specificity of these imaging techniques.

For instance, Gambhir et al. [60] have found that the average sensitivity and specificity of FDG-PET across all oncology applications ranges from 88 up to 93% based on the evaluation of scans of 14, 264 patients. In cervical cancer, Rose et al. [61] have suggested that FDG-PET can detect pelvic lymph nodes with a reported sensitivity of 85–90% and a specificity of 95–100%. With respect to the staging of mediastinal nodal metastasis in patients with NSCLC, the sensitivity and specificity of FDG-PET were found to be 91 and 75%, respectively [62]. For the detection of locally recurrent colorectal tumors, FDG-PET showed 98% sensitivity and 90% specificity [63].

While functional imaging modalities have been in use since the mid-1970s, the application of these in radiotherapy has been stimulated by their potential use in selective boosting strategies. Again, the specificity and sensitivity of the employed functional imaging is of importance since these factors will have a definite impact on the expected tumor control probability as well as on expected normal tissue complication probability. In the following section, we present a brief review of the application of functional or molecular imaging in selective boosting.

Theragnostic Imaging in Risk-Adaptive Radiotherapy

As the integration of biological information into radiotherapy advances, we will include more and more cellular/molecular information as well as physiological information into the treatment planning process. The term “theragnostic imaging” has been coined by Bentzen [28] to describe this process. Bentzen [28] has defined theragnostics as “a method by which the radiation dose can be delivered in the four dimensions of space and time to achieve the optimum outcome after radiotherapy.” It is conceivable that theragnostic imaging might show high-risk tumor subvolumes within the target volume. High-risk tumor characteristics that can potentially be detected using theragnostic imaging include hypoxia, cellular proliferation, and angiogenesis. Increased cellular proliferation and hypoxia have been identified as adverse prognostic factors. In particular, hypoxia has been noted to exist in nonsmall cell lung cancer (NSCLC), squamous-cell carcinoma of H & N (HNSCC) (a hypoxic fraction of up to 80%), and cervical cancer (a hypoxic fraction of up to 50%) [64]. Furthermore, Brizel et al. [65] have found that tumor hypoxia is associated with an increase in the incidence of distant metastasis besides notably poorer local control. As a theragnostic imaging modality for hypoxia, ^{18}F-FMISO-PET, ^{60}Cu-ATSM-PET, and BOLD-MRI have been widely investigated. With regard to tumor proliferation (i.e., overall treatment time) – an important issue for HNSCC – the most promising marker is ^{18}F-labeled fluorothymine (FLT) [66]. These theragnostic-imaging modalities could be used to decide by how much to boost as well as where to boost. As mentioned above, current approaches for using theragnostic imaging in selective boosting can be categorized into two groups: dose painting by number (i.e., voxel intensity-based boosting) [22, 67, 68] and selective boosting of tumor subvolumes (i.e., subvolume-based boosting) [17, 23, 24, 27] – both of these strategies are being introduced into clinical practice [22, 24, 25]. In either of these two approaches to theragnostics, the diagnostic accuracy (sensitivity and specificity) is crucial to achieve optimum clinical outcome.

The Impact of Imaging Sensitivity on Risk-Adaptive Radiotherapy

Selective boosting based on theragnostic imaging has been proposed as promising strategy for locally advanced tumor sites. However, the theragnostic imaging accuracy (sensitivity and specificity) for high-risk subvolumes has not been adequately studied. Sensitivity is the probability of correctly identifying a voxel as a disease-bearing voxel, while specificity is the probability that a voxel identified as nondisease-bearing is truly a normal voxel (cf. Fig. 3). As shown in Fig. 3, there is an inverse relationship between sensitivity and specificity, that is, either one can be increased by decreasing the other. Therefore, it is important to evaluate the impact of sensitivity and specificity

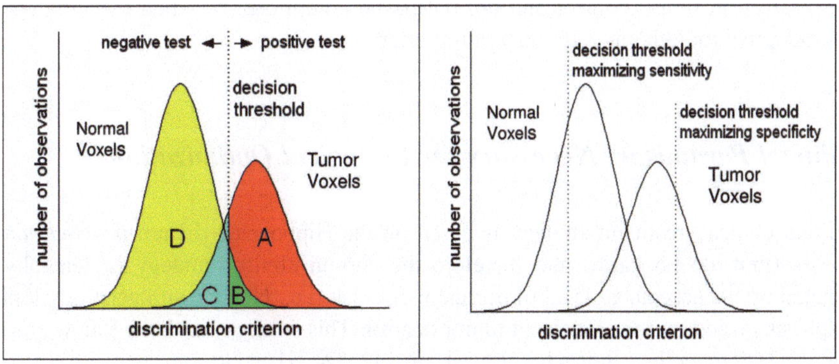

Fig. 3 Shows sensitivity (true positive fraction = $A/(A + C)$) and specificity (true negative faction $D/(B + D)$) for tumor voxels (red bell-shaped curve) and normal tissue voxels (yellow bell-shaped curve). The diagram on the right shows the interplay between sensitivity and specificity for decision-making. (Diagrams adapted from Šámal [69])

of a theragnostic imaging modality on a given selective-boosting strategy in which they are employed for target definition, in order to quantify the optimal trade-off between these image qualities for a given selective boosting strategy.

To illustrate the possible impact of sensitivity on TCP, we have performed a number of risk-adaptive optimizations and have calculated the overall TCP for a range of sensitivity scenarios (100–50%) employing an intermediate $\gamma_{50} = 4$. In the risk adaptive radiotherapy concept presented above, it was assumed that we have a sensitivity of 100%. To gain an understanding of the effect of misclassifying high-risk tumor voxels as low-risk tumor voxels (i.e., a loss of sensitivity), we have considered the scenario of a very high-risk nodule ($D_{50} = 84.5$ Gy) that is embedded in an intermediate remainder PTV ($D_{50} = 64.5$ Gy).

In Table 1, we have collected the TCP estimates that correspond to DVH for high-risk tumor subvolume (nodule) and a remainder PTV (rPTV) if the sensitivity ranges from 100 to 50%. Miss-classified high-risk tumor voxels are randomly distributed in the low-risk rPTV and the TCP of those volumes was estimated using the mean dose received by the rPTV. To minimize TCP model dependency, we have employed two TCP models: The logistic model and the linear quadratic Poisson model that was reparameterized such that D_{50} and γ_{50} can be used as the clinical parameters that determine the shape of the dose–response curve (cf. Table 1 in [36]). A sensitivity of 80% and higher shows some benefit employing risk-adaptive radiotherapy for an intermediate slope value ($\gamma_{50} = 4$), when comparing with that of the MSKCC-IMRT dose-escalation trial (prescription dose = 86.5 Gy) (cf. [70]). With regard to using a steep slope ($\gamma_{50} = 8$), we found that a sensitivity of 85% and higher showed a higher overall TCP than the MSKCC-IMRT dose escalation trial (prescription dose = 86.5 Gy). On the other hand, if a population-based low slope ($\gamma_{50} = 2$) is employed, we find that risk-adaptive radiotherapy is almost equivalent to the MSKCC-IMRT dose escalation trial in terms of overall TCP, regardless of sensitivity. As pointed out by Tomé and Fowler [71], if a 1% tumor subvolume is under-dosed by more than 20%, it will start to derive the overall TCP. Therefore, a detailed understanding of the effects of theragnostic accuracy (i.e., sensitivity and specificity) on tumor control and normal tissue complications when carrying out risk-adaptive radiotherapy strategy is important.

Clinical Parameters Necessary for Biological Optimization

Current clinical treatment strategy is based on the Hippocratic dictum *primum non nocere* (first, do no harm) and therefore the chosen clinical strategy is generally dictated by the acceptable level of normal tissue risk (i.e., NTCP) with generally less emphasis placed on the associated tumor control. This strategy has been followed in many NTCP modeling studies for clinical data [42, 72–77] and to some extent has also governed many of the clinical dose–response studies for human tumors [55, 78].

The first NTCP modeling study based on clinical data was started by Burman and coworkers using the LKB model in 1991 [72]. Recently, new NTCP parameters (D_{50}, m, n) from patients' data are emerging for a range of OAR. To give a few

Table 1 The loss of overall tumor control probability (TCP) for each sensitivity level for a gamma (γ_{50}) = 4

	Nodule (TCP (%))		Missing Ran. Vol. (TCP (%))		rPTV (TCP (%))		Overall TCP (%)		IMRT Dose-Escalation 86.5 Gy (TCP (%))	
Sen (%)	LQ-Poisson	Logistic	LQ-Poisson	Logistic	LQ-Poisson	Logistic	LQ-Poisson	Logistic	LQ-Poisson	Logistic
100	96.46	97.40	0.00	0.00	95.23	96.25	95.36	96.37	93.99	93.85
99	96.46	97.40	42.3	42.51	95.23	96.25	95.28	96.29	93.94	93.80
95	96.46	97.40	42.3	42.51	95.23	96.25	94.93	95.93	93.72	93.58
90	96.46	97.40	42.3	42.51	95.23	96.25	94.46	95.45	93.42	93.29
85	96.46	97.40	42.3	42.51	95.23	96.25	93.93	94.91	93.09	92.96
80	96.46	97.40	42.3	42.51	95.23	96.25	93.34	94.31	92.73	92.58
75	96.46	97.40	42.3	42.51	95.23	96.25	92.67	93.64	92.31	92.17
70	96.46	97.40	42.3	42.51	95.23	96.25	91.92	92.87	91.84	91.69
65	96.46	97.40	42.3	42.51	95.23	96.25	91.06	91.99	91.29	91.14
60	96.46	97.40	42.3	42.51	95.23	96.25	90.06	90.98	90.66	90.51
55	96.46	97.40	42.3	42.51	95.23	96.25	88.90	89.79	89.92	89.77
50	96.46	97.40	42.3	42.51	95.23	96.25	87.52	88.40	89.04	88.89

When we use an intermediate slope value ($\gamma_{50} = 4$), risk-adaptive radiotherapy strategy is of benefit from 85% sensitivity when comparing with that of IMRT dose escalation trial (prescription dose = 86.5 Gy) that has been advanced by the Memorial Sloan-Kettering Cancer Center (MSKCC) (cf. [70]). *Sen* sensitivity of theragnostic imaging, *Nodule* high-risk tumor subvolume, *Missing Ran. Vol.* miss-classified high-risk tumor subvolumes that are randomly distributed within rPTV, *rPTV* the remainder of PTV when we exclude the nodule volume from PTV, *LQ-Poisson* a linear quadratic Poisson model, *Logistic* a Logistic model examples, Dawson et al. [73, 74] have evaluated the data of 204 patients with hepatic malignancies using the LKB model and obtained the values: $n = 0.97$, $m = 0.12$, $D_{50} = 39.8$ Gy (for patients with primary liver cancer), $D_{50} = 45.8$ Gy (for patients with liver metastases) for radiation-induced liver disease. With regard to late rectal bleeding, Rancati and colleagues [42] fitted NTCP parameters (D_{50}, m, n) and compared the predicted values using three standard NTCP models: Lyman, Logistic, and Poisson. Their results are as follows (for Lyman, Logistic, and Poisson model, respectively): $D_{50} = 81.9$ Gy, 82.2 Gy, and 87.7 Gy, *slope parameter* = 0.19 (m), 7.85 (k), and 0.51 (γ), $n = 0.23$, 0.24, and 0.23. In the case of thoracic irradiation (e.g., Nonsmall cell lung cancer (NSCLC)), radiation pneumonitis (RP) is a major dose-limiting toxicity. Therefore, a number of NTCP modeling studies for RP have been published along with studies that aim to quantify the impact of clinical parameters such as age and smoking, as well as that of dosimetric and spatial parameters on RP (cf. Refs. [75, 76], and references therein). With regard to acute esophagitis, which becomes an issue during concurrent chemo-radiation therapy for locally advanced NSCLC, Chapet and colleagues [77] have recently published new NTCP parameters (i.e., $D_{50} = 51$, $m = 0.32$, and $n = 0.44$) using the toxicity data obtained form 101 NSCLC patients.

New model parameter values for normal tissue complications are emerging as seen above. However, apart from the literature review by Burman and colleagues in 1991 [72] that has been carried out before the advent of the 3D conformal radiation therapy era, subsequent clinical studies have been rarely reviewed for NTCP parameters. The same is true regarding TCP parameters, which have not been reviewed in the literature since the work of Okunieff and colleagues in 1995 [78].

To push biological optimization forward it is necessary to compile the newest model parameters for dose-limiting complications in normal structures, and as mentioned above, new model parameters for normal tissue complication probabilities have started to emerge.

However, with regard to tumor control probability, novel clinical studies are necessary and first attempts at carrying them out are being made by a number of groups (cf. Refs. [22, 24, 25]). First, the clinical correlation studies between TCP and risk level from theragnostic image intensity will need to be established. As mentioned before, Thorwarth and colleagues [35] have shown one possible way to obtain personal TCP parameters from image intensity. Secondly, trials on selective boosting will need to be carried out and a correlation between expected outcomes and observed clinical outcomes will need to be established. These trials will provide the necessary information to make biological optimization a clinical reality.

Summary

Biological optimization can be based on the possible risk characteristics for local recurrence in *tumor sub-volumes* rather than individual tumor voxels and treatment plans may be optimized using *biological objective functions that are region-specific.*

To this end, risk characteristics for local recurrence should be identified and quantified using functional imaging or functional imaging in combination with biopsy data. However, the diagnostic accuracy (sensitivity and specificity) of these functional imaging techniques will have a definite impact on any optimization strategy that uses such imaging information as input. Therefore, a detailed understanding of the effects of theragnostic accuracy (i.e., sensitivity and specificity) on tumor control and normal tissue complications is crucial to achieve optimum clinical outcome.

References

1. Thomlinson RH, Gray LH. The histological structure of some human lung cancers and the possible implications for radiotherapy. Br J Cancer 1955; 9:539–549.
2. Weichselbaum RR, Beckett MA, Schwartz JL, Dritschilo A. Radioresistant tumor cells are present in head and neck carcinoma that recur after radiotherapy. Int J Radiat Oncol Biol Phys 1988; 15:575–579.
3. Bentzen SM. Repopulation in radiation oncology: perspectives of clinical research. Int J Radiat Biol 2003; 79:581–585.
4. Marks JE, Bedwinek JM, Lee F, et al. Dose–response analysis for nasopharyngeal carcinoma: an historical perspective. Cancer 1982; 50:1042–1050.
5. Vikram B, Mishra UB, Strong EW, et al. Patterns of failure in carcinoma of the nasopharynx: I. Failure at the primary site. Int J Radiat Oncol Biol Phys 1985; 11:1455–1459.
6. Bentzen SM. Radiobiological considerations in the design of clinical trials. Radiother Oncol 1994; 32:1–11.
7. Hanks GE, Hanlon AL, Schultheiss TE, et al. Dose escalation with 3D conformal treatment: five year outcomes, treatment optimization, and future directions. Int J Radiat Oncol Biol Phys 1998; 41:501–510.
8. Zelefsky MJ, Leibel SA, Gaudin PB, et al. Dose escalation with three-dimensional conformal radiation therapy affects the outcome in prostate cancer. Int J Radiat Oncol Biol Phys 1998; 41:491–500.
9. Kong FM, Ten Haken RK, Schipper MA, et al. High dose radiation improved local tumor control and overall survival in inoperable/unresectable non-small cell lung cancer: Longterm results from radiation dose escalation study. Int J Radiat Oncol Biol Phys 2005; 63:324–333.
10. Willner J, Baier K, Caragiani E, et al. Dose, volume, and tumor control prediction in primary radiotherapy of non-small-cell lung cancer. Int J Radiat Oncol Biol Phys 2002; 52:382–389.
11. Rengan R, Rosenzweig KE, Venkatraman E, et al. Improved local control with higher doses of radiation in large-volume stage III non-small-cell lung cancer. Int J Radiat Oncol Biol Phys 2004; 60:741–747.
12. Dawson LA, McGinn CJ, Grazia A, et al. Escalated focal liver radiation and concurrent hepatic artery fluorodeoxyuridine for unresectable intrahepatic malignancies. J Clin Oncol 2000; 18:2210–2218.
13. Park HC, Seong J, Han KH, Dose–response relationship in local radiotherapy for hepatocellular carcinoma. Int J Radiat Oncol Biol Phys 2002; 54:150–155.
14. Wadsley JC, Bentzen SM. Investigation of relationship between change in locoregional control and change in overall survival in randomized controlled trials of modified radiotherapy in head-and-neck cancer. Int J Radiat Oncol Biol Phys 2004; 60:1405–1409.
15. Thames HD, Schultheiss TE, Hendry JH, et al. Can modest escalations of dose be detected as increased tumor control? Int J Radiat Oncol Biol Phys 1992; 22:241–246.
16. Bartelink H, Horiot JC, Poortmans P, et al. Recurrence rates after treatment of breast cancer with standard radiotherapy with or without additional radiation. N Eng J Med 2001; S345:1378–1387.

17. Tomé WA, Fowler JF. Selective boosting of tumor subvolumes. Int J Radiat Oncol Biol Phys 2000; 48:593–599.
18. Goitein M, Niemierko A, Okunieff P. The probability of controlling an inhomogeneously irradiated tumor. In: Kaulner K, Carey B, Crellin A, et al., editors. Quantitative imaging in oncology Proceedings of the 19th LH Gray Conference: London: British Institute of Radiology; 1995. p. 25–32.
19. Deasy J. Tumor control probability models for nonuniform dose distributions. In: Paliwal BR, Fowler JF, Herbert DE, et al., editors. Volume & Kinetics in Tumor Control & Normal Tissue Complication. Madison, WI: Medical Physics Publishing; 1997. p. 65–85.
20. Popple RA, Ove R, Shen S. Tumor control probability for selective boosting of hypoxic subvolumes, including the effect of reoxygenation. Int J Radiat Oncol Biol Phys 2002; 54:921–927.
21. Hong TS, Tomé WA, Chappell RJ, et al. The impact of daily setup variations on head-and-neck intensity-modulated radiation therapy. Int J Radiat Oncol Biol Phys 2005; 61:779–788.
22. Vanderstraeten B, Duthoy W, De Gersem W, et al. [18F]fluoro-deoxy-glucose positron emission tomography ([18F]FDG-PET) voxel intensity-based intensity-modulated radiation therapy (IMRT) for head and neck cancer. Radiother Oncol 2006; 79:249–258.
23. De Meerleer G, Villeirs G, Bral S, et al. The manetic resonance detected intraprostatic lesion in prostate cancer: planning and delivery of intensity-modulated radiotherapy. Radiother Oncol 2005; 75:325–333.
24. Chao KSC, Bosch WR, Mutic S, Lewis JS, et al. A novel approach to overcome hypoxic tumour resistance: Cu-ATSM-guided intensity-modulated radiation therapy. Int J Radiat Oncol Biol Phys 2001; 49:1171–1182.
25. van Lin EN, Fütterer JJ, Heijmink SW, et al. IMRT boost dose planning on dominant intraprostatic lesions: gold marker-based three-dimensional fusion of CT with dynamic contrast-enhanced and 1H-spectroscopic MRI. Int J Radiat Oncol Biol Phys 2006; 65:291–303.
26. De Ruysscher D, Wanders S, Minken A, et al. Effects of radiotherapy planning with a dedicated combined PET-CT-simulator of patients with non-small cell lung cancer on dose limiting normal tissues and radiation dose-escalation: a planning study. Radiother Oncol 2005; 77:5–10.
27. Xing L, Cotrutz C, Hunjan S, et al. Inverse planning for functional image-guided intensity-modulated radiation therapy. Phys Med Biol 2002; 47:3567–3578.
28. Bentzen SM. Theragnostic imaging for radiation oncology: dose-painting by numbers. Lancet Oncol 2005; 6:112–117.
29. Källman P, Lind BK, Brahme A. An algorithm for maximizing the probability of complication free tumor control in radiation therapy. Phys Med Biol 1992; 37:871–890.
30. Söderström S, Gustafsson A, Brahme A. Optimization of the dose delivery in few field techniques using radiobiological objective functions. Med Phys 1993; 20:1201–1210.
31. Kim Y, Tomé WA. Risk-adaptive optimization: selective boosting of high-risk tumor subvolumes. Int J Radiat Oncol Biol Phys 2006; 66:1528–1542.
32. Munro TR, Gilbert CW. The relation between tumour lethal doses and the radiosensitivity of tumour cells. Br J Radiol 1961; 34:246–251.
33. Holthusen H. Erfahrungen über die Verträglichkeitsgrenze für Röntgenstrahlen und deren Nutzanwendung zur Verhütung von Schäden. Strahlentherapie 1936; 57:254–269.
34. Tanderup K, Olsen DR, Grau C. Dose painting: art or science? Radiother Oncol 2006; 79: 245–248.
35. Thorwarth D, Eschmann SM, Scheiderbauer J, et al. Kinetic analysis of dynamic 18F-fluoromisonidazole PET correlates with radiation treatment outcome in head-and-neck cancer. BMC Cancer 2005; 5:152.
36. Bentzen SM, Tucker SL. Quantifying the position and steepness of radiation dose–response curves. Int J Radiat Biol 1997; 71:531–542.
37. Kutcher GJ, Burman C. Calculation of complication probability factors for non-uniform normal tissue irradiation: the effective volume method. Int J Radiation Oncology Biol Phys 1989; 16:1623–1630.

38. Niemierko A. A generalized concept of equivalent uniform dose (EUD). Med Phys 1999; 26:1100.
39. Niemierko A. Reporting, and analyzing dose distributions: a concept of equivalent uniform dose. Med Phys 1997; 24:103–110.
40. Kreyszig E. Advanced Engineering Mathematics. Sixth edition, John Wiley & Sons, New York, USA. 1985.
41. Suit HD, Shalek RJ, Wette R. Radiation response of C3H mouse mammary carcinoma evaluated in terms of cellular radiation sensitivity. In Cellular Radiation Biology. Baltimore. Williams & Wilkins 1965. pp 514–530.
42. Rancati T, Fiorino C, Gagliardi G, et al. Fitting late rectal bleeding data using different NTCP models: results from an Italian multi-centric study (AIROPROS0101). Radiother Oncol 2004; 73: 21–32.
43. Lyman JT. Complication probability as assessed from dose–volume histogram. Radiat Res Suppl 1985; 8:S13–S19.
44. Fowler J. Normal tissue complication probabilities: how well do the models work? Phys Med 2001; XVII:24–34.
45. Ågren AK, Brahme A, Turesson I. Optimization of uncomplicated control for head and neck tumors. Int J Radiat Oncol Biol Phys 1990; 19:1077–1085.
46. Romeijn HE, Dempsey JF, Li JG. A unifying framework for multi-criteria fluence map optimization models. Phys Med Biol 2004; 49:1991–2013.
47. American Cancer Society. Cancer Facts and Figures 2005. Atlanta: American Cancer Society; 2005.
48. Cellini N, Morganti AG, Mattiucci GC, et al. Analysis of intraprostatic failures in patients treated with hormonal therapy and radiotherapy: implications for conformal therapy planning. Int J Radiat Oncol Biol Phys 2002; 53:595–599.
49. Kuban DA, El-Mahdi AM, Schellhammer PF. Potential benefit of improved local tumor control in patient with prostate carcinoma. Cancer 1995; 75:2373–2382.
50. Zagars GK, von Eschenbach AC, Ayala AG, et al. The influence of local control on metastatic dissemination of prostate cancer treated by external beam megavoltage radiation therapy. Cancer 1991; 68:2370–2377.
51. Fuks Z, Leibel SA, Wallner KE, et al. The effect of local control on metastatic dissemination in carcinoma of the prostate: long-term results in patients treated with 125-I implantation. Int J Radiat Oncol Biol Phys 1991; 21:537–547.
52. Fowler J, Chappell R, Ritter MA. Is alpha/beta for prostate tumors really low? Int J Radiation Oncology Biol Phys 2001; 50:1021–1031.
53. Bentzen SM, Ritter MA. The alpha/beta ratio for prostate cancer: What is it, really? Radiother Oncol 2005; 76:1–3.
54. Zagars GK, Schultheiss TE, Peters LP. Inter-tumor heterogeneity and radiation dose control curves. Radiother Oncol 1987; 8:353–362.
55. Levegrün SA, Jackson MJ, Zelefsky ES, et al. Risk group dependence of dose–response for biopsy outcome after three-dimensional conformal radiation therapy of prostate cancer. Radiother. Oncol. 2002; 63:11–26.
56. Gregoire V. Is there any future in radiotherapy planning without the use of PET: unraveling the myth. Radiother Oncol 2004; 73:261–263.
57. Antoch G, Saoudi N, Kuehl H, et al. Accuracy of whole-body dual-modality fluorine-18-2-fluoro-2-deoxy-D-glucose positron emission tomography and computed tomography (FDG-PET/CT) for tumor staging in solid tumors: comparison with CT and PET. J Clin Oncol 2004; 22:4357–4368.
58. Apisarnthanarax S, Chao KSC. Current imaging paradigms in radiation oncology. Radiat Res 2005; 163:1–25.
59. Jerusalem G, Hustinx R, Beguin Y, et al. PET scan imaging in oncology. Eur J Cancer 2003; 39:1525–1534.
60. Gambhir SS, Czernin J, Schwimmer DH, et al. A tabulated summary of the FDG PET literature. J Nucl Med 2001; 42:1S–93S.

61. Rose PG, Adler LP, Rodriguez M, et al. Positron emission tomography for evaluating paraaortic nodal metastasis in locally advanced cervical cancer before staging: a surgicopathologic study. J Clin Oncol 1999; 17:41–45.
62. Pieterman RM, van Putten JW, Meuzelaar JJ, et al. Preoperative staging of non-small-cell lung cancer with positron-emission tomography. N Engl J Med 2000; 343:254–261.
63. Staib L, Schirrmeister H, Reske SN, Beger HG. Is 18F-fluorodeoxyglucose positron emission tomography in recurrent colorectal cancer a contribution to surgical decision making? Am J Surg 2000; 180:1–5.
64. Van de Wiele C, Lahorte C, Oyen W, et al. Nuclear medicine imaging to predict response to radiotherapy: a review. Int J Radiation Oncology Biol Phys 2003; 55:5–15.
65. Brizel DM, Scully SP, Harrelson JM, et al. Tumor oxygenation predicts for the likelihood of distant metastases in human soft tissue sarcoma. Cancer Res 1996; 56:941–943.
66. Shields AF, Grierson JR, Dohmen BM, et al. Imaging proliferation in vivo with 18F FLT and positron emission tomography. Nat Med 1998; 4:1334–1336.
67. Alber M, Paulsen F, Eschmann SM, Machulla HJ. On biologically conformal boost dose optimization. Phys Med Biol 2003; 48:N31–N35.
68. Das SK, Miften MM, Zhou S, et al. Feasibility of optimizing the dose distribution in lung tumours using fluorine-18-fluorodeoxyglucose positron emission tomography and single photon emission computed tomography guided dose prescriptions. Med Phys 2004; 31:1452–1461.
69. Šámal M, Statistical decision theory. In regional training workshop, advanced image processing of SPECT studies, Tygerberg Hospital. 2004.
70. Burman CM, Zelefsky MJ, Leibel SA. Treatment planning, dose delivery, and outcome of IMRT For localized prostate cancer. In: Samuel Hellman et al., A Practical Guide To Intensity-Modulated Radiation Therapy. Madison, WI: Medical Physics Publishing; 2003. p. 169–190.
71. Tomé WA, Fowler JF. On cold spots in tumor subvolumes. Med Phys 2002; 29:1590–1598.
72. Burman C, Kutcher GJ, Emami B, et al. Fitting of normal tissue tolerance data to an analytic function. Int J Radiat Oncol Biol Phys 1991; 21:123–135.
73. Dawson LA, Normolle D, Balter JM, et al. Analysis of radiation-induced liver disease using the Lyman NTCP model. Int J Radiat Oncol Biol Phys 2002; 53:810–821.
74. Dawson LA, Ten Haken RK. Partial volume tolerance of the liver to radiation. Semin Radiat Oncol 2005; 15:279–283.
75. Rodrigues G, Lock M, D'Souza D, et al. Prediction of radiation pneumonitis by dose–volume histogram parameters in lung cancer-a systematic review. Radiother Oncol 2004; 71:127–138.
76. Hope AJ, Lindsay PE, Naqa IE, et al. Modeling radiation pneumonitis risk with clinical, dosimetric, and spatial parameters. Int J Radiat Oncol Biol Phys 2006; 65:112–124.
77. Chapet O, Kong F, Lee JS, et al. Normal tissue complication probability modeling for acute esophagitis in patients treated with conformal radiation therapy for non-small cell lung cancer. Radiother Oncol 2005; 77:176–181.
78. Okunieff P, Morgan D, Niemierko A, Suit HD, Radiation dose–response of human tumors. Int J Radiat Oncol Biol Phys 1995; 32:1227–1237.

Section IV
Clinical Advances

13
Combined Chemoradiotherapy Advances

Gordon Wong and Minesh P. Mehta

Introduction

Management of locally advanced cancers has changed dramatically in the past few decades. Stepwise improvements have been made in surgical techniques, radiation delivery and fractionation, and systemic agents. In addition, multimodality treatment approaches have been increasingly used to improve outcomes in patients with locoregionally advanced disease.

The addition of chemotherapy can enhance the response to definitive radiation [1]. There are many theories regarding the exact nature of the additive effect of combined modality treatment, although no definitive evidence exists about the exact mechanisms of interaction. Combining chemotherapy and radiation can alter cell cycle kinetics, reduce and/or kill hypoxic cells, reduce accelerated repopulation, increase apoptosis, address microscopic systemic disease, increase susceptibility to radiation-induced cell kill, decrease cellular repair of sublethal and potentially lethal radiation damage. Cisplatin and 5-fluorouracil (5-FU) are two of the most studied cytotoxic agents in combination with radiation. Cisplatin reacts with cellular DNA to form intrastrand and interstrand crosslinks, causing inhibition of DNA replication and RNA transcription as well as activation of apoptosis. Concurrent cisplatin and radiation can lead to multiple interactions including inhibition of repair of radiation-induced DNA lesions, radiation-induced increased cellular cisplatin uptake, and increased toxic platinum intermediates in the presence of radiation-induced free radicals. 5-FU is an antimetabolite that inhibits DNA synthesis and DNA repair. Theories regarding the interaction of 5-FU and radiation involve disruption of cell cycle regulation, decreased radiation-induced DNA repair, and radiation-related increased thymidine phosphorylase activity. Continued investigations are being conducted evaluating models of interactions between radiation and cytotoxic or targeted agents. Similar mechanisms related to increased interaction in tumor control can also lead to enhanced toxicity of treatment. Skin and mucosal toxicity rates can dramatically rise with multimodality therapy. In addition, myelogenous toxicities from chemotherapy alone may also cause complications which could prevent or delay completion of definitive treatment.

M.P. Mehta et al. (eds.), *Radiation Oncology Advances.*

Published evidence supports the use of combined chemoradiation in many disease sites. There is level I evidence in support of concurrent chemoradiation for gliomas, head and neck cancer, nonsmall cell lung cancer, and cervical cancer. Level II evidence has been published for esophageal, rectal, anal, and bladder cancers. This section will outline the major clinical trials in these disease sites, except for gliomas which will be addressed in a separate chapter.

Head and Neck Cancers

Surgery and radiation have traditionally been the definitive treatment modalities for locally advanced head and neck cancer. However, Cosmesis and organ function are often compromised with surgery, and single modality outcomes for these patients remain poor. The addition of chemotherapy to radiation has improved locoregional control and survival in locally advanced head and neck cancer in the definitive and postoperative settings. Chemoradiation has also offered an organ-preserving treatment alternative to primary surgical resection for locally advanced larynx and hypopharynx cancers.

Multiple randomized phase III studies have compared definitive radiation to concurrent chemoradiation in the treatment of locally advanced head and neck cancer (see Table 1). Wendt et al. reported a German randomized trial comparing 70.2 Gy given in three courses with or without concurrent cisplatin and fluorouracil [2]. The combined modality arm had an increased 3 year overall survival and locoregional control rate, as well as increased acute toxicities, mainly mucositis and leukopenia. The Cleveland Clinic Foundation randomized patients to radiation alone or concurrent chemoradiation for stage III/IV head and neck cancer [3]. Concurrent chemoradiation improved the response rate, disease-free survival, and primary site preservation, but did not impact overall survival. A combined Eastern Cooperative Oncology Group (ECOG) and Southwest Oncology Group (SWOG) study randomized patients to radiation alone, concurrent chemoradiation with cisplatin, or concurrent split course radiation with cisplatin and 5-FU [4]. In the split course arm, surgery was allowed for patients who were resectable after the first 30 Gy and two courses of chemotherapy. Acute toxicities were greatest in patients who received concurrent chemoradiation with continuous treatment. However, this arm also demonstrated an improved 3 year overall and disease-specific survival over radiation alone. The split course arm outcome was between the first and second arms, and not statistically significant from either two arms. The French Head and Neck Oncology and Radiotherapy Group (GORTEC) trial also compared radiation alone to concurrent chemoradiation using cisplatin and fluorouracil in patients with locally advanced oropharyngeal carcinomas [5]. The 5 year results showed an improvement in overall survival, disease-free survival, and locoregional control. The acute toxicities, as in previous studies, were elevated in the combined modality arm.

Altered fractionation allows the potential advantage of increasing the total tumor dose, minimizing repopulation, and decreasing late toxicities. Hyperfractionation

Table 1 Selected studies of chemoradiation in locally advanced head and neck cancer

Author/study	Eligibility	Treatment regimen	*n*	Outcome	*p*
Wendt, German (1998)	III/IV H&N	70.2 Gy in 3 RT courses	140	24% 3 year OS, 17% 3 year LRC	$p < 0.003$ for OS
		70.2 Gy with concurrent cisplatin, 5-FU	130	48% 3 year OS, 36% 3 year LRC	$p < 0.004$ for LRC
Adelstein, CCF (2000)	III/IV H&N	66–72 Gy	50	48% 5 year OS, 51% 5 year DFS	
		66–72 Gy with concurrent cisplatin, 5-FU	50	50% 5 year OS, 62% 5 year DFS	$p = 0.55$ OS, $p = 0.04$ DFS
Adelstein, Intergroup (2003)	III/IV H&N	70 Gy alone	95	23% 3 year OS, 12.6 med surv, 33% 3 year DFS	CCRT vs. RT $p = 0.014$ OS, $p = 0.01$ DFS
		70 Gy with cisplatin	87	37% 3 year OS, 51% 3 year DFS	
		60–70 Gy split course with cisplatin and 5-FU	89	27% 3 year OS, 41% 3 year DFS	Split course, p = ns
Denis, GORTEC (2004)	III/IV Oropharynx	70 Gy	113	16% 5 year OS, 15% 5 year DFS, 25% 5 year LRC	
		70 GY with cisplatin, 5-FU	109	22% 5 year OS, 27% 5 year DFS, 48% 5 year LRC	$p = 0.05$ OS, $p = 0.01$ DFS, $p = 0.002$ LRC
Brizel, Duke	III/IV H&N	75 Gy, 1.25 Gy BID	60	34% 3 year OS, 41% 3 year DFS, 44% 3 year LRC	
		75 Gy, 1.25 Gy BID, with cisplatin, 5-FU	56	55% 3 year OS, 61% 3 year DFS, 70% 3 year LRC	$p = 0.07$ OS, $p = 0.08$ DFS, $p = 0.01$ LRC

(continued)

Table 1 (continued)

Author/study	Eligibility	Treatment regimen	*n*	Outcome	*p*
Jeremic, Yugoslavian trial (2000)	III/IV H&N	77 Gy, 1.1 Gy BID	53	25% 5 year OS, 25% 5 year DFS, 36% 5 year LRC	
		77 Gy, 1.1 Gy BID with cisplatin	55	46% 5 year OS, 46% 5 year DFS, 50% 5 year LRC	$p = 0.0075$ OS, $p = 0.0068$ DFS, $p = 0.041$ LRC
VA Larynx trial (1991)	III/IV Larynx	Sx and adjuvant XRT 50–74.2 Gy	166	68% 2 year OS	
		Cisplatin and 5-FU × 3, RT 66–76 Gy	166	68% 2 year OS, 64% LP	$p = 0.9846$ OS
Intergroup R91–11 (2003)	III/IV Larynx	Induction cisplatin 5-FU, RT 70 Gy	173	75% 2 year LP, 61% 2 year LRC	CCRT vs. seq $p = 0.005$ LP, $p = 0.004$ LRC; CCRT vs. RT $p < 0.001$ LP, $p < 0.001$ LRC
		RT 70 Gy with concurrent cisplatin	172	88% 2 year LP, 78% 2 year LRC	
		RT alone 70 Gy	173	70% 2 year LP, 56% 2 year LRC	
Lefebvre, EORTC (1996)	III/IV hypopharynx	Sx and adjuvant XRT 64 Gy	94	43% 3 year OS	
		Induction cisplatin and 5-FU, RT 70 Gy	100	57% 3 year OS, 42% 3 year LP, 35% 5 year LP	$p =$ ns OS
Bauchaud (1996)	Postop III/IV H&N s/p Sx w/ECE	RT 65–74 Gy	44	46% 2 year OS, 13% 5 year OS, 23% LRC	$p = 0.05$ OS, $p = 0.08$ LRC
		RT 65–74 Gy with concurrent cisplatin	39	72% 2 year OS, 36% 5 year OS, 41% LRC	

Cooper, RTOG 9501 (2004)	Postop III/IV H&N s/p Sx w/ECE, N2 dz, micro+ margins	RT 60–66 Gy	210	72% 2 year LRC	$p = 0.01$ LRC
		RT 60–66 Gy with concurrent cisplatin	206	82% 2 year LRC, no OS difference	
Bernier, EORTC 22931 (2004)	Postop III/IV H&N	RT 66 Gy	167	40% 5 year OS, 36% 5 year DFS, 31% 5 year LRF	$p = 0.02$ OS, $p = 0.04$ DFS, $p = 0.001$ LRF
		RT 66 Gy with concurrent cisplatin	167	53% 5 year OS, 47% 5 year DFS, 18% 5 year LRF	
Al-Sarraf, Intergroup 0099 (1998)	III/IV nasopharynx	70 Gy	68	47% 3 year OS, 24% 3 year DFS	$p = 0.005$ OS, $p < 0.001$ DFS
		70 Gy with concurrent cisplatin, 3 cycles adj cisplatin, 5-FU	78	78% 3 year OS, 69% 3 year DFS	

RT radiation therapy, *OS* overall survival, *DFS* disease-free survival, *LRC* locoregional control, *LP* larynx preservation rate, *CCRT* concurrent chemoradiation therapy, *ECE* extracapsular extension and accelerated fractionation with concomitant boost shown improvement in control rates as compared to conventional radiation fractionation of 1.8 to 2 Gy per fraction [6]. Subsequent trials have compared these improvements in radiation schedules to combined modality therapy. Brizel and colleagues published the results of the Duke study randomizing patients to twice-daily radiation given 1.25 Gy twice daily to 70 Gy with concurrent and adjuvant cisplatin and fluorouracil or to 75 Gy alone [7]. Combined modality treatment improved 3-year locoregional control and a trend toward overall and disease-free survival, without a significant difference in rates of acute toxicities. Jeremic et al. reported a Yugoslavian trial comparing 1.1 Gy twice daily to 77 Gy with or without cisplatin [8]. Acute myelogenous toxicities were greater with chemotherapy. Overall survival, disease-free survival and locoregional control at five years were all improved with combined modality treatment.

In head and neck cancer, organ preservation is also an important endpoint. Quality of life after definitive treatment can be drastically altered when comparing primary surgery to chemoradiation. The Veteran Affairs (VA) larynx trial enrolled patients with locally advanced laryngeal cancer to receive primary surgery and adjuvant radiation vs. induction chemotherapy and radiation [9]. Patients without complete or partial response following the 2 cycles of induction chemotherapy (15%) underwent laryngectomy and adjuvant radiation. The 2-year overall survival was equivalent for both arms; however, 64% of patients in the chemoradiation arm did not require laryngectomy. An Intergroup R91–11 study then investigated the optimal sequencing of radiation in a 3-arm locally advanced larynx trial including induction chemotherapy followed by radiation, concurrent chemoradiation, or radiation alone [10]. Larynx preservation and locoregional control rates were highest in the concurrent arm, although overall survival was similar for all arms. The rate of acute toxicities was increased in the concurrent arm, mainly involving mucositis. The European Organization for Research and Treatment of Cancer (EORTC) group investigated larynx preservation multimodality approach in patients with locally advanced hypopharynx cancer, conducted in a similar fashion to the VA larynx trial [11]. Induction chemotherapy yielded a 54% complete and 32% partial response rate. Approximately half of the patients had successful larynx preservation at 3 years, with a lower rate of distant metastasis and similar rates of locoregional control and overall survival compared to the surgery arm.

Multiple meta-analyses have been performed to determine the benefit of chemotherapy in the treatment of head and neck cancer. The Meta-Analysis of Chemotherapy in Head and Neck Cancer (MACH-NC) collaborative group reviewed individual patient data in 63 trials from 1965 to 1993 [12]. A recent update included an additional 24 trials performed between 1994 and 2000 [13]. The initial report showed a small overall survival benefit with the addition of chemotherapy. This benefit was most significant for concomitant chemotherapy with a hazard ratio of 0.81 and absolute benefit of 8% at 5 years, also confirmed in the updated report. The benefit was not significant for neoadjuvant or adjuvant treatment. Differences in monochemotherapy vs. polychemotherapy were not seen, but the survival was improved in platinum-based regimens.

Combined modality adjuvant treatment has also been used to improve disease control following definitive surgical resection with high risk features. Bauchaud et al. reported the results of a randomized trial of postoperative locally advanced head and neck patients with extracapsular nodal disease comparing adjuvant radiation to chemoradiation [14]. The concomitant arm had a significantly improved overall survival, disease-free survival, and locoregional control. Acute toxicities were not reported, and late complications were not significantly different. The Radiation Therapy Oncology Group (RTOG) 9501 study, also supported by ECOG and SWOG, randomized postoperative patients with multiple positive lymph nodes, extracapsular nodal disease, and/or microscopically positive margins to radiation or chemoradiation [15]. The 2-year outcomes showed improved locoregional control and disease-free survival, but not an overall survival benefit. The acute grade 3 or higher toxicities were increased in the concurrent arm with 77% compared to 34%, including myelogenous, mucosal, and gastrointestinal toxicities. The EORTC 22931 trial compared the same treatment arms to patients with locally advanced disease or early stage disease with extranodal spread, positive margins, vascular tumor embolism, or specific nodal metastasis [16]. Acute toxicities were increased with chemoradiation, although late complications were similar. The combined modality arm, similar to the previous study showed a locoregional control and disease-free survival benefit, but additionally demonstrated a significant improvement in overall survival.

Nasopharyngeal carcinoma is considered a separate entity from the other head and neck sites. It was not included in nearly all of the previously mentioned studies, and there have been many trials investigating the optimal treatment approach. Due to the location of the nasopharynx and proximity to the base of skull, primary radiation has been the traditional treatment approach. The Intergroup 0099 trial initiated a shift toward combined modality therapy as the first trial to show a survival benefit [17]. This study evaluated the effect of adding concurrent and adjuvant chemotherapy to radiation in patients with stage III or IV nasopharyngeal carcinoma. The combined modality arm had an increased response rate and survival, in addition to increased acute myelogenous and gastrointestinal toxicities. However, there was criticism of the poor outcome in the control arm of the study compared to historical controls, specifically in radiation alone series from Southeast Asia where nasopharyngeal carcinomas are endemic. A follow-up study conducted in Taiwan confirmed that an overall and disease-free survival advantage of concurrent chemoradiation over radiation alone in an endemic population [18]. In this trial significant improvements were seen in control rates of local and distant recurrences, but not for regional recurrence. Lee et al. reported the results of a Hong Kong trial comparing radiation alone to concurrent and adjuvant chemotherapy, given in the same fashion as the Intergroup trial [19]. The results showed an increased locoregional control and disease-free survival, without significant benefit in distant control or overall survival. Combined modality also increased acute and late toxicities including mucositis, leukopenia, and hearing loss. A meta-analysis reviewed nasopharyngeal trials comparing radiation with or without chemotherapy [20]. Neoadjuvant and concurrent chemotherapy improved locoregional control and distant metastasis. An overall survival benefit was seen with concurrent chemotherapy, but not for neoadjuvant or adjuvant treatment.

Management for locally advanced head and neck cancer has incorporated concurrent chemoradiation as the treatment approach in the definitive and postoperative settings. This aggressive treatment approach requires good patient performance status as the acute toxicities are enhanced with multimodality treatment. Systemic targeted therapy has also shown to benefit patients with locally advanced disease [21]. This is further discussed in another chapter. Future studies are evaluating the timing of chemotherapy, the combination of chemotherapy and altered fractionation, and the addition of targeted therapy to chemoradiation.

Nonsmall Cell Lung Carcinoma

Stage III, locally advanced, unresectable NSCLC has traditionally been treated with definitive radiation. However, overall outcome remains poor with 5-year survival estimates of 5–10% with radiation alone. Investigators looked to multimodality therapy to improve upon these outcomes. Chemoradiation has been studied in many randomized trials investigating the benefit of sequential and concurrent chemotherapy, ultimately shifting the treatment approach to combined chemoradiation.

Numerous trials have compared radiation alone to sequential chemotherapy and radiation. Early trials did not show significant improvement, likely related to trial design and choice of chemotherapy regimens. Two recent major trials, the cancer and leukemia group B (CALGB) and the Intergroup studies, showed improved survival with combined modality therapy (see Table 2). The CALGB study randomized patients to thoracic radiation with or without induction cisplatin and vinblastine chemotherapy [22, 23]. The addition of induction chemotherapy increased the median survival from 9.6 to 13.7 months. Increased hospitalizations and severe weight loss were seen in the combined modality arm, although no treatment-related deaths occurred. The results of the CALGB study were confirmed in the Intergroup trial, a combined RTOG 88–08 and ECOG 4588 protocol. This protocol used the same two treatment arms as in the CALGB trial in addition to a hyperfractionation arm [24]. Combined modality therapy had a significantly increased median survival over both radiation alone arms. The chemotherapy arm did not have any increased acute grade 4 toxicities, although there were three treatment-related deaths compared to one death in the hyperfractionation arm and none in the conventional radiation arm.

Concurrent chemotherapy has had mixed results in randomized trials. Enhanced interaction through concurrent administration of chemotherapy and radiation can potentially lead to improved tumor control. However, this also increases acute toxicity during treatment. Multiple trials investigating concurrent chemotherapy with cisplatin, carboplatin, and multiagent regimens did not show significant improvement [25–28]. However, three trials showed a significant survival benefit (see Table 2). An EORTC trial compared split course radiation alone to concurrent administration

Table 2 Selected NSCLC trials of chemotherapy and radiation

Author/study	Treatment regimen	*n*	Outcome	*p*
CALGB, Dillman (1996)	RT alone 60 Gy	77	9.6 mo med surv	
	induction cisplatin and vinblastine followed by RT 60 Gy	78	13.7 mo med surv	0.012
Intergroup, Sause (1995)	RT alone 60 Gy	149	11.4 mo med surv	
	Hyperfractionated RT 1.2 Gy BID to 69.6 Gy	152	12.3 mo med surv	
	Induction cisplatin and vinblastine followed by RT 60 Gy	151	13.8 mo med surv	0.03
	Split course RT, 30 Gy/10 fx, 3 week rest, 25 Gy/10 fx	114	46% 1 year, 13% 2 year OS	
EORTC, Shaake-Koning (1992)	Split course RT with concurrent weekly cisplatin 30 mg/m^2	110	44% 1 year, 19% 2 year OS	
	Split course RT with concurrent daily cisplatin 6 mg/m^2	107	54% 1 year, 26% 2 year OS	0.04 for chemo vs. RT alone
Jeremic I (1995)	Hyperfractionated RT 1.2 Gy BID to 64.8 Gy	61	8 mo med surv	0.0027 vs. RT alone
	Hyperfractionated RT + wkly carboplatin (100 mg) and etoposide	52	18 mo med surv	
	Hyperfractionated RT + wkly carboplatin (200 mg) and etoposide	56	13 mo med surv	
Jeremic II (1996)	Hyperfractionated RT 1.2 Gy BID to 69.6 Gy	66	14 mo med surv	
	Hyperfractionated RT + daily carboplatin and etoposide	65	22 mo med surv	0.021
Furuse (1999)	Cisplatin, vindesine, mitomycin followed by RT 56 Gy	158	13.3 mo med surv	
	Concurrent cisplatin, vindesine, mitomycin with RT 56 Gy	156	16.5 mo med surv	0.04
	Induction cisplatin, vinorelbine followed by RT 66 Gy	104	13.8 mo med surv	
GLOT, Pierre (2001)	Concurrent cisplatin, etoposide with RT 66 Gy, then adj cisplatin, vinorelbine	103	15 mo med surv	0.41
LAMP, Belani (2005)	Induction paclitaxel, carboplatin, then RT 63 Gy	91	13.0 mo med surv	Not significant when compared to historic controls not reported

(continued)

Table 2 (continued)

Author/study	Treatment regimen	n	Outcome	p
	Induction and concurrent paclitaxel, carboplatin with RT 63 Gy	74	12.7 mo med surv	
	Concurrent and consolidation paclitaxel, carboplatin with RT 63 Gy	92	16.3 mo med surv	
RTOG 9410, Curran (2003)	Induction cisplatin and vinblastine, then RT 60 Gy		14.6 mo med surv	
	Concurrent cisplatin, vinblastine with RT 60 Gy	595	17.0 mo med surv	0.046 vs. seq
	Concurrent cisplatin and etoposide with RT 1.2 Gy BID to 69.6 Gy	total	15.2 mo med surv	0.296 vs. seq
Czech, Zemanova (2002)	Concurrent cisplatin, vinorelbine with RT 60 Gy	102	20.4 mo med surv	
	Induction cisplatin, vinorelbine, RT 60 Gy	total	13.0 mo med surv	0.0216

of either daily or weekly cisplatin [29]. The concurrent treatment improved overall survival with divergence of the survival curves apparent at 2 years. Toxicities were mild with few grade 3 or higher events. The chemotherapy arms had increased nausea, vomiting, and leukopenia. Jeremic reported the results of two trials comparing 64.8 Gy hyperfractionated radiation alone with or without concurrent chemotherapy [30, 31]. The first trial compared radiation alone to concurrent weekly carboplatin and etoposide, given at two different doses of carboplatin. The lower dose carboplatin arm had the best overall survival although not significantly different than the high dose carboplatin arm. The acute toxicities did not differ among the three arms. However, late grade 3 or 4 toxicities were increased in the chemotherapy arms. The second trial compared a higher dose of hyperfractionated radiation (69.6 Gy) alone to a higher dose than the first trial to concurrent daily carboplatin and etoposide, showing an improvement in median survival from 14 to 22 months, without significant differences in toxicity.

The next set of trials compared sequential chemotherapy and radiation to concurrent chemoradiation. Furuse reported the results of comparing induction and concurrent chemotherapy with cisplatin, vindesine, and mitomycin [32]. Concurrent combined modality treatment increased median survival from 13.3 to 16.5 months. This arm also had an increased rate of myelosuppresion, although only one treatment-related death was seen compared to three in the sequential arm. The groupe Lyon-Saint-Etienne d'Oncologie Thoracique (GLOT) trial randomized locally advanced patients to receive either induction cisplatin and vinorelbine followed by radiation or concurrent cisplatin and etoposide with radiation and adjuvant cisplatin and vinorelbine [33]. Toxicities included significant neutropenia in both arms, and increased dysphagia and esophagitis in the concurrent arm. A trend toward increased survival was observed in the concurrent arm, although not statistically significant. The locally advanced multimodality protocol (LAMP) phase 2 trial compared paclitaxel and carboplatin with radiation given in one of three ways: sequentially, induction and concurrent, or concurrent and consolidation [34]. The latter arm had the longest median survival of 16.1 months, and similar to other trials had the highest rate of esophagitis (28%). Zemanova reported the results of a Czech trial of concurrent vs. sequential multimodality treatment [35]. The concurrent arm had improved survival and experienced greater myelosuppression, nausea/vomiting, and esophagitis. RTOG 9410 was a three arm study comparing induction or concurrent cisplatin and vinblastine with conventional radiation, and cisplatin and etoposide concurrently with hyperfractionated radiation [36]. Concurrent chemoradiation with standard fractionation improved median survival compared with sequential treatment. The hyperfractionation arm did not demonstrate a significant difference in survival.

The current standard of care for patients with locally advanced unresectable nonsmall cell lung carcinoma is concurrent chemoradiation. This combined modality approach increases the risk of mucosal, myelogenous, and pulmonary toxicities. Trials are underway investigating various chemotherapy drug regimens and the role of induction and consolidative chemotherapy.

Cervical Carcinoma

Locally advanced cervical cancer has been historically managed with primary radiation. In patients with bulky locally advanced lesions, high rates of local failure occur following RT alone. Multiple randomized trials have attempted neoadjuvant chemotherapy before definitive radiation, showing no advantage to sequential multimodality treatment. Two of these trials actually showed a survival decrement with this regimen [37, 38]. However, subsequent trials using concurrent chemoradiation has led to a significant improvement in overall survival.

The encouraging early studies evaluating hydroxyurea, 5-FU, and cisplatin led to five major prospective randomized trials of chemoradiation (see Table 3). The Gynecologic Oncology Group (GOG) conducted two trials of patients with IIB-IVA cervical cancer, comparing various concurrent regimens of radiation with hydroxyurea (HU), cisplatin, and/or 5-FU [39, 40]. GOG 85 showed improved local control, progression-free survival, and overall survival with less myelogenous toxicity in the cisplatin/5-FU arm over those treated with HU. GOG 120 compared radiation combined with one of three chemotherapy regimens of cisplatin, cisplatin/5-FU/HU, or HU. The two cisplatin arms had improved disease-free and overall survival rates over the HU arm. Toxicities were greatest in the cispatin/5-FU/HU arm compared to the single agent arms. GOG 123 enrolled patients with bulky (≥4 cm) IB cervical primaries to undergo radiation with or without cisplatin, followed by extrafascial hysterectomy [41]. Trimodality therapy increased acute toxicities, mostly hematologic and gastrointestinal, but also improved rates of progression-free and overall survival. The RTOG 9001 trial compared extended field radiation to pelvic radiation combined with cisplatin and 5-FU in patients diagnosed with stage IIB-IVA, bulky (≥5 cm) IB-IIA, or biopsy-proven pelvic nodal disease [42]. The chemoradiation arm experienced greater acute toxicities, but had superior rates of locoregional control, distant control, and disease-free survival. Overall survival was improved for all patients, but subset analysis did not show significance in overall survival for stage III and IVA patients. The SWOG 8797 trial investigated postoperative radiation vs. chemoradiation in patients with IA2-IIA cervical cancer status postradical hysterectomy and pelvic lymph node dissection with positive lymph nodes, positive margins, and/or microscopic involvement of the parametrium [43]. Improved disease-free and overall survival were seen in the chemoradiation arm, and similarly showed increased acute hematologic toxicities.

The results of these five clinical trials led to an NCI clinical announcement in February, 1999 for “strong consideration” to be given for chemoradiation in the treatment of cervical cancer [44]. Subsequent chemoradiation trials have supported the use of combined modality therapy with noncisplatin-based drug regimens [45]. One trial, conducted by the NCIC, did not show a benefit of chemoradiation over radiation alone [46]. Criticisms of this study included lack of surgical staging, increased rates of anemia in the cisplatin arm, and smaller size of study compared to the positive trials.

Table 3 Selected studies of chemoradiation in cervical cancer

Author/study	Eligibility	Median f/u	Treatment regimen	N	PFS (%)	OS (%)
Whitney, GOG 85, (1999)	IIB–IVA	8.7 years	RT 61.2 to 81 Gy with HU	191	47	43
			RT 61.2 to 81 Gy with cisplatin and 5-FU	177	57	55
Rose, GOG 120, (1999)	IIB–IVA	35 months	RT 61.2 to 81 Gy with HU	177	47	50
			RT 61.2 to 81 Gy with cisplatin, 5-FU, and HU	173	64	67
			RT 61.2 to 81 Gy with cisplatin	176	67	66
Keys, GOG 123, (1999)	Bulky IB	36 months	RT 75 Gy => Extrafascial Hysterectomy	186	63	74
			RT 75 Gy + cisplatin => Extrafascial Hysterectomy	183	79	83
Morris, RTOG 9001 (1999)	IIB-IVA or Bulky IB-IIA or LN+	43 months	RT 85 Gy (extended field)	193	40	58
			RT 85 Gy with cisplatin, 5-FU	195	67	73
Peters, SWOG 8797	IA2-IIB postop, LN+, margin+, or parametrium+	42 months	RT45–49.3 Gy	116	63	71
			RT 45–49.3 Gy with cisplatin, 5-FU	127	80	81

All PFS and OS are significant ($p \leq 0.05$) compared to control arm

Chemoradiation is currently the standard of care for bulky or locally advanced cervical cancer. Future studies are evaluating the optimal radiation dose, varying techniques with incorporation of brachytherapy, chemotherapy regimen, and sequencing of multimodality therapy.

Esophageal Carcinoma

Esophageal carcinoma often presents with locally advanced disease and is associated with a very poor survival and control rates. Surgery is the preferred definitive treatment, but multimodality approaches have been studied to improve locoregional control and survival. Radiation, chemotherapy, and combined chemoradiation have been evaluated in the neoadjuvant and adjuvant setting with mixed results. For unresectable patients, definitive chemoradiation has become the standard treatment option.

Adjuvant treatment with chemotherapy and radiation has been investigated in multiple trials (see Table 4). With small improvements in select trials, the focus in the US has shifted toward a trimodality approach. The Dublin trial, reported by Walsh et al. randomized patients with esophageal carcinoma to definitive surgery with or without neoadjuvant 5-FU, cisplatin, and radiation to 40 Gy [47, 48]. Thirteen (22%) of the 58 patients in the multimodality arm had a pathologic complete response. The median survival and overall survival were significantly improved in the neoadjuvant arm. Criticism of this trial notes a low 6% 3-year overall survival in the surgery alone arm; however, 80% of patients were lymph node positive. Bosset et al. reported the results of the addition of neoadjuvant chemoradiation to surgery in patients with stage I and II squamous cell esophageal carcinomas [49]. Patients in the multimodality arm had a 26% pathologic complete response rate and increased rate of disease-free survival, locoregional control, and cause-specific survival, but without any improvement in overall survival. The University of Michigan conducted a randomized trial of surgery alone vs. preoperative chemoradiation followed by surgery in patients with esophageal or gastroesophageal junction carcinomas. Neoadjuvant treatment included cisplatin, 5-FU, and vinblastine with twice daily radiation to 45 Gy. The multimodality arm showed improved locoregional control and a nonsignificant 3-year overall survival difference of 30% compared to 16% in the surgery-alone arm, without significant change in disease-free or cause-specific survival. Patients who experienced a pathologic complete response had a higher survival probability than those with residual disease following neoadjuvant treatment.

The Intergroup 0113 trial is the only major positive study published evaluating adjuvant chemoradiation. This trial was mainly a gastric trial, but also included gastroesophageal junction lesions, which constituted 20% of patients enrolled [50]. Patients were randomized postoperatively to observation or adjuvant chemoradiation. Median, relapse-free, and overall survival, as well as locoregional control were significantly improved in the adjuvant arm. The inclusion of gastroesophageal

Table 4 Selected studies in esophageal carcinoma

Author/study	Eligibility	Treatment regimen	*n*	Outcome
Walsh, Dublin (1996)	M0 Esoph CA	Surgery	55	12 mo med surv, 6% 3 year OS
		Preop 5-FU, cisplatin, RT 40 Gy	58	17 mo med surv, 32% 3 year OS
Bosset (1997)	Stage I/II	Surgery	139	18.6 med surv, 36% 3 year OS
	SCCA	Preop Cisplatin and RT 37 Gy	143	18.6 med surv, 34% 3 year OS
Urba, U of Michigan (2001)		Surgery alone	50	16% 3 year OS, 39% LF
	I–IVA Esoph,GEJ CA	Preop Cisplatin, 5-FU, vinblastine, BID RT 45 Gy	47	30% 3 year OS (ns), 19% LF
Macdonald, Int 0116 (2001)	IB–IVM0 AdenoCA Gastric, GEJ Postop	Surgery alone	275	27 mo med surv, 41% 3 year OS, 29% LF
		Postop 5-FU, leucovorin, XRT 45 Gy	281	36 mo med surv, 50% 3 year OS, 19% LF
Herskovic, RTOG 8501 (1992)	T1–3N0-1M0 Esoph CA	RT 64 Gy	62	9.3 mo med surv, 10% 2 year OS, 0% 3 year OS
		RT 50 Gy + 5-FU, cisplatin	61	14.1 mo med surv, 38% 2 year OS, 30% 3 year OS
Minsky, Int 0123	T1–4N0-1M0 Esoph CA	RT 50.4 Gy + 5-FU, cisplatin	109	18.1 mo med surv, 40% 2 year OS
		RT 64.8 Gy + 5-FU, cisplatin	109	13 mo med surv, 31% 2 year OS (both ns)
		RT 40 Gy (preop) or 60 Gy (def)	60	9.2 mo med surv, 8% 3 year OS
Smith, ECOG EST-1282 (1998)	Stage I/II SCCA Esoph	RT 40 Gy (preop) or 60 Gy (def) + 5-FU, MMC	59	14.8 mo med surv, 13% 3 year OS

AdenoCA Adenocarcinoma, *SCCA* Squamous cell carcinoma, Gastroesophageal junction
All endpoints are statistically significant ($p \leq 0.05$), unless otherwise specified

junction primaries allows for application of adjuvant multimodality treatment to distal esophageal adenocarcinomas.

For unresectable patients, primary radiation has been the next treatment option, although results remain poor with single modality. The RTOG 8501 protocol enrolled unresectable patients to undergo chemoradiation or radiation alone [51–53]. Severe acute toxicities were greater in the chemoradiation arm, mainly hematologic and mucosal toxicities. The rates of persistent, recurrent, and distant disease were lower in the multimodality arm, and the overall survival rate was significantly improved. An additional 69 nonrandomized patients were treated in the chemoradiation arm. This cohort of patients had similar outcomes to the randomized chemoradiation patients and confirmed the results of the original trial. The Eastern Cooperative Oncology Group (ECOG) EST1282 trial compared radiation with or without 5-FU and mitomycin C in patients with Stage I–II squamous cell esophageal carcinoma [54]. The protocol allowed for evaluation for potential surgical resection after 40 Gy. Surgical resection was evenly distributed between both arms. The chemoradiation arm had increased acute toxicities, including two life-threatening toxicities compared to the radiation-alone arm. The median and overall survival rates were significantly improved with multimodality therapy. The Intergroup 0123 (R-9405) evaluated the role of radiation dose escalation from 50.4 to 64.8 Gy with concurrent chemotherapy with 5-FU and cisplatin [55]. No significant differences in disease control or survival were seen with radiation dose escalation.

Multimodality approaches have improved survival and locoregional control. These improvements are modest, with significant gains to be made for long term local control and overall survival. Ongoing trials are optimizing cytotoxic and targeted systemic therapies in an attempt to improve these endpoints for patients diagnosed with esophageal carcinoma.

Rectal Adenocarcinoma

Surgery is the primary modality of treatment for patients with invasive rectal cancer. Locoregional recurrence is seen in 25–50% of stage II/III patients, and can be associated with significant morbidity. For these patients whose tumors that invade through the muscularis (T3-4) or have nodal involvement, treatment has been augmented with neoadjuvant or adjuvant multimodality treatment to decrease disease recurrence and to increase the likelihood of sphincter sparing resections. Traditionally, low lying rectal lesions necessitated an abdominal perineal resection. However, with preoperative treatment, select patients with good neoadjuvant response may be able to undergo sphincter sparing surgery.

Multiple trials have randomized patients undergoing definitive surgery to adjuvant treatment with radiation, chemotherapy, or combined chemoradiation. The Gastrointestinal Tumor Study Group (GITSG) 7175 trial enrolled patients with

Dukes B2 or C disease and compared postoperative treatments of radiation (44–48 Gy), chemotherapy (5-FU and semustine), chemoradiation (44 Gy with 5-FU followed by 5-FU and semustine), or observation [56]. The combined modality arm had the highest rate of acute toxicities at 61%, but had the lowest rate of disease recurrence (33%). Disease recurrence was highest in the observation arm (55%). No significant overall survival improvement was seen among the four treatment arms, although trend toward improvement was shown for combined adjuvant treatment over observation. The National Surgical Adjuvant Breast and Bowel Project (NSABP) R-01 trial randomized patients postoperatively with Dukes B or C rectal carcinoma to observation, chemotherapy with 5-FU, semustine, and vincristine (MOF), or radiation (46–53 Gy) [57]. The chemotherapy arm showed a disease-free and overall survival benefit at 5 years, whereas adjuvant radiation had a locoregional benefit only. The following trial, NSABP R-02, was a four arm trial investigating the benefit of radiation to adjuvant chemotherapy for postoperative patients with Dukes B or C rectal carcinoma [58]. Female patients received 5-FU and leucovorin with or without radiation to 50.4 Gy. Male patients received either 5-FU and leucovorin or MOF chemotherapy with or without pelvic radiation. The addition of radiation did not affect DFS or OS, but decreased locoregional relapse from 13% to 8% ($p = 0.02$) at 5 years. In the male patients, 5-FU and leucovorin showed an improved disease-free survival over the MOF regimen. The North Central Cancer Treatment Group investigated the addition of 5-FU and semustine chemotherapy to postoperative radiation of 45–50.4 Gy [59]. Combined chemoradiation had a significant improvement in recurrence rate, disease-free and overall survival, with manageable increased acute toxicities. With the results of these early trials, the NIH consensus conference published recommendations for patients with stage II/III rectal cancer patients to undergo adjuvant chemoradiation [60].

Investigators have also studied the role of neoadjuvant treatment. Following the results of preoperative radiation, subsequent protocols have compared preoperative chemoradiation to neoadjuvant radiation alone and to postoperative chemoradiation. The EORTC 22921 trial compared neoadjuvant radiation vs. chemoradiation prior to surgery and found increased pathologic downstaging with combined modality [49]. No results of tumor control or survival have been published at this time. NSABP R-03 was closed early due to poor accrual [61]; however, results published early showed preoperative chemoradiation may downstage tumors prior to resection and allow for higher likelihood of sphincter preserving procedures. The German rectal trial also compared preoperative vs. postoperative chemoradiation [62]. No difference was seen in overall or disease-free survival, but the neoadjuvant arm had improved locoregional control, decreased acute toxicity, and increased sphincter preserving surgery.

The current treatment for T3-4 and/or node positive rectal carcinoma is surgical resection with either neoadjuvant or adjuvant chemoradiation. Neoadjuvant treatment is generally preferred with lower toxicities and higher rate of sphincter preservation with pathologic downstaging. Current trials are investigating the optimal chemotherapy regimen and delivery for further improvement.

Anal Squamous Cell Carcinoma

Anal cancers have been treated with abdominoperineal resection with resultant permanent colostomy. Although not directly compared with prospective randomized clinical trials, radiation has been utilized for definitive treatment. The addition of chemotherapy to radiation has been shown to decrease colostomy rates and increase disease-free survival in patients with anal squamous cell carcinoma.

Definitive chemoradiation was first reported in a series published by Wayne State. In an attempt to improve upon surgical outcomes, neoadjuvant radiation to 30 Gy with concurrent 5-FU and mitomycin (MMC) was delivered [63]. In a report of the first three patients enrolled, one patient experienced a complete clinical response and refused surgery. The other two patients had an abdominoperineal resection and were found to have complete pathologic response. The initial protocol requiring surgery was changed after five out of the first six patients who had resections and complete pathologic response. This led to the use of chemoradiation and reserving surgical resection as salvage therapy for biopsy-proven persistent or recurrent disease. In the report of 45 patients treated in this manner, there was an 84% pathologic complete response rate [64].

Three randomized trials have evaluated the efficacy of definitive chemoradiation. The Intergroup (RTOG/ECOG) study reported by Flam et al. [65, 66] evaluated the chemotherapy regimen of 5-FU vs. 5-FU and MMC given concurrently with radiation. Posttreatment biopsies were performed, and patients with positive biopsies received additional radiation and chemotherapy. The 5-FU and MMC arm had higher colostomy-free survival (71% vs. 59%, $p = 0.014$) and disease-free survival (73% vs. 51%, $p = 0.003$). Acute toxicities were increased at 23% vs. 7% for the multidrug regimen, although late toxicities were similar. The EORTC trial randomized patients to radiation alone or with concurrent 5-FU and MMC [67]. The combined modality arm had an increased complete response rate (80% vs. 54%), an 18% advantage in 5 year locoregional control, and a 32% improvement in 5 year colostomy-free rate, without an effect on overall survival. Overall, the acute and late toxicities were not different, with the exception of increased anal ulcers in the chemoradiation group. The United Kingdom Coordinating Committee on Cancer Research (UKCCCR) protocol also compared definitive radiation alone to chemoradiation with 5-FU and MMC [68]. The chemoradiation arm similarly showed improved locoregional control and cause-specific survival, without an impact on overall survival. Acute, but not late, toxicities were greater in the combined modality treatment, including six chemotherapy-related deaths.

Chemoradiation has become the definitive treatment for anal cancers. More recent nonrandomized trials have shown similar efficacy of cisplatin and fluorouracil with reduced toxicities [69, 70]. Radiation dose–response has also been evaluated, showing the importance of continuous course radiation to at least 54 Gy [71, 72]. Current investigations are studying the optimum chemotherapy regimen and radiation fractionation schedule.

Muscle Invasive Bladder Cancer

Definitive management for bladder cancer is surgical resection involving local excision alone for early superficial lesions and radical cystectomy with pelvic lymph node dissection for more advanced lesions. Muscle invasive bladder cancer treatment has evolved in the past few decades in investigating bladder-sparing approaches. Although no study has directly compared this approach to radical cystectomy, available data has shown its effectiveness in organ preservation and survival.

Following a report showing safety and efficacy of chemoradiation in inoperable patients [73], the National Cancer Institute of Canada (NCIC) conducted one of the earliest randomized trials, evaluating the addition of cisplatin to definitive or preoperative radiation, which significantly reduced pelvic recurrence rate with the addition of chemotherapy [74]. Multiple RTOG and institutional studies have been conducted investigating the outcome of definitive chemoradiation. Outcomes of selected trials are shown in Table 5 [75–82]. These trials were designed to evaluate the efficacy of bladder sparing approaches, but not at the sacrifice of survival. Patients were routinely with monitored cystoscopy and cytology. Those without a complete response to initial treatment or with subsequent local recurrence proceeded to undergo definitive surgical resection. The success of the trials and institutional experiences has been based on the selection of appropriate patients for organ preservation.

Table 5 Selected trials of definitive chemoradiation for muscle invasive bladder carcinoma

Bladder sparing studies	Treatment	*n*	CR	5 year OS	5 year Surv w/intact bladder
RTOG 8512 (1993)	RT + CP	42	66%	52%	42%
RTOG 8802 (1996)	TURBT, MCV, RT + CP	91	75%	51%	44% (4 year)
RTOG 8903 (1998)	TURBT, +/–MCV, RT + CP	123	59%	50%	38%
U. Paris (1997)	TURBT, 5-FU, RT (3 Gy BID days 1,3,15,17) + CP	120	77%	63%	NA
Erlangen (2002)	TURBT, RT +/–cisplatin/ carboplatin/cis+5FU	415	72%	50% (31% 10 year)	42% (27% 10 year)
MGH (2003)	TURBT, +/– MCV, RT + CP	190	71% T2, 57% T3-4a	54% (36% 10 year)	45%
RTOG 95-06	TURBT, 5FU, RT (3 Gy BID days 1,3,15,17) + CP	34	67%	83% (3 year)	66% (3 year)
RTOG 97-06	TURBT, RT(BID, concomitant boost) + CP, adj MCV	47	74%	61% (3 year)	48% (3 year)

TURBT Transurethral resection of bladder tumor, *RT* Radiation therapy, *MCV* methotrexate, cisplatin, and vinblastine, *CP* cisplatin

No prospective randomized study has prospectively compared definitive chemoradiation to radical cystectomy and pelvic lymph node dissection. However, the 5 year overall survival in the bladder preservation trials is similar to published surgical series [83, 84]. With chemoradiation, approximately 40% of patients have successful bladder preservation at 5 years. Current trials in muscle invasive bladder cancer are evaluating the optimal chemotherapy regimen and radiation fractionation schedules.

Conclusion

Combined modality treatments have improved outcomes in locally advanced cancers. The addition of concurrent chemotherapy to radiation for gliomas, head and neck, lung, cervical, esophageal, rectal, anal, and bladder cancers have made stepwise improvements. The price of these improvements is the acute toxicities of treatment, which are mainly mucosal and hematologic. Patients must be carefully selected to undergo concurrent combined modality therapy to avoid severe treatment-related toxicity and morbidity. Caution must be taken in applying the results of clinical trials into practice, as many of the patients seen in consultation do not meet the rigorous requirements of enrollment onto a protocol. Many ongoing studies continue to investigate optimal treatment approaches to improve disease control, survival, and quality of life.

References

1. Wilson GD, Bentzen SM, Harari PM. Biologic basis for combining drugs with radiation. Semin Radiat Oncol 2006;16(1):2–9.
2. Wendt TG, Grabenbauer GG, Rodel CM, et al. Simultaneous radiochemotherapy versus radiotherapy alone in advanced head and neck cancer: a randomized multicenter study. J Clin Oncol 1998;16(4):1318–24.
3. Adelstein DJ, Lavertu P, Saxton JP, et al. Mature results of a phase III randomized trial comparing concurrent chemoradiotherapy with radiation therapy alone in patients with stage III and IV squamous cell carcinoma of the head and neck. Cancer 2000;88(4):876–83.
4. Adelstein DJ, Li Y, Adams GL, et al. An intergroup phase III comparison of standard radiation therapy and two schedules of concurrent chemoradiotherapy in patients with unresectable squamous cell head and neck cancer. J Clin Oncol 2003;21(1):92–8.
5. Denis F, Garaud P, Bardet E, et al. Final results of the 94–01 French Head and Neck Oncology and Radiotherapy Group randomized trial comparing radiotherapy alone with concomitant radiochemotherapy in advanced-stage oropharynx carcinoma. J Clin Oncol 2004;22(1):69–76.
6. Fu KK, Pajak TF, Trotti A, et al. A Radiation Therapy Oncology Group (RTOG) phase III randomized study to compare hyperfractionation and two variants of accelerated fractionation to standard fractionation radiotherapy for head and neck squamous cell carcinomas: first report of RTOG 9003. Int J Radiat Oncol Biol Phys 2000;48(1):7–16.
7. Brizel DM, Albers ME, Fisher SR, et al. Hyperfractionated irradiation with or without concurrent chemotherapy for locally advanced head and neck cancer. N Engl J Med 1998;338(25):1798–804.

8. Jeremic B, Shibamoto Y, Milicic B, et al. Hyperfractionated radiation therapy with or without concurrent low-dose daily cisplatin in locally advanced squamous cell carcinoma of the head and neck: a prospective randomized trial. J Clin Oncol 2000;18(7):1458–64.
9. Induction chemotherapy plus radiation compared with surgery plus radiation in patients with advanced laryngeal cancer. The Department of Veterans Affairs Laryngeal Cancer Study Group. N Engl J Med 1991;324(24):1685–90.
10. Forastiere AA, Goepfert H, Maor M, et al. Concurrent chemotherapy and radiotherapy for organ preservation in advanced laryngeal cancer. N Engl J Med 2003;349(22):2091–8.
11. Lefebvre JL, Chevalier D, Luboinski B, et al. Larynx preservation in pyriform sinus cancer: preliminary results of a European Organization for Research and Treatment of Cancer phase III trial. EORTC Head and Neck Cancer Cooperative Group. J Natl Cancer Inst 1996;88(13):890–9.
12. Pignon JP, Bourhis J, Domenge C, et al. Chemotherapy added to locoregional treatment for head and neck squamous-cell carcinoma: three meta-analyses of updated individual data. MACH-NC Collaborative Group. Meta-Analysis of Chemotherapy on Head and Neck Cancer. Lancet 2000;355(9208):949–55.
13. Bourhis J, Amand C, Pignon JP. Update of the MACH-NC (Meta-Analysis of Chemotherapy in Head & Neck Cancer) database focused on concomitant chemoradiotherapy. In: Proc Am Soc Clin Onc 22: 5505; 2004.
14. Bachaud JM, Cohen-Jonathan E, Alzieu C, et al. Combined postoperative radiotherapy and weekly cisplatin infusion for locally advanced head and neck carcinoma: final report of a randomized trial. Int J Radiat Oncol Biol Phys 1996;36(5):999–1004.
15. Cooper JS, Pajak TF, Forastiere AA, et al. Postoperative concurrent radiotherapy and chemotherapy for high-risk squamous-cell carcinoma of the head and neck. N Engl J Med 2004;350(19):1937–44.
16. Bernier J, Domenge C, Ozsahin M, et al. Postoperative irradiation with or without concomitant chemotherapy for locally advanced head and neck cancer. N Engl J Med 2004;350(19):1945–52.
17. Al-Sarraf M, LeBlanc M, Giri PG, et al. Chemoradiotherapy versus radiotherapy in patients with advanced nasopharyngeal cancer: phase III randomized Intergroup study 0099. J Clin Oncol 1998;16(4):1310–7.
18. Lin JC, Jan JS, Hsu CY, et al. Phase III study of concurrent chemoradiotherapy versus radiotherapy alone for advanced nasopharyngeal carcinoma: positive effect on overall and progression-free survival. J Clin Oncol 2003;21(4):631–7.
19. Lee AW, Lau WH, Tung SY, et al. Preliminary results of a randomized study on therapeutic gain by concurrent chemotherapy for regionally-advanced nasopharyngeal carcinoma: NPC-9901 Trial by the Hong Kong Nasopharyngeal Cancer Study Group. J Clin Oncol 2005;23(28):6966–75.
20. Langendijk JA, Leemans CR, Buter J, et al. The additional value of chemotherapy to radiotherapy in locally advanced nasopharyngeal carcinoma: a meta-analysis of the published literature. J Clin Oncol 2004;22(22):4604–12.
21. Bonner JA, Harari PM, Giralt J, et al. Radiotherapy plus cetuximab for squamous-cell carcinoma of the head and neck. N Engl J Med 2006;354(6):567–78.
22. Dillman RO, Herndon J, Seagren SL, et al. Improved survival in stage III non-small-cell lung cancer: seven-year follow-up of cancer and leukemia group B (CALGB) 8433 trial. J Natl Cancer Inst 1996;88(17):1210–5.
23. Dillman RO, Seagren SL, Propert KJ, et al. A randomized trial of induction chemotherapy plus high-dose radiation versus radiation alone in stage III non-small-cell lung cancer. N Engl J Med 1990;323(14):940–5.
24. Sause WT, Scott C, Taylor S, et al. Radiation Therapy Oncology Group (RTOG) 88–08 and Eastern Cooperative Oncology Group (ECOG) 4588: preliminary results of a phase III trial in regionally advanced, unresectable non-small-cell lung cancer. J Natl Cancer Inst 1995;87(3):198–205.

25. Blanke C, Ansari R, Mantravadi R, et al. Phase III trial of thoracic irradiation with or without cisplatin for locally advanced unresectable non-small-cell lung cancer: a Hoosier Oncology Group protocol. J Clin Oncol 1995;13(6):1425–9.
26. Clamon G, Herndon J, Cooper R, et al. Radiosensitization with carboplatin for patients with unresectable stage III non-small-cell lung cancer: a phase III trial of the Cancer and Leukemia Group B and the Eastern Cooperative Oncology Group. J Clin Oncol 1999;17(1):4–11.
27. Soresi E, Clerici M, Grilli R, et al. A randomized clinical trial comparing radiation therapy v radiation therapy plus cis-dichlorodiammine platinum (II) in the treatment of locally advanced non-small cell lung cancer. Semin Oncol 1988;15(6 Suppl 7):20–5.
28. Trovo MG, Minatel E, Franchin G, et al. Radiotherapy versus radiotherapy enhanced by cisplatin in stage III non-small cell lung cancer. Int J Radiat Oncol Biol Phys 1992;24(1):11–5.
29. Schaake-Koning C, van den Bogaert W, Dalesio O, et al. Effects of concomitant cisplatin and radiotherapy on inoperable non-small-cell lung cancer. N Engl J Med 1992;326(8):524–30.
30. Jeremic B, Shibamoto Y, Acimovic L, et al. Randomized trial of hyperfractionated radiation therapy with or without concurrent chemotherapy for stage III non-small-cell lung cancer. J Clin Oncol 1995;13(2):452–8.
31. Jeremic B, Shibamoto Y, Acimovic L, et al. Hyperfractionated radiation therapy with or without concurrent low-dose daily carboplatin/etoposide for stage III non-small-cell lung cancer: a randomized study. J Clin Oncol 1996;14(4):1065–70.
32. Furuse K, Fukuoka M, Kawahara M, et al. Phase III study of concurrent versus sequential thoracic radiotherapy in combination with mitomycin, vindesine, and cisplatin in unresectable stage III non-small-cell lung cancer. J Clin Oncol 1999;17(9):2692–9.
33. Pierre F, Maurice P, Gilles R, et al. A Randomized Phase III Trial of Sequential Chemo-Radiotherapy Versus Concurrent Chemo-Radiotherapy in Locally Advanced Non Small Cell Lung Cancer (NSCLC) (GLOT-GFPC NPC 95–01 study). In: Proc Am Soc Clin Onc 20:1246; 2001.
34. Belani CP, Choy H, Bonomi P, et al. Combined chemoradiotherapy regimens of paclitaxel and carboplatin for locally advanced non-small-cell lung cancer: a randomized phase II locally advanced multi-modality protocol. J Clin Oncol 2005;23(25):5883–91.
35. Zemanova M, Petruzelka L, Havel L, et al. Concurrent versus sequential radiochemotherapy with vinorelbine plus cisplatin (V-P) in locally advanced non-small cell lung cancer. A randomized phase II study. In: Proc Am Soc Clin Onc 21:1159; 2002.
36. Curran W, Scott C, Langer C, et al. Long-term benefit is observed in a phase III comparison of sequential vs concurrent chemo-radiation for patients with unresected stage III nsclc: RTOG 9410. In: Proc Am Soc Clin Onc 22:2499; 2003.
37. Souhami L, Gil RA, Allan SE, et al. A randomized trial of chemotherapy followed by pelvic radiation therapy in stage IIIB carcinoma of the cervix. J Clin Oncol 1991;9(6):970–7.
38. Tattersall MH, Lorvidhaya V, Vootiprux V, et al. Randomized trial of epirubicin and cisplatin chemotherapy followed by pelvic radiation in locally advanced cervical cancer. Cervical Cancer Study Group of the Asian Oceanian Clinical Oncology Association. J Clin Oncol 1995;13(2):444–51.
39. Rose PG, Bundy BN, Watkins EB, et al. Concurrent cisplatin-based radiotherapy and chemotherapy for locally advanced cervical cancer. N Engl J Med 1999;340(15):1144–53.
40. Whitney CW, Sause W, Bundy BN, et al. Randomized comparison of fluorouracil plus cisplatin versus hydroxyurea as an adjunct to radiation therapy in stage IIB-IVA carcinoma of the cervix with negative para-aortic lymph nodes: a Gynecologic Oncology Group and Southwest Oncology Group study. J Clin Oncol 1999;17(5):1339–48.
41. Keys HM, Bundy BN, Stehman FB, et al. Cisplatin, radiation, and adjuvant hysterectomy compared with radiation and adjuvant hysterectomy for bulky stage IB cervical carcinoma. N Engl J Med 1999;340(15):1154–61.
42. Morris M, Eifel PJ, Lu J, et al. Pelvic radiation with concurrent chemotherapy compared with pelvic and para-aortic radiation for high-risk cervical cancer. N Engl J Med 1999;340(15):1137–43.

43. Peters WA, 3rd, Liu PY, Barrett RJ, 2nd, et al. Concurrent chemotherapy and pelvic radiation therapy compared with pelvic radiation therapy alone as adjuvant therapy after radical surgery in high-risk early-stage cancer of the cervix. J Clin Oncol 2000;18(8):1606–13.
44. National Cancer Institute: NCI Clinical Announcement. Bethesda, MD, United States Department of Health adn Human Services, Public Health service, National Institutes of Health, February 1999. In.
45. Wong LC, Ngan HY, Cheung AN, et al. Chemoradiation and adjuvant chemotherapy in cervical cancer. J Clin Oncol 1999;17(7):2055–60.
46. Pearcey R, Brundage M, Drouin P, et al. Phase III trial comparing radical radiotherapy with and without cisplatin chemotherapy in patients with advanced squamous cell cancer of the cervix. J Clin Oncol 2002;20(4):966–72.
47. Walsh TN, Grennell M, Mansoor S, et al. Neoadjuvant treatment of advanced stage esophageal adenocarcinoma increases survival. Dis Esophagus 2002;15(2):121–4.
48. Walsh TN, Noonan N, Hollywood D, et al. A comparison of multimodal therapy and surgery for esophageal adenocarcinoma. N Engl J Med 1996;335(7):462–7.
49. Bosset JF, Calais G, Mineur L, et al. Enhanced tumorocidal effect of chemotherapy with preoperative radiotherapy for rectal cancer: preliminary results–EORTC 22921. J Clin Oncol 2005;23(24):5620–7.
50. Macdonald JS, Smalley SR, Benedetti J, et al. Chemoradiotherapy after surgery compared with surgery alone for adenocarcinoma of the stomach or gastroesophageal junction. N Engl J Med 2001;345(10):725–30.
51. Al-Sarraf M, Martz K, Herskovic A, et al. Progress report of combined chemoradiotherapy versus radiotherapy alone in patients with esophageal cancer: an intergroup study. J Clin Oncol 1997;15(1):277–84.
52. Cooper JS, Guo MD, Herskovic A, et al. Chemoradiotherapy of locally advanced esophageal cancer: long-term follow-up of a prospective randomized trial (RTOG 85–01). Radiation Therapy Oncology Group. Jama 1999;281(17):1623–7.
53. Herskovic A, Martz K, al-Sarraf M, et al. Combined chemotherapy and radiotherapy compared with radiotherapy alone in patients with cancer of the esophagus. N Engl J Med 1992;326(24):1593–8.
54. Smith TJ, Ryan LM, Douglass HO, Jr., et al. Combined chemoradiotherapy vs. radiotherapy alone for early stage squamous cell carcinoma of the esophagus: a study of the Eastern Cooperative Oncology Group. Int J Radiat Oncol Biol Phys 1998;42(2):269–76.
55. Minsky BD, Pajak TF, Ginsberg RJ, et al. INT 0123 (Radiation Therapy Oncology Group 94–05) phase III trial of combined-modality therapy for esophageal cancer: high-dose versus standard-dose radiation therapy. J Clin Oncol 2002;20(5):1167–74.
56. Thomas PR, Lindblad AS. Adjuvant postoperative radiotherapy and chemotherapy in rectal carcinoma: a review of the Gastrointestinal Tumor Study Group experience. Radiother Oncol 1988;13(4):245–52.
57. Fisher B, Wolmark N, Rockette H, et al. Postoperative adjuvant chemotherapy or radiation therapy for rectal cancer: results from NSABP protocol R-01. J Natl Cancer Inst 1988;80(1):21–9.
58. Wolmark N, Wieand HS, Hyams DM, et al. Randomized trial of postoperative adjuvant chemotherapy with or without radiotherapy for carcinoma of the rectum: National Surgical Adjuvant Breast and Bowel Project Protocol R-02. J Natl Cancer Inst 2000;92(5):388–96.
59. Krook JE, Moertel CG, Gunderson LL, et al. Effective surgical adjuvant therapy for high-risk rectal carcinoma. N Engl J Med 1991;324(11):709–15.
60. NIH consensus conference. Adjuvant therapy for patients with colon and rectal cancer. Jama 1990;264(11):1444–50.
61. Hyams DM, Mamounas EP, Petrelli N, et al. A clinical trial to evaluate the worth of preoperative multimodality therapy in patients with operable carcinoma of the rectum: a progress report of National Surgical Breast and Bowel Project Protocol R-03. Dis Colon Rectum 1997;40(2):131–9.

62. Sauer R, Becker H, Hohenberger W, et al. Preoperative versus postoperative chemoradiotherapy for rectal cancer. N Engl J Med 2004;351(17):1731–40.
63. Nigro ND, Vaitkevicius VK, Considine B, Jr. Combined therapy for cancer of the anal canal: a preliminary report. Dis Colon Rectum 1974;17(3):354–6.
64. Leichman L, Nigro N, Vaitkevicius VK, et al. Cancer of the anal canal. Model for preoperative adjuvant combined modality therapy. Am J Med 1985;78(2):211–5.
65. Flam M, John M, Pajak TF, et al. Role of mitomycin in combination with fluorouracil and radiotherapy, and of salvage chemoradiation in the definitive nonsurgical treatment of epidermoid carcinoma of the anal canal: results of a phase III randomized intergroup study. J Clin Oncol 1996;14(9):2527–39.
66. John M, Flam M, Berkey B, et al. Five year results and analyses of a phase III randomized RTOG/ECOG chemoradiation protocol for anal cancer. In: Proc Am Soc Clin Onc 17:989; 1998.
67. Bartelink H, Roelofsen F, Eschwege F, et al. Concomitant radiotherapy and chemotherapy is superior to radiotherapy alone in the treatment of locally advanced anal cancer: results of a phase III randomized trial of the European Organization for Research and Treatment of Cancer Radiotherapy and Gastrointestinal Cooperative Groups. J Clin Oncol 1997;15(5):2040–9.
68. Epidermoid anal cancer: results from the UKCCCR randomised trial of radiotherapy alone versus radiotherapy, 5-fluorouracil, and mitomycin. UKCCCR Anal Cancer Trial Working Party. UK Co-ordinating Committee on Cancer Research. Lancet 1996;348(9034):1049–54.
69. Gerard JP, Ayzac L, Hun D, et al. Treatment of anal canal carcinoma with high dose radiation therapy and concomitant fluorouracil-cisplatinum. Long-term results in 95 patients. Radiother Oncol 1998;46(3):249–56.
70. Hung A, Crane C, Delclos M, et al. Cisplatin-based combined modality therapy for anal carcinoma: a wider therapeutic index. Cancer 2003;97(5):1195–202.
71. Constantinou EC, Daly W, Fung CY, et al. Time-dose considerations in the treatment of anal cancer. Int J Radiat Oncol Biol Phys 1997;39(3):651–7.
72. Nigh SS, Smalley SR, D. AM, et al. Conservative therapy for anal carcinoma: an analysis of prognostic factors (abstract). In J Radiat Oncol Biol Phys 1991;21(Suppl 1):224.
73. Shipley WU, Prout GR, Jr., Einstein AB, et al. Treatment of invasive bladder cancer by cisplatin and radiation in patients unsuited for surgery. Jama 1987;258(7):931–5.
74. Coppin CM, Gospodarowicz MK, James K, et al. Improved local control of invasive bladder cancer by concurrent cisplatin and preoperative or definitive radiation. The National Cancer Institute of Canada Clinical Trials Group. J Clin Oncol 1996;14(11):2901–7.
75. Hagan MP, Winter KA, Kaufman DS, et al. RTOG 97–06: initial report of a phase I-II trial of selective bladder conservation using TURBT, twice-daily accelerated irradiation sensitized with cisplatin, and adjuvant MCV combination chemotherapy. Int J Radiat Oncol Biol Phys 2003;57(3):665–72.
76. Housset M, Dufour B, Maulard-Durdux C, et al. Concomitant fluorouraacil (5-FU)-cisplatin (CDDP) and bifractionated split course radiation therapy (BSCRT) for invasive bladder cancer. In: Proc Am Soc Clin Onc 16:1139; 1997.
77. Kaufman DS, Winter KA, Shipley WU, et al. The initial results in muscle-invading bladder cancer of RTOG 95–06: phase I/II trial of transurethral surgery plus radiation therapy with concurrent cisplatin and 5-fluorouracil followed by selective bladder preservation or cystectomy depending on the initial response. Oncologist 2000;5(6):471–6.
78. Rodel C, Grabenbauer GG, Kuhn R, et al. Combined-modality treatment and selective organ preservation in invasive bladder cancer: long-term results. J Clin Oncol 2002;20(14):3061–71.
79. Shipley WU, Kaufman DS, Tester WJ, et al. Overview of bladder cancer trials in the Radiation Therapy Oncology Group. Cancer 2003;97(8 Suppl):2115–9.
80. Shipley WU, Winter KA, Kaufman DS, et al. Phase III trial of neoadjuvant chemotherapy in patients with invasive bladder cancer treated with selective bladder preservation by combined radiation therapy and chemotherapy: initial results of Radiation Therapy Oncology Group 89–03. J Clin Oncol 1998;16(11):3576–83.

81. Tester W, Caplan R, Heaney J, et al. Neoadjuvant combined modality program with selective organ preservation for invasive bladder cancer: results of Radiation Therapy Oncology Group phase II trial 8802. J Clin Oncol 1996;14(1):119–26.
82. Tester W, Porter A, Asbell S, et al. Combined modality program with possible organ preservation for invasive bladder carcinoma: results of RTOG protocol 85–12. Int J Radiat Oncol Biol Phys 1993;25(5):783–90.
83. Dalbagni G, Genega E, Hashibe M, et al. Cystectomy for bladder cancer: a contemporary series. J Urol 2001;165(4):1111–6.
84. Stein JP, Lieskovsky G, Cote R, et al. Radical cystectomy in the treatment of invasive bladder cancer: long-term results in 1,054 patients. J Clin Oncol 2001;19(3):666–75.

14 Cytoprotection for Radiation-Associated Normal Tissue Injury

Jingfang Mao, Oluwatoyosi A. Fatunase, and Lawrence B. Marks

One of the cornerstones of radiation therapy is the delivery of therapeutic radiation doses to the target tissue, yet minimization of dose to surrounding normal tissue. In practice, there is always some dose delivered to surrounding normal tissue. Pure restriction of dose to the target volume, without any incidental irradiation of normal tissue, is physically impossible for most situations. Furthermore, the normal tissue effects of radiation are typically increased when concurrent chemotherapy and radiotherapy (RT) are used [1]. Concurrent chemoradiotherapy has been demonstrated to be superior, with regard to local control and/or survival, compared to single modality alone [2], in multiple disease sites such as the head and neck [3–6], lung [7–10], and pelvis [11–15]. Therefore, it is incumbent upon physicians to do what is possible to minimize the risks associated with incidental irradiation of normal tissues.

Several approaches have been used to minimize radiation-induced normal tissue injury. First, 3D imaging and treatment planning software are critical in the planning process. These tools allow the user to visualize the target tissues and define beam orientations/apertures that minimize dose delivered to normal tissues. Nevertheless, despite these tools, there is always some dose delivered to the surrounding normal tissues. Sophisticated treatment planning/delivery tools, such as intensity-modulated radiation therapy tend to reduce and redistribute incidental radiation [16] and hence reduce/alter, but not eliminate, the risks to normal tissues.

A complementary approach is to use pharmacologic agents that mitigate radiation-induced normal tissue effects. In this chapter, we briefly review the biologic rationale for commonly used pharmacologic agents, and summarize the available randomized clinical trials regarding the application of these agents in human patients.

Biologic Rationale of Cytoprotectors

Radiation-induced cell death is thought, at least in part, to involve with the creation of free radicals. These radicals then react with cellular macromolecules (e.g., DNA, RNA, proteins, membrane) to cause cell dysfunction and death. These reactions take place in tumor and normal cells. The radiation damage to a cell is

M.P. Mehta et al. (eds.), *Radiation Oncology Advances.*

potentiated (enhanced) or mitigated (reduced) depending on the presence of several factors that impact on the biochemistry of these radicals, such as oxygen or sulfhydryl compounds [17].

Pharmacologic agents that can scavenge free-oxygen radicals have been proposed as radiation protectors. The most commonly used agent is amifostine (Ethyol, WR-2721; MedImmune, Inc., Gaithersburg, MD). In brief, amifostine is thought to provide selective protection to the normal cells, over the tumor cells, based on differences in the biochemistry of the two cell types.

Cytoprotection is believed to result from elimination of free radicals by amifostine's dephophorylated active metabolite WR-1065 [18]. Dephosphorylisation of amifostine is either caused by spontaneous nonenzymatic hydrolysis or by a catalyzed process involving alkaline phosphatase, with an optimal pH at 8–9 [19]. Inside the cell, WR-1065 is further metabolized to the disulfide, WR-33278, that may also cause radioprotection by enhancement of the DNA repair process [20–22]. The alkaline phosphatase is not as abundant in tumor tissues as in normal tissues. Further, the better vascularization and the higher pH in the normal tissues (vs. tumor cells) afford selective protection of normal cells [23–30]. Extensive uptake of amifostine is seen in salivary glands, kidneys, and intestinal mucosa [19].

Pilocarpine is a cholinergic agonist that has been suggested to palliate RT-associated xerostomia. It is a naturally occurring, cholinergic, parasympathicomimetic alkaloid [31], with predominantly muscarinic action. It is postulated to stimulate cholinergic receptors on the surfaces of the exocrine glands [32], causing salivary secretion, both in individuals with normal salivary gland function and in those with impaired salivary flow [33, 34].

Theoretically, the increased salivary flow provided from such agents would require their continued use, as the agents do not directly prevent cell death. Nevertheless, some authors suggest that continuous stimulation of the salivary glands *during* RT could prevent/diminish the incidence of radiation-induced xerostomia [35–37]. Therefore, the utility of pilocarpine administrated prior to, or during, RT has been studied.

Keratinocyte growth factor (KGF) is another radioprotective agent that has been studied in humans. KGF is a heparin-bound growth factor, produced by fibroblasts and microvascular endothelium within a variety of tissues (e.g., lung, skin, stomach, bladder) [38]. KGF appears to stimulate proliferation and differentiation of specific epithelial tissues that express KGF receptors [38]. KGF receptors have been detected within many tissues and organs [39] such as epithelial cells of the gastrointestinal tract [40], hepatocytes [40], pulmonary type II pneumocytes [41], mammary gland [42], transitional urothelial cells [43], pancreatic ductal epithelium [44], hair follicles [45, 46], and keratinocytes in all stratified squamous epithelia [47]. Therefore, KGF has been postulated to play an important role in the repair of radiation-induced injury in multiple tissues [47]. Such reparative agents can be given *after* RT, while specific protectors (e.g., amifostine) must be given *during* RT, to be effective.

Since amifostine has been the most commonly used cytoprotective agent in humans, its toxicity and efficacy are reviewed in detail. The information below is derived mainly from randomized clinical trials in human patients receiving RT +/– amifostine. Most of these trials were randomized but not blinded. This endpoint consideration, like many of the endpoints used in these studies, was subjective.

Assessment of Amifostine in Patients with Head and Neck Cancer

The primary normal tissue toxicities in patients receiving RT for head and neck cancers are acute mucositis and acute/late xerostomia. The results from several trials testing the efficacy of amifostine in such patients are summarized in Table 1. In general, these data suggest that amifostine can protect against these effects [1, 49–52, 54], except studies from Buentzel et al. and Buntzel et al. [48, 54].

Assessment of Amifostine in Patients with Thoracic Tumors

There are seven randomized trials of amifostine in patients with thoracic cancer treated with thoracic radiation therapy ± chemotherapy (Table 2).

Lung Injury

Four trials evaluated the potential protective effects of amifostine against RT-induced lung injury [55, 57–59]. A statistically significant protective effect of amifostine against pneumonitis has been reported in three of these studies, two from Greece [55, 59] and one from M.D. Anderson Cancer Center [58]. Gopal et al. also studied the effects of amifostine on pulmonary function in a subset of 23 patients treated on their randomized trial of concurrent chemotherapy/RT, with or without amifostine [62]. The subgroup receiving amifostine had average reduction in DLCO of 24% vs. 42% ($p = 0.004$) in the controls; thus also supporting the protective effect of the drug.

The largest trial, from the RTOG [57], demonstrated no difference in pneumonitis rates with or without amifostine. However, patients in this study received RT twice a day, but amifostine only once a day, resulting in a potential protection for only half of the treatments. There was also a high patient dropout rate of 19% in the treatment arm (due largely to amifostine toxicity and patient's refusal), and 52% did not receive the full intended dose of amifostine.

The two trials from Greece also assessed radiation-induced fibrosis via thoracic CT scan 6 months post therapy. Both studies reported a lower incidence of fibrosis in the amifostine group than in the control group. In the 2001 report [55], the rates of radiologic fibrosis were 9% vs. 19%, with and without the drug, respectively ($p<0.05$). In the 2003 report, the corresponding rates were 29% vs. 50% ($p = 0.16$) [59].

Table 1 Randomized trials testing the efficacy of amifostine on RT-induced injury in patients with head and neck cancer

First author year	Number of patients	RT dose (Gy)[a]	Chemo-therapy[b]	Amifostine usage		Grade ≥3 acute mucositis rate (%)			Acute grade ≥2 xerostomia rate (%)			Late grade ≥2 xerostomia rate (%)		
				Dose (mg)	Timing (min)	Amif	Contr	*p*	Amif	Contr	*p*	Amif	Contr	*p*
Buentzel [48] 2005	132	60–70	Yes	300/m² *IV*	right pre-CRT	39	22	0.7	39	34	0.7	39	24	0.06
Wasserman [1] 2005	303	50–70	No	200/m² *IV* 200/m² *IV*	within 30 pre-RT 15–30 pre-RT	–	–	–	19	36	0.05	–	–	–
Vacha [49] 2003	56	60–70	Yes	250 *IV*	15 pre-RT	–	–	0.002[c]	–	–	–	–	–	0.005[c]
Antonadou [50] 2002	50	60–74	Yes	300/m² *IV*	30 pre-RT	–	–	–	27	74	0.0001	64	96	0.01
Bourhis [51] 2000	26	64[d]	No	150/m² *IV*	15–30 pre-RT	–	–	–	–	–	–	8[e]	67[e]	0.02
Brizel [52] 2000	315	50–70	No	200/m² *IV*	15–30 pre-RT	51	78	<0.0001	34	57	0.002	35	39	0.5
Koukourakis [53] 2000	39	64–70	No	500 *SC*	20 pre-RT	58	75	0.3	–	–	–	0	30	–
Buntzel [54] 1998	39	60	Yes	500 *IV*	right pre-ChT only	12	100	0.0001	17	55	0.05	0	86	0.0001

CRT chemoradiotherapy; *Amif* amifostine group; *Contr* control group

[a]All dose at 1.8–2 Gy QD, except as noted

[b]Concurrent Chemotherapy: all carboplatin

[c]In terms of WHO toxicity criteria Grade 4, if RTOG criteria used, the *p* value is not significant

[d]BID

[e]In favor of amifostine group

Table 2 Randomized trials assessing the efficacy of amifostine on RT-induced injury in patients with lung cancer

First author year	Institution	Number of patients	RT dose (Gy)	Chemo-therapy	Amifostine usage		Acute grade≥2 pneumonitis rate (%)			Lung fibrosis rate (%)			Severe esophagus toxicity rate (%)		
					Dose (mg)	Timing (min)	Amif	Contr	*p*	Amif	Contr	*p*	Amif	Contr	*p*
Movsas [57] 2005	RTOG	242	69.6 (1.2 bid)	ind + conc	500 *IV* Mon.–Thu.	pre-afternoon RT	27	28	NS	–	–	–	30[a]	34[a]	NS
Komaki [58] 2004	M.D. Anderson Cancer Center	62	69.6 (1.2 bid)	conc	500 *IV*[d]	20–30 pre-ChT 30–60 pre-RT	0[a]	16[a]	0.02	–	–	–	16[a]	35[a]	0.02
Antonadou [59] 2003	Metaxa Cancer Center, Greece	73	60–67 (2 qd)	conc	300/m² *IV*	15 pre-ChT/RT	30	67	0.009	29	50	0.16	39[a]	84[a]	<0.001
Leong [60] 2003	Singapore	60	60–66 (2 qd)	ind + conc	740/m² *IV*	pre-ChT	–	–	–	–	–	–	43[b]	70[b]	0.08
Senzer [61] 2002	Sammons Cancer Center	100	64.8 (1.8 qd)	conc + post	500 *IV*	15–30 pre-ChT	–	–	–	–	–	–	11[a]	12[a]	NS
					200/m² *IV*	15–30 pre-RT									
Antonadou [55] 2001	Metaxa Cancer Center, Greece	146	55–60 (2 qd)	none	340/m² *IV*	15 pre-RT	12	52	<0.001	28	53	<0.05	4[b]	42[b]	<0.0001
Koukourakis [53] 2000[c]	University Hospital of Iraklion, Greece	60	50–64 (2 qd)	not specified	500 *SC*	20 pre-RT	–	–	–	–	–	–	20[b]	54[b]	0.05[b]

RTOG Radiation Therapy Oncology Group; *ind* induction, *conc* concurrent; *ChT* chemotherapy; *Amif* amifostine group; *Contr* control group; *NS* nonsignificant

[a]Grade 3 or greater

[b]Grade 2 or greater

[c]Three patients with thymoma and one with neuroendocrine tumor included

[d]Amifostine was only given the first 2 days of each week. It was given 20–30 min before chemotherapy (60–90 min before 1st fraction RT) on the days when cisplatin was administered (Days 1, 8, 29, and 36), 30–60 min before RT when no cisplatin was given

Esophageal Injury

The data from the seven studies assessing the impact of amifostine on RT-induced esophageal injury are summarized in Table 2. The data are divergent. Four studies reported a significant reduction in esophageal injury with the addition of amifostine [53, 55, 58, 59]. These include the three that were positive for lung injury [55, 58, 59], as well as an additional study from the Greek group [53].

Three other studies did not report statistically significant benefits regarding esophageal injury. The RTOG study (with its caveats noted above in the lung section) was essentially negative for esophagitis [57]. Several esophageal endpoints were considered. For the Area Under the Curve (AUC) that reflects the severity and duration of swallowing symptoms during RT, the amifostine arm was superior to the control ($p = 0.025$). However, for all other metrics (e.g., the incidences of acute grade ≥2 pneumonitis, grade ≥3 esophagitis, and late toxicities of esophagus, lung, heart, etc.), there were no meaningful differences. The dose of amifostine used in the Sammons Cancer Center [61] study was relatively low compared to that used in some of the other trials. In the trial from Singapore [60], a nearly statistically significant finding was obtained ($p = 0.08$) in a relatively small study (60 patients). Thus, the nonsignificant p value may be due to the limited number of patients (i.e., low power).

Assessment of Amifostine in Patients with Pelvic Tumors

Four trials have studied the impact of amifostine during RT for a variety of pelvic tumors (Table 3) [53, 63–65]. In general, the addition of amifostine appeared to reduce the rate of *acute* GU and GI toxicity. Three of the studies reported statistically significant differences regarding toxicity [53, 63–65]. The Kligerman et al. study is small (n = 100) and statistically negative [65]. However, 6% of patients in nonamifostine group experienced moderate or severe acute GU reactions vs. none of the patients in amifostine arm ($p = 0.06$).

Assessment of Amifostine in Patients with Tumors at Other Sites

Koukourakis et al. from Greece conducted a trial in 92 patients with breast cancer [66]. Patients were enrolled to hypofractionated accelerated radiotherapy (46 Gy in 12 fractions, 1 fraction/day, 5 fractions/week) with amifostine or conventional radiotherapy without amifostine under the same inclusion and exclusion criteria. The NTD (normalized total dose) corrected for overall treatment time were estimated to be comparable (62.8 Gy vs. 62–64 Gy). The addition of the drug appeared

Table 3 Randomized trials assessing the efficacy of amifostine on RT-induced injury in patients with pelvic cancers[a]

First author year	Number of patients	RT dose (Gy)[b]	Amifostine usage		Toxicity rate (%)											
					Acute GU			Late GU			Acute lower GI			Late lower GI		
			Dose (mg)	Timing (min)	Amif	Contr	*p*	Amif	Contr	*p*	Amif	Contr	*p*	Amif	Contr	*p*
Athanassiou [63] 2003	205	50–70	340/m² *IV*	15–30 pre-RT	9[c]	38[c]	<0.05	1[c]	1[c]	NS	12[c]	45[c]	<0.05	1[c]	4[c]	NS
Kouvaris [64] 2003	36	66–86[d]	500 *IV*	20–30 pre-RT	11[c]	44[c]	0.06	–	–	–	11[e]	89[e]	0.007	–	–	–
Koukourakis [53] 2000	36	50–70	500 *SC*	20 pre-RT	0[c]	100[c]	0.0006[f]	–	–	–	13	50	<0.05	–	–	–
Kligerman [65] 1992	100[g]	52–59	340/m² *IV*	15 pre-RT	0[h]	6[h]	0.06	0[h]	6[h]	NS	0[h]	6[h]	NS	0[h]	6[h]	NS

GU genitourinary; *GI* gastrointestinal; *Amif* amifostine group; *Contr* control group; *NS* nonsignificant

[a]Diseases included rectal, bladder, prostate, and gynecologic cancer in trial from Athanassiou [63] et al. 2003; prostate and gynecologic cancer in trial from Kouvaris [64] et al. 2003; bladder, gynecologic, rectal cancer, sarcoma, and pancreas in trial from Koukourakis [53] et al. 2000; and epidermoid carcinoma of the uterine cervix in trail from Kligerman [65] et al. 1992

[b]All dose at 1.8–2.25 Gy QD

[c]Grade2 or greater

[d]For gynecologic tumor: external beam irradiation to 50 Gy, and additional 16–36 Gy by brachytherapy; for prostate cancer: external beam irradiation to 68 Gy

[e]Results are the same using either WHO or EORTC-RTOG criteria

[f]Only evaluated in 14 patients with bladder cancer (7 treated with amifostine, and 7 not)

[g]Late toxicity was evaluated in 72 patients

[h]Moderate and severe toxicity (mild toxicity excluded); Data estimated from data presented in the tables in the original paper

to reduce the rate of acute skin toxicity (50% vs. 100%, $p < 0.001$), acute radiographic and/or symptomatic pneumonitis (1% vs. 3%, $p = 0.6$), and lung fibrosis (0% vs. 3%, $p = 0.03$). Two-year local relapse-free survival was similar in the amifostine and control groups (84% vs. 76%, $p = 0.35$).

Impact of Amifostine on Tumor Control and Survival

One of the concerns to applying radiation protectors such as amifostine, is their potential tumor-protective effect. In randomized studies noted above, there appeared to be no demonstrable effect of amifostine on tumor-control metrics (Tables 4–6).

Amifostine-Related Toxicity

The most-often reported toxicities of amifostine are hypotension, nausea/vomiting, allergic reaction, and asthenia. There are six randomized trials comparing the incidences of side effects between the amifostine and control arms (Table 7). Three of them are conducted in patients with head and neck cancer, three in patients with lung cancer. The differences in five of them reached statistical significance [48, 52, 57, 58, 60]. The rates of hypotension varied from 14–70%, and appeared to possibly be related to the dose of drug delivered.

Other reported adverse effects include anemia [48], leukopenia [48], dysgeusia [58], sneezing [58, 60], dizziness [60], chills [60], hiccups [60], and skin rash [67]. Overall, the rates of toxicity leading to IV amifostine interruption caused by its toxicity varied from 0 to 38% [51, 55, 58, 59, 63–66]. There are no clear trends to relate the rate of drug toxicity with either tumor site or chemotherapy use. Most of amifostine-related side effects resolved with discontinuation of the drug [23].

Administration of Amifostine

Most of the studies described intravenous (IV) amifostine used at approximately 500 mg or 340 mg/m^2, delivered 15–30 min prior to RT, for over 3–15 min period of time. Due to the toxicities of the IV route, investigators have also administrated the drug subcutaneously (SC) or intrarectally [53, 68–70].

Subcutaneous amifostine appears to be logistically easier to deliver than IV. Most importantly, the rates of hypotension induced by amifostine appear to be lower with SC (Table 8) than with IV (Table 7). Nevertheless, SC administration has its own toxicity profile (Table 8).

Table 4 The impact of amifostine on tumor control and survival in randomized trials of patients with head and neck cancer

First author year	Number of patients	RT dose (Gy)[a]	Conc. chemo-therapy[b]	Amifostine usage		Local response/control rate (%)				Survival rate (%)			
				Dose (mg)	Timing (min)	Endpoint	Amif	Contr	*p*	Endpoint	Amif	Contr	*p*
Buentzel [48] 2005	132	60–70	Yes	300/m² *IV*	right pre-CRT	1 year LRC	62	73	0.2	1 year OS	75	77	0.9
				200/m² *IV*	within 30 pre-RT					1 year PFS	64	72	0.5
Wasserman [1] 2005	303	50–70	No	200/m² *IV*	15–30 pre RT	2 years LRC	54	58	0.5	2 years OS	72	67	0.2
										2 years PFS	56	59	1
Antonadou [50] 2002	50	60–74	Yes	300/m² *IV*	30 pre RT	CR	91	78	0.4	1.5 years PFS	82	74	–
						0.5 year LRC	95	87	0.6				
Bourhis [51] 2000	26	64[c]	No	150/m² *IV*	15–30 pre RT	1.25 years LRC	46	46	–	–	–	–	–
Brizel [52] 2000	315	50–70	No	200/m² *IV*	15–30 pre-RT	2 years LRC	58	63	–	2 years DFS	53	57	–
										2 years OS	71	66	–
Koukourakis [53] 2000	39	64–70	No	500 *SC*	20 pre-RT	CR	58	54	–	–	–	–	–
Buntzel [54] 1998	39	60	Yes	500 *IV*	right pre-ChT only	CR	72	43	0.07	1 year DFS	79	64	–

CRT chemoradiotherapy; *ChT* chemotherapy; *Amif* amifostine group; *Contr* control group; *LRC* local regional control; *CR* complete response; *OS* overall survival, *PFS* progression-free survival, *DFS* disease-free survival

[a]All dose at 1.8–2 Gy QD, except as noted

[b]Concurrent Chemotherapy: all carboplatin

[c]BID

Table 5 The impact of amifostine on tumor response and survival in randomized trials of patients with thoracic tumors

First author year	Number of patients	RT dose (Gy)	Chemo-therapy	Amifostine usage		CR + PR rates (%)			Median survival (months)		
				Dose (mg)	Timing (min)	Amif	Contr	*p*	Amif	Contr	*p*
Movsas [57] 2005	242	69.6 (1.2 bid)	ind + conc	500 *IV* Mon.–Thu.	pre-afternoon RT	–	–	–	17	18	NS
Komaki [58] 2004	62	69.6 (1.2 bid)	conc	500 *IV*[a]	20–30 pre-ChT	–	–	–	19	20	NS
Antonadou [59] 2003	73	60–67 (2 qd)	conc	$300/m^2$ *IV*	15 pre-ChT/RT	89	82	NS	–	–	–
Leong [60] 2003	60	60–66 (2 qd)	ind + conc	$740/m^2$ *IV*	pre-ChT	57	60	NS	13	15	NS
Senzer [61] 2002	100	64.8 (1.8 qd)	conc + post	500 *IV*	15–30 pre-ChT weekly	26	25	NS	–	–	–
				$200/m^2$ *IV*	15–30 pre-RT daily						
Antonadou [55] 2001	146	55–60 (2 qd)	none	$340/m^2$ *IV*	15 pre-RT	75	76	NS	–	–	–
Koukourakis [53] 2000	60	50–64 (2 qd)	not specified	500 *SC*	20 pre-RT	34	21	0.5	–	–	–

ind induction; *conc* concurrent; *ChT* chemotherapy; *Amif* amifostine group; *Contr* control group; *NS* nonsignificant

[a] Amifostine was only given the first 2 days of each week. It was given 20–30 min before chemotherapy (60–90 min before 1st fraction RT) on the days when cisplatin was administered (Days 1, 8, 29, and 36), 30-60 min before RT when no cisplatin was given

Table 6 The impact of amifostine on tumor control and survival in randomized trials of patients with pelvic cancers[a]

First author year	Number of patients	RT dose (Gy)[b]	Amifostine usage		CR + PR rate (%)			Survival rate (%)			
			Dose (mg)	Timing (min)	Amif	Contr	*p*	Endpoints	Amif	Contr	*p*
Athanassiou [63] 2003	205	50–70	340/m² *IV*	15–30 pre-RT	98	97	NS	–	–	–	–
Kouvaris [64] 2003	36	50[c]	500 *IV*	20–30 pre-RT	–	–	NS	Freedom from relapse	100	100	NS
Kligerman [65] 1992	100	52.2–59.4	340/m² *IV*	15 pre-RT	54	42	NS	Crude survival[d]	77	66	NS

Amif amifostine group; *Contr* control group; *NS* nonsignificant

[a]Diseases included rectal, bladder, prostate, and gynecologic cancer in trial from Athanassiou [63] et al. 2003; prostate and gynecologic cancer in trial from Kouvaris [64] et al. 2003; and rectal cancer in trail from Kligerman [65] et al. 1992

[b]All dose at 1.8–2.25 Gy QD

[c]For gynecologic tumor: external beam irradiation to 50 Gy, and additional brachytherapy of 16–36 Gy; for prostate cancer: external beam irradiation to 68 Gy

[d]Mean 1-year follow-up

Table 7 Toxicity rates in randomized trials using IV amifostine (%)

First-author year	Number of patients	Site	Amif. dose (mg)	Pre-medications	Hypotension			Nausea			Vomiting			Other toxicity			Rates of amifostine interruption (%)
					Amif	Contr	*p*	Amif	Contr	*p*	Amif	Contr	*p*	Amif	Contr	*p*	
Buentzel [48] 2005	132	Head and neck	200–300/m^2	Hydration antiemetic	39	17	0.006	6[i]	6[i]	NS	12[i]	3[i]	0.1	3[g]	0[g]	NS	30[a]
Antonadou [50] 2002	45	Head and neck	300/m^2	Antiemetic dexamethasone hydration	14	0	0.1	5[j]	0[j]	NS	–	–	–	–	–	–	–
Brizel [52] 2000	315	Head and neck	200/m^2	Antiemetic	15	2	<0.0001	44	16	<0.0001	37	7	<0.0001	5[g]	0[g]	0.003	21[b,c,d,e]
Movsas [57] 2005	242	Lung	500	Ondansetron/ Granisetron[k]	16	7	<0.001	33	21	0.03	25	14	0.007	–	–	–	–
Komaki [58] 2004	62	Lung	500	–	65	3	<0.001	–	–	–	–	–	–	13[h]	0[h]	0.04	2[f]
Leong [60] 2003	60	Lung	740/m^2	Dexamethasone diphenhydr-amine granisetron	70	30	0.002	–	–	–	30	0	<0.001	77[h]	7[h]	<0.001	2[c]

Amif amifostine group; *Contr* control group; *NS* nonsignificant
Reasons for interruption: (a) vomiting, (b) nausea, (c) hypotension, (d) allergic reaction, (e) others, (f) myocardial infarction caused by hypertension
Other toxicities caused by amifostine: (g) allergic reaction, (h) sneezing, (i) Grade 3 or 4, (j) Vomiting included, (k) Dexamethasone and cimetadine were used only pre-chemotherapy

Table 8 Toxicity reported with subcutaneous amifostine

First author year	Number of patients	Tumor site	Radiation dose (Gy)	Chemo-therapy	Amif. dose (Mg)	Rate of amifostine related toxicity (%)						Rates of amifostine interruption (%)
						Hypotension	Nausea	Vomiting	Allergic reaction	Asthenia	Other reaction	
Anne [71] 2002	54	Head and neck	50–70	No	500				7		Injection site reaction 32,	35
Bardet [67] 2002	54	Head and neck	50–70	No	500	0	13			0	Skin rash 16	
Braaksma [72] 2002	54	Head and neck	66–72	Conc	500		43				Anaphylaxis 10	19
Koukourakis [68] 2002	25	Lung	64	Conc	500	0		8	0			0
Kouloulias [69] 2005	53	Pelvic	50–72	Nono	500		11			15^{b}		15
Koukourakis [53] 2000	70	Head and neck, lung, pelvic	50–70	None	500	3^{a}	29	3	9	29^{c}	Xerostomia 12^{d} headache 16	14

conc concurrent; *Amif* amifostine

[a]Grade 1

[b]Grade2–3

[c]Grade 2–3: 16%

[d]Patients with head and neck cancer were excluded

The bioavailability of subcutaneously delivered amifostine, *compared* to IV, is approximately 40% at 30 min, 67% at 60 min, and 97% at 240 min. Preliminary tissue studies in monkeys indicated that amifostine levels in lung, kidney, and parotid gland tissue were slightly higher 30 min after SC amifostine than after IV amifostine but were generally comparable after 60 min [86].

Bardet et al. compared the efficacy of amifostine between IV and SC routes in 54 patients with head and neck cancer. The rates of grade ≥2 acute xerostomia and grade ≥2 mucositis were comparable between them (23% vs. 19%, 69% vs. 68%, respectively) [67]. The rates of acute toxicity were similar in terms of nausea/vomiting (12% vs. 13%) and skin rash (15% vs. 17), however, higher in IV group than in SC group in terms of hypotension (6% vs. 0%) and asthenia (4% vs. 0%). These results indicate that tolerance is better with SC than IV administration, particularly because of the absence of hypotension. Another ongoing study in patients with lung cancer is comparing the utility of IV to SC amifostine [73].

While the majority of studies demonstrating the potential efficacy of amifostine used the IV route, there are data to support the activity of SC amifostine. Koukourakis et al. randomized 140 patients irradiated for head and neck, lung, and pelvic cancer to SC amifostine vs. control [53]. Amifostine appeared to reduce the severity of oral, esophageal, and rectal toxicity, and prevent the delay of radiotherapy.

Intrarectal administration has been considered to deliver a high concentration of amifostine to the local rectal area for mucosal protection. A phase I clinical trial conducted by Ben-Josef et al. in patients with prostate cancer suggested that intrarectal application of amifostine was well-tolerated [70]. With a median follow-up time of 21 months, only 5 of 29 patients (17%) had rectal bleeding related to RT (mostly grade 1 or 2, no grade 3). This compared favorably to historical controls [74, 75]. The degree of protection appeared to be dose–dependent, with most of the symptomatic patients receiving the lower dose of 500–1,000 mg (vs. the higher dose of 1,500–2,500 mg: 7 of 14 [50%] vs. 2 of 13 [15%], $p = 0.03$). Their preliminary efficacy data are encouraging and suggest that intrarectal administration of amifostine may reduce radiation damage [70]. Another phase I/II trial was conducted in early 1990s at Duke University Medical Center [76]. Twenty-four patients undergoing radiotherapy received 100–450 mg amifostine daily, in enema form, 45 min before RT. The endpoint was the degree of damage to the rectal mucosa, determined by rectal biopsy, compared to a nonrandomized control group of similarly irradiated patients who did not receive amifostine. This study showed that amifostine could be administered safely in enema form in this dose range. The degree of the cellular damage detected by biopsy was slightly less severe in the amifostine than in the control group, however, this difference was not significant.

A phase II randomized study conducted by Kouloulias et al. compared intrarectal with subcutaneous application of amifostine in patients with prostate or gynecologic cancer [69]. Intrarectal amifostine was feasible and well tolerated with no amifostine-related toxicity in 26 patients. The rates of acute radiation-induced rectal mucositis were lower in the intrarectal group than in the SC group (15% vs. 48%, $p = 0.04$). Conversely, rates of acute urinary toxicity were higher in intrarectal arm than in SC arm (43% vs. 11%, $p = 0.03$). This result can be explained by the higher distribution of amifostine in the administered local area using intrarectal application and the higher systemic distribution using subcutaneous route compared to intrarectal route.

Thus, intrarectal amifostine appears to be a promising manner to selectively protect the rectal mucosa.

Other Cytoprotectors

Five trials testing the efficacy of pilocarpine as a cytoprotector are summarized in Table 9. The differences in the endpoints used in these studies make it difficult to compare the result from the different studies. Overall, the data do not demonstrate efficacy of pilocarpine.

Brizel et al. reported a phase II randomized study of recombinant human keratinocyte growth factor (rHuKGF) in head and neck cancer [81]. Sixty-six patients received standard radiotherapy (70 Gy at 2 Gy QD) and 33 received hyperfractionated irradiation (72 Gy at 1.25 Gy BID). Concurrent chemotherapy was given to all patients. Ninety patients were evaluable for efficacy. In patients treated with hyperfractionated RT, the mucositis duration, area under curves (AUC) of all grades of mucositis and AUC of pharyngeal toxicity were lower in the study group than the control group (34 days vs. 57 days, $p = 0.05$ [for the mucositis duration]; 101 vs. 148, $p = 0.01$ [for AUC of all grades of mucositis]; 114 vs. 158, $p = 0.02$ [for AUC of pharyngeal toxicity]). No significant difference of unstimulated saliva production was found between study and placebo groups (0.5 g vs. 0.3 g). However, no clear trends were found between study and control groups in patients treated with daily RT, indicating that standard RT may require a different dose schedule than hyperfractionated RT.

Pentoxifylline inhibits platelet aggregation and reduces tumor necrosis factor, and has been suggested to ameliorate radiation-induced normal tissue damage. In a prospective double-blinded control trial, 40 patients were randomized to receive 400 mg of pentoxifylline vs. placebo during radiotherapy for breast or lung cancer [82]. The pentoxifylline-treated patients experienced lesser rates of subjective symptoms, reductions in PFTs, and abnormalities on regional perfusion scans. Similarly, another prospective randomized study involving 78 patients irradiated for head and neck cancer showed that late skin changes and soft tissue fibrosis were reduced in patients receiving pentoxifylline, compared to the control group ($p < 0.05$) [83].

Additionally, a variety of other radioprotective agents are being evaluated in preclinical models, including Glycagon-like peptide-2 [84], and heat shock proteins 70 (HSP 70) [85].

There have been a variety of protective agents suggested to mitigate injury due to chemotherapy. A complete review of these is beyond the scope of this review and are summarized elsewhere [9, 18, 47].

Table 9 Double-blinded randomized, placebo-controlled trials[m] testing the efficacy of pilocarpine on RT-induced injury in head and neck cancer

First author year	Number of patients	Mean parotid dose (Gy)	Pilocarpine administration[i]		Subjective score: Endpoints	Timing (post-RT)	Ratio[j] (contr/pilo)	p	Objective score: Endpoints	Timing (post-RT)	Ratio[j] (contr/pilo)	p
Gornitsky [32] 2004	58	≥50	Five times daily Qid	with RT ~ 5 weeks post-RT[p]	Change of xerostomia[a]	5 weeks	0.5	0.02[l]	Change of saliva not unstimulated[e]	5 weeks	1.0[k]	NS
					Change of global QOL[d]		0.2	NS	Change of saliva stimulated[e]		0.9[k]	NS
[i]Fisher [77] 2003	249	≥50	Qid	3 days pre RT ~3 months post-RT	Saliva amount[b]	3 months	0.9	NS	–	–	–	–
						6 months	1.4	NS				
Haddad [78] 2002	39	58	tid	with RT ~3 months post-RT	Xerostomia[a]	6 months	1.4	0.02	Xerostomia grade[f]	6 months	1.2	0.01
Warde [31] 2002	130	>50	tid	with RT ~1 month post-RT	Xerostomia[c]	6 months	1.0[o]	NS	Rate of grade 3 mucositis[g]	1 month	0.9	NS
					QOL[d]		1.0[o]	NS				
Mateos [79] 2001	49	≥50	tid	1 day pre RT ~12 months post-RT	Xerostomia[d]	Immediately	1	NS	Decrease in parotid excretion[h]	immediately	1.2	<0.001
						6 months	0.8	NS		6 months	1.2	NS

Pilo pilocarpine arm; *Contr* control arm; *QOL* quality of life; *NS* nonsignificant

Assessing methods used for subjective and objective scores: (a) VAS (Visual Analog Scale questionnaire) or VAS modified for xerostomia, (b) UW-QOL (University of Washington Quality of Life questionnaire), (c) LAS (Linear Analog Scale Questionnaire), (d) HNRQ-QOL (McMaster University Head and Neck QOL questionnaire), (e) SAXON Test [80], (f) LENT SOMA scale, (g) RTOG (Radiation Therapy Oncology Group) acute morbidity scoring criteria, (h) Dynamic salivary scintigraphy, (i) Each administration of pilocarpine was given as a 5 mg pill, (j) Values greater than 1 are in favor of pilocarpine group except on noted, (k) Values less than 1 are in favor of pilocarpine group, (l) p Value and data set are based on intention to treat analysis. However, results are not significant with the secondary analysis, (m) All are double-blinded randomized, placebo-controlled trials excepted on noted, (n) Nondouble-blinded, (o) Nonrandomized, prospective, controlled but no placebo, (p) Patients in both pilocarpine and placebo arms received this post-RT pilocarpine administration

Conclusion

Amifostine appears to protect several normal tissues from radiation-induced injury, without reducing the antitumor effects of the RT. Acute morbidity, particularly hypotension, remains a challenge for IV administration. Alternative routes of administration, such as SC or intrarectal, may reduce these morbidities and hence improve the therapeutic ratio. Additional evaluation of these and other cytoprotectors are warranted.

Acknowledgment The authors thank Drs. David M. Brizel and Zeljko Vujaskovic for background materials and suggestions.

References

1. Wasserman TH, Brizel DM, Henke M, et al. Influence of intravenous amifostine on xerostomia, tumor control, and survival after radiotherapy for head-and- neck cancer: 2-year follow-up of a prospective, randomized, phase III trial. Int J Radiat Oncol Biol Phys 2005; 63(4):985–990.
2. Brizel DM. Strategies for Protecting Normal Tissue in the Treatment of Head and Neck Cancer. Totowa, NJ: Humana Press, Inc.; 2005.
3. Wendt TG, Grabenbauer GG, Rodel CM, et al. Simultaneous radiochemotherapy versus radiotherapy alone in advanced head and neck cancer: a randomized multicenter study. J Clin Oncol 1998; 16(4):1318–1324.
4. Maguire PD, Meyerson MB, Neal CR, et al. Toxic cure: hyperfractionated radiotherapy with concurrent cisplatin and fluorouracil for Stage III and IVA head-and-neck cancer in the community. Int J Radiat Oncol Biol Phys 2004; 58(3):698–704.
5. Dobrowsky W, Naude J. Continuous hyperfractionated accelerated radiotherapy with/without mitomycin C in head and neck cancers. Radiother Oncol 2000; 57(2):119–124.
6. Denis F, Garaud P, Bardet E, et al. Final results of the 94-01 French Head and Neck Oncology and Radiotherapy Group randomized trial comparing radiotherapy alone with concomitant radiochemotherapy in advanced-stage oropharynx carcinoma. J Clin Oncol 2004; 22(1): 69–76.
7. Dillman RO, Seagren SL, Propert KJ, et al. A randomized trial of induction chemotherapy plus high-dose radiation versus radiation alone in stage III non-small-cell lung cancer. N Engl J Med 1990; 323(14):940–945.
8. Rowell NP, O'Rourke N P. Concurrent chemoradiotherapy in non-small cell lung cancer. Cochrane Database Syst Rev 2004(4):CD002140.
9. Schiller JH. Lung cancer: therapeutic modalities and cytoprotection. Lung 1998; 176(3):145–164.
10. Byhardt RW, Scott C, Sause WT, et al. Response, toxicity, failure patterns, and survival in five Radiation Therapy Oncology Group (RTOG) trials of sequential and/or concurrent chemotherapy and radiotherapy for locally advanced non-small-cell carcinoma of the lung. Int J Radiat Oncol Biol Phys 1998; 42(3):469–478.
11. Ryu HS, Chun M, Chang KH, Chang HJ, Lee JP. Postoperative adjuvant concurrent chemoradiotherapy improves survival rates for high-risk, early stage cervical cancer patients. Gynecol Oncol 2005; 96(2):490–495.

12. Lam CW, Chen WT, Liu MT, et al. Effect of preoperative concurrent chemoradiotherapy in locally advanced low rectal cancer after radical resection surgery. Int Surg 2005; 90(1):53–59.
13. Morris M, Eifel PJ, Lu J, et al. Pelvic radiation with concurrent chemotherapy compared with pelvic and para-aortic radiation for high-risk cervical cancer. N Engl J Med 1999; 340(15): 1137–1143.
14. Rose PG, Bundy BN, Watkins EB, et al. Concurrent cisplatin-based radiotherapy and chemotherapy for locally advanced cervical cancer. N Engl J Med 1999; 340(15):1144–1153.
15. Peters WA 3rd, Liu PY, Barrett RJ 2nd, et al. Concurrent chemotherapy and pelvic radiation therapy compared with pelvic radiation therapy alone as adjuvant therapy after radical surgery in high-risk early-stage cancer of the cervix. J Clin Oncol 2000; 18(8):1606–1613.
16. Kocak Z, Yu X, Zhou SM, et al. The impact of pre-radiotherapy surgery on radiation-induced lung injury. Clin Oncol (R Coll Radiol) 2005; 17(4):210–216.
17. Nair CK, Parida DK, Nomura T. Radioprotectors in radiotherapy. J Radiat Res (Tokyo) 2001; 42(1):21–37.
18. Capizzi RL. The preclinical basis for broad-spectrum selective cytoprotection of normal tissues from cytotoxic therapies by amifostine. Semin Oncol 1999; 26(2 Suppl 7):3–21.
19. Andreassen CN, Grau C, Lindegaard JC. Chemical radioprotection: a critical review of amifostine as a cytoprotector in radiotherapy. Semin Radiat Oncol 2003; 13(1):62–72.
20. Holwitt EA, Koda E, Swenberg CE. Enhancement of topoisomerase I-mediated unwinding of supercoiled DNA by the radioprotector WR-33278. Radiat Res 1990; 124(1):107–109.
21. Peters GJ, van der Vijgh WJ. Protection of normal tissues from the cytotoxic effects of chemotherapy and radiation by amifostine (WR-2721): preclinical aspects. Eur J Cancer 1995; 31A(Suppl 1):S1–S7.
22. Savoye C, Swenberg C, Hugot S, et al. Thiol WR-1065 and disulphide WR-33278, two metabolites of the drug ethyol (WR-2721), protect DNA against fast neutron-induced strand breakage. Int J Radiat Biol 1997; 71(2):193–202.
23. Culy CR, Spencer CM. Amifostine: an update on its clinical status as a cytoprotectant in patients with cancer receiving chemotherapy or radiotherapy and its potential therapeutic application in myelodysplastic syndrome. Drugs 2001; 61(5):641–684.
24. Tannehill SP, Mehta MP. Amifostine and radiation therapy: past, present, and future. Semin Oncol 1996; 23(4 Suppl 8):69–77.
25. Travis EL. The oxygen dependence of protection by aminothiols: implications for normal tissues and solid tumors. Int J Radiat Oncol Biol Phys 1984; 10(9):1495–1501.
26. Valles EG, de Castro CR, Castro JA. Radioprotectors as late preventive agents against carbon tetrachloride induced liver necrosis: protection by 2-(3-aminopropylamino) ethylphosphorothioic acid (WR2721). Exp Mol Pathol 1995; 63(2):101–109.
27. Wasserman TH. Radiotherapeutic studies with amifostine (Ethyol). Semin Oncol 1994; 21(5 Suppl 11):21–25.
28. Tresher M NL, Shepman A, et al. Effects of modulating agent WR-2721 and its main metabolites on the formaiton and stability of cisplatin/DNA adducts in vitro. Bio Chem Pharmacol 1992; 33:1013.
29. Small W Jr. Cytoprotection/radioprotection with amifostine: potential role in cervical cancer and early findings in the Radiation Therapy Oncology Group C-0116 trial. Semin Oncol 2003; 30(6 Suppl 18):68–71.
30. Grdina DJ, Murley JS, Kataoka Y. Radioprotectants: current status and new directions. Oncology 2002; 63(Suppl 2):2–10.
31. Warde P, O'Sullivan B, Aslanidis J, et al. A Phase III placebo-controlled trial of oral pilocarpine in patients undergoing radiotherapy for head-and-neck cancer. Int J Radiat Oncol Biol Phys 2002; 54(1):9–13.
32. Gornitsky M, Shenouda G, Sultanem K, et al. Double-blind randomized, placebo-controlled study of pilocarpine to salvage salivary gland function during radiotherapy of patients with

head and neck cancer. Oral Surg Oral Med Oral Pathol Oral Radiol Endod 2004; 98(1):45–52.
33. Fox PC, Atkinson JC, Macynski AA, et al. Pilocarpine treatment of salivary gland hypofunction and dry mouth (xerostomia). Arch Intern Med 1991; 151(6):1149–1152.
34. Wiseman LR, Faulds D. Oral pilocarpine: a review of its pharmacological properties and clinical potential in xerostomia. Drugs 1995; 49(1):143–155.
35. Wolf A AJ, Macynski AA, et al. Pretherapy interventions to modify salivary dysfunction. Monogr 1990; 9:87–90.
36. Valdez JH WA, Atkinson JC, et al. Use of pilocarpine during head and neck radiation therapy to reduce xerostomia and salivary dysfunction. Cancer 1993; 71:1148–1151.
37. Rode M, Smid L, Budihna M, Soba E, Rode M, Gaspersic D. The effect of pilocarpine and biperiden on salivary secretion during and after radiotherapy in head and neck cancer patients. Int J Radiat Oncol Biol Phys 1999; 45(2):373–378.
38. Baumann M, Krause M, Zips D, et al. Molecular targeting in radiotherapy of lung cancer. Lung Cancer 2004; 45 Suppl 2:S187–S197.
39. MacDonald KP, Hill GR. Keratinocyte Growth Factor (KGF) in hematology and oncology. Curr Pharm Des 2002; 8(5):395–403.
40. Housley RM, Morris CF, Boyle W, et al. Keratinocyte growth factor induces proliferation of hepatocytes and epithelial cells throughout the rat gastrointestinal tract. J Clin Invest 1994; 94(5):1764–1777.
41. Ulich TR, Yi ES, Longmuir K, et al. Keratinocyte growth factor is a growth factor for type II pneumocytes in vivo. J Clin Invest 1994; 93(3):1298–1306.
42. Ulich TR, Yi ES, Cardiff R, et al. Keratinocyte growth factor is a growth factor for mammary epithelium in vivo. The mammary epithelium of lactating rats is resistant to the proliferative action of keratinocyte growth factor. Am J Pathol 1994; 144(5):862–868.
43. Yi ES, Shabaik AS, Lacey DL, et al. Keratinocyte growth factor causes proliferation of urothelium in vivo. J Urol 1995; 154(4):1566–1570.
44. Yi ES, Yin S, Harclerode DL, et al. Keratinocyte growth factor induces pancreatic ductal epithelial proliferation. Am J Pathol 1994; 145(1):80–85.
45. Rubin JS, Osada H, Finch PW, Taylor WG, Rudikoff S, Aaronson SA. Purification and characterization of a newly identified growth factor specific for epithelial cells. Proc Natl Acad Sci USA 1989; 86(3):802–806.
46. Danilenko DM, Ring BD, Pierce GF. Growth factors and cytokines in hair follicle development and cycling: recent insights from animal models and the potentials for clinical therapy. Mol Med Today 1996; 2(11):460–467.
47. Danilenko DM. Preclinical and early clinical development of keratinocyte growth factor, an epithelial-specific tissue growth factor. Toxicol Pathol 1999; 27(1):64–71.
48. Buentzel J, Micke O, Adamietz IA, Monnier A, Glatzel M, de Vries A. Intravenous amifostine during chemoradiotherapy for head-and-neck cancer: a randomized placebo-controlled phase III study. Int J Radiat Oncol Biol Phys 2005.
49. Vacha P, Fehlauer F, Mahlmann B, et al. Randomized phase III trial of postoperative radiochemotherapy +/– amifostine in head and neck cancer. Is there evidence for radioprotection? Strahlenther Onkol 2003; 179(6):385–389.
50. Antonadou D, Pepelassi M, Synodinou M, Puglisi M, Throuvalas N. Prophylactic use of amifostine to prevent radiochemotherapy-induced mucositis and xerostomia in head-and-neck cancer. Int J Radiat Oncol Biol Phys 2002; 52(3):739–747.
51. Bourhis J, De Crevoisier R, Abdulkarim B, et al. A randomized study of very accelerated radiotherapy with and without amifostine in head and neck squamous cell carcinoma. Int J Radiat Oncol Biol Phys 2000; 46(5):1105–1108.
52. Brizel DM, Wasserman TH, Henke M, et al. Phase III randomized trial of amifostine as a radioprotector in head and neck cancer. J Clin Oncol 2000; 18(19):3339–3345.
53. Koukourakis MI, Kyrias G, Kakolyris S, et al. Subcutaneous administration of amifostine during fractionated radiotherapy: a randomized phase II study. J Clin Oncol 2000; 18(11): 2226–2233.

54. Buntzel J, Schuth J, Kuttner K, Glatzel M. Radiochemotherapy with amifostine cytoprotection for head and neck cancer. Support Care Cancer 1998; 6(2):155–160.
55. Antonadou D, Coliarakis N, Synodinou M, et al. Randomized phase III trial of radiation treatment + /– amifostine in patients with advanced-stage lung cancer. Int J Radiat Oncol Biol Phys 2001; 51(4):915–922.
56. Buntzel J, Kuttner K, Frohlich D, Glatzel M. Selective cytoprotection with amifostine in concurrent radiochemotherapy for head and neck cancer. Ann Oncol 1998; 9(5):505–509.
57. Movsas B, Scott C, Langer C, et al. Randomized trial of amifostine in locally advanced non-small-cell lung cancer patients receiving chemotherapy and hyperfractionated radiation: radiation therapy oncology group trial 98-01. J Clin Oncol 2005; 23(10): 2145–2154.
58. Komaki R, Lee JS, Milas L, et al. Effects of amifostine on acute toxicity from concurrent chemotherapy and radiotherapy for inoperable non-small-cell lung cancer: report of a randomized comparative trial. Int J Radiat Oncol Biol Phys 2004; 58(5):1369–1377.
59. Antonadou D, Throuvalas N, Petridis A, Bolanos N, Sagriotis A, Synodinou M. Effect of amifostine on toxicities associated with radiochemotherapy in patients with locally advanced non-small-cell lung cancer. Int J Radiat Oncol Biol Phys 2003; 57(2):402–408.
60. Leong SS, Tan EH, Fong KW, et al. Randomized double-blind trial of combined modality treatment with or without amifostine in unresectable stage III non-small-cell lung cancer. J Clin Oncol 2003; 21(9):1767–1774.
61. Senzer N. A phase III randomized evaluation of amifostine in stage IIIA/IIIB non-small cell lung cancer patients receiving concurrent carboplatin, paclitaxel, and radiation therapy followed by gemcitabine and cisplatin intensification: preliminary findings. Semin Oncol 2002; 29(6 Suppl 19):38–41.
62. Gopal R SG, Tucher S, Liao Z, Kelly J, Stevens C, Komaki R. The effects of radaition therapy, chemotherapy and the radioprotector amifostine o the diffusion capacity of patients with non-small cell lung cancer (NSCLC). Int J Radiat Oncol Biol Phys 2001; 51(3 Suppl 1):22.
63. Athanassiou H, Antonadou D, Coliarakis N, et al. Protective effect of amifostine during fractionated radiotherapy in patients with pelvic carcinomas: results of a randomized trial. Int J Radiat Oncol Biol Phys 2003; 56(4):1154–1160.
64. Kouvaris J, Kouloulias V, Malas E, et al. Amifostine as radioprotective agent for the rectal mucosa during irradiation of pelvic tumors. A phase II randomized study using various toxicity scales and rectosigmoidoscopy. Strahlenther Onkol 2003; 179(3):167–174.
65. Kligerman MM, Liu T, Liu Y, Scheffler B, He S, Zhang Z. Interim analysis of a randomized trial of radiation therapy of rectal cancer with/without WR-2721. Int J Radiat Oncol Biol Phys 1992; 22(4):799–802.
66. Koukourakis MI, Giatromanolaki A, Kouroussis C, et al. Hypofractionated and accelerated radiotherapy with cytoprotection (HypoARC): a short, safe, and effective postoperative regimen for high-risk breast cancer patients. Int J Radiat Oncol Biol Phys 2002; 52(1): 144–155.
67. Bardet E, Martin L, Calais G, et al. Preliminary data of the GORTEC 2000–02 phase III trial comparing intravenous and subcutaneous administration of amifostine for head and neck tumors treated by external radiotherapy. Semin Oncol 2002; 29(6 Suppl 19):57–60.
68. Koukourakis MI, Romanidis K, Froudarakis M, et al. Concurrent administration of Docetaxel and Stealth liposomal doxorubicin with radiotherapy in non-small cell lung cancer: excellent tolerance using subcutaneous amifostine for cytoprotection. Br J Cancer 2002; 87(4): 385–392.
69. Kouloulias VE, Kouvaris JR, Pissakas G, et al. Phase II multicenter randomized study of amifostine for prevention of acute radiation rectal toxicity: topical intrarectal versus subcutaneous application. Int J Radiat Oncol Biol Phys 2005; 62(2):486–493.
70. Ben-Josef E, Han S, Tobi M, et al. Intrarectal application of amifostine for the prevention of radiation-induced rectal injury. Semin Radiat Oncol 2002; 12(1 Suppl 1):81–85.

71. Schraube P, Schell R, Wannenmacher M, Drings P, Flentje M. [Pneumonitis after radiotherapy of bronchial carcinoma: incidence and influencing factors]. Strahlenther Onkol 1997; 173(7):369–378.
72. Braaksma M, Levendag P. Tools for optimal tissue sparing in concomitant chemoradiation of advanced head and neck cancer: subcutaneous amifostine and computed tomography-based target delineation. Semin Oncol 2002; 29(6 Suppl 19):63–70.
73. Mehta V. Open label multicenter trial of subcutaneous amifostine (Ethyol) in the prevention of radiation induced esophagitis and pneumonitis in patients with measurable, unresectable non-small cell lung cancer. Semin Oncol 2004; 31(6 Suppl 18):42–46.
74. Gerard JP, Xie C, Carrie C, et al. Curative external beam radiotherapy for prostate carcinoma: results in 231 patients treated in Lyon. Aust N Z J Surg 1999; 69(10):707–711.
75. Skwarchuk MW, Jackson A, Zelefsky MJ, et al. Late rectal toxicity after conformal radiotherapy of prostate cancer (I): multivariate analysis and dose–response. Int J Radiat Oncol Biol Phys 2000; 47(1):103–113.
76. Montana GS, Anscher MS, Mansbach CM 2nd, et al. Topical application of WR-2721 to prevent radiation-induced proctosigmoiditis. A phase I/II trial. Cancer 1992; 69(11): 2826–2830.
77. Fay M, Tan A, Fisher R, Mac Manus M, Wirth A, Ball D. Dose–volume histogram analysis as predictor of radiation pneumonitis in primary lung cancer patients treated with radiotherapy. Int J Radiat Oncol Biol Phys 2005; 61(5):1355–1363.
78. Haddad P, Karimi M. A randomized, double-blind, placebo-controlled trial of concomitant pilocarpine with head and neck irradiation for prevention of radiation-induced xerostomia. Radiother Oncol 2002; 64(1):29–32.
79. Mateos JJ, Setoain X, Ferre J, et al. Salivary scintigraphy for assessing the protective effect of pilocarpine in head and neck irradiated tumours. Nucl Med Commun 2001; 22(6):651–656.
80. Kohler PF, Winter ME. A quantitative test for xerostomia. The Saxon test, an oral equivalent of the Schirmer test. Arthritis Rheum 1985; 28(10):1128–1132.
81. Brizel D, Le Q, Rosenthal D, et al. Phase 2 study of recombinant human keratinocyte growth factor (rHuKGF) in head and neck cancer treated with standard (SRT) or hyperfractionated irradiation (HRT) and concurrent chemotherapy (CT). Int J Radiat Biol Phys 2002; 54(2 Suppl):285–286.
82. Ozturk B, Egehan I, Atavci S, Kitapci M. Pentoxifylline in prevention of radiation-induced lung toxicity in patients with breast and lung cancer: a double-blind randomized trial. Int J Radiat Oncol Biol Phys 2004; 58(1):213–219.
83. Aygenc E, Celikkanat S, Kaymakci M, Aksaray F, Ozdem C. Prophylactic effect of pentoxifylline on radiotherapy complications: a clinical study. Otolaryngol Head Neck Surg 2004; 130(3):351–356.
84. Booth C, Booth D, Williamson S, Demchyshyn LL, Potten CS. Teduglutide ([Gly2]GLP-2) protects small intestinal stem cells from radiation damage. Cell Prolif 2004; 37(6):385–400.
85. Ito YH, Ippongi S, Nakano M, Kurabe T, Kazaoka Y, Ishiguchi T. [Bioprotection by local and whole-body preheating–bioprotection of damage to mice tongue from burning by local preheating of oral cavity and of radiation damage of small intestine from whole-body preheating]. Nippon Igaku Hoshasen Gakkai Zasshi 2005; 65(3):255–262.
86. Cassatt DR, Fazenbaker CA, Kifle G, Bachy CM. Preclinical studies on the radioprotective efficacy and pharmacokinetics of subcutaneously administered amifostine. Semin Oncol 2002; 29(6 Suppl 19):2–8.

Index

D

H

I

J

K

L

R

V

W

X

Y

Z

Cancer Treatment and Research

Steven T. Rosen, M.D., ***Series Editor*** *(continued from page ii)*

Figlin, R. A. (ed.): *Kidney Cancer. 2003.* *ISBN 1-4020-7457-3.*
Kirsch, M.; Black, P. McL. (ed.): *Angiogenesis in Brain Tumors. 2003.*
ISBN 1-4020-7704-1.
Keller, E.T., Chung, L.W.K. (eds): *The Biology of Skeletal Metastases. 2004.*
ISBN 1-4020-7749-1.
Kumar, R. (ed.): *Molecular Targeting and Signal Transduction. 2004.*
ISBN 1-4020-7822-6.
Verweij, J., Pinedo, H.M. (eds): *Targeting Treatment of Soft Tissue Sarcomas. 2004.*
ISBN 1-4020-7808-0.
Finn, W.G., Peterson, L.C. (eds.): *Hematopathology in Oncology. 2004.*
ISBN 1-4020-7919-2.
Farid, N. (ed.): *Molecular Basis of Thyroid Cancer. 2004.* *ISBN 1-4020-8106-5.*
Khleif, S. (ed.): *Tumor Immunology and Cancer Vaccines. 2004.* *ISBN 1-4020-8119-7.*
Balducci, L., Extermann, M. (eds): *Biological Basis of Geriatric Oncology. 2004.*
ISBN
Abrey, L.E., Chamberlain, M.C., Engelhard, H.H. (eds): *Leptomeningeal Metastases. 2005.*
ISBN 0-387-24198-1
Platanias, L.C. (ed.): *Cytokines and Cancer. 2005.* *ISBN 0-387-24360-7.*
Leong, S.P.L., Kitagawa, Y., Kitajima, M. (eds): *Selective Sentinel Lymphadenectomy for Human Solid Cancer. 2005.* *ISBN 0-387-23603-1.*
Small, Jr. W., Woloschak, G. (eds): *Radiation Toxicity: A Practical Guide. 2005.*
ISBN 1-4020-8053-0.
Haefner, B., Dalgleish, A. (eds): *The Link Between Inflammation and Cancer. 2006.*
ISBN 0-387-26282-2.
Leonard, J.P., Coleman, M. (eds): *Hodgkin's and Non-Hodgkin's Lymphoma. 2006.*
ISBN 0-387-29345.
Leong, S.P.L. (ed): *Cancer Clinical Trials: Proactive Strategies. 2006.*
ISBN 0-387-33224-3.
Meyers, C. (ed): *Aids-Associated Viral Oncogenesis. 2007.*
ISBN 978-0-387-46804-4.
Ceelen, W.P. (ed): *Peritoneal Carcinomatosis: A Multidisciplinary Approach. 2007.*
ISBN 978-0-387-48991-9.
Leong, S.P.L. (ed): *Cancer Metastasis and the Lymphovascular System: Basis for rational therapy. 2007.* *ISBN 978-0-387-69218-0.*
Raizer, J., Abrey, L.E. (eds): *Brain Metastases. 2007.* *ISBN 978-0-387-69221-0.*
Woodruff, T., Snyder, K.A. (eds): *Oncofertility. 2007.* *ISBN 978-0-387-72292-4.*
Mehta, M., Bentzen, S., Harari, P., Tomé, W. (eds): *Radiaton Oncology Advances. 2008.*
ISBN 978-0387-36743-9.

MIX
Papier aus verantwortungsvollen Quellen
Paper from responsible sources
FSC® C105338

If you have any concerns about our products,
you can contact us on
ProductSafety@springernature.com

In case Publisher is established outside the EU,
the EU authorized representative is:
Springer Nature Customer Service Center GmbH
Europaplatz 3, 69115 Heidelberg, Germany

Printed by Libri Plureos GmbH
in Hamburg, Germany